Cooking for Halflings
~ & ~
Monsters

111 Comfy, Cozy Recipes for Fantasy-Loving Souls

| Astrid Tuttle Winegar  Geneva Harstine |
| Author　　　　　　　　　　　　　　Illustrator |

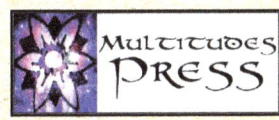

Cooking for Halflings & Monsters © 2016 Astrid Tuttle Winegar. All rights reserved. No part of this book may be used or reproduced in any manner whatsoever, including Internet usage, without written permission from the author, except in the case of brief quotations embodied in critical articles and reviews.

Second Edition © 2017
Second Printing

Paperback edition:
ISBN 978-0-9994179-0-4
EBook edition:
ISBN 978-0-9994179-2-8

Printed in U.S.A.
Illustrations © 2016 Geneva Harstine
Photographs © 2016 Astrid Tuttle Winegar
Cover Design © 2017 Lara Sookoo of Moonzilla Studios

For more information, please see: www.astridwinegar.com

DEDICATION

To my husband Bob, ever patient and indulgent.

To my wonderful daughters, Chloë and Callista.

To Janis Ann Briggs, who should have been one of
my recipe testers!
We all miss you so much.

To my father, Richard S. Tuttle, who never had much
interest in literature, yet was kind and quirky and a firm
believer in the healthful aspects of eating many cookies
during one's lifetime.

To my mother, Esther A. Tuttle, who always encouraged
me to cook. You were a powerful force of nature and
I miss you every day.

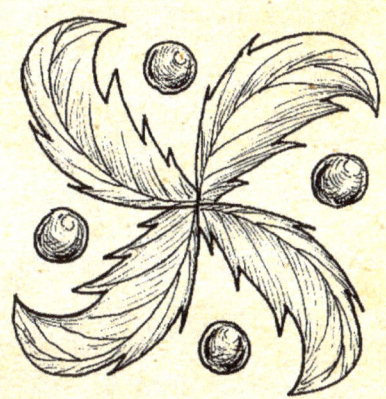

TABLE OF CONTENTS

INTRODUCTION | i
    A Fantasy Tale | i
    A Few Personal & Realistic Details | i
    Academics | ii
    My Brief & Sketchy Biography | iii
    Cooking Experience | iv
    My Geography & Family | iv
    Notes About Optional Green Chile Additions | vi

A FEW NOTES ON METHODOLOGY | IX
    What Drives the Cookbook | ix
    Recipes | xi
    Skill Levels | xii
    Environmental | xiii
    Ingredients | xiii
    Why 111? | xiv

MUSINGS ABOUT DIETING & WATER | XVII

A SUMMATION | XIX

ESSENTIAL SEASONING MIXES | XX

CHAPTER ONE — HALFLING HIDEAWAY | 1

CHAPTER TWO — THE INN OF THE DOUGHTY HERO | 27

CHAPTER THREE — COUNCIL CATERING | 55

CHAPTER FOUR — QUEST DEPOT: SUPPLIES FOR THE SEEMINGLY HOPELESS ENTERPRISE | 79

CHAPTER FIVE — THE EPIC-UREAN | 105

Chapter Six — Glitnír's Hall | 147

Chapter Seven — Monstrous Morsels: The Hot Spot for Egregious Enemies | 171

Chapter Eight — Nympha Nemorosa | 201

A Typical Fantasy Meal | 229

Menu Suggestions | 231

Practical Matters | 235
   Altitude | 235
   Substitutions | 235
   Measuring & Baking | 236
   Salt & Butter | 237
   Herbs & Spices | 237
   Mushrooms | 240
   Pie Crusts | 240
   A Listing of Kitchen Utensils | 241
      Cooking Utensils & Miscellaneous Items | 241
      Small & Large Appliances | 242
      Pots & Pans | 243
      Baking Pans & More Miscellaneous Items | 243
   Conversion Charts | 244
      Dry Ingredients by Weight | 244
      Liquid Ingredients by Volume | 245
      Lengths & Widths | 245
      Temperatures | 246

Conclusion | 249

Acknowledgments/The Fellowship of the Recipe Testers | 251

Works Cited and Sourced | 252

Index | 255

Author's Biography | 267

Illustrator's Biography | 267

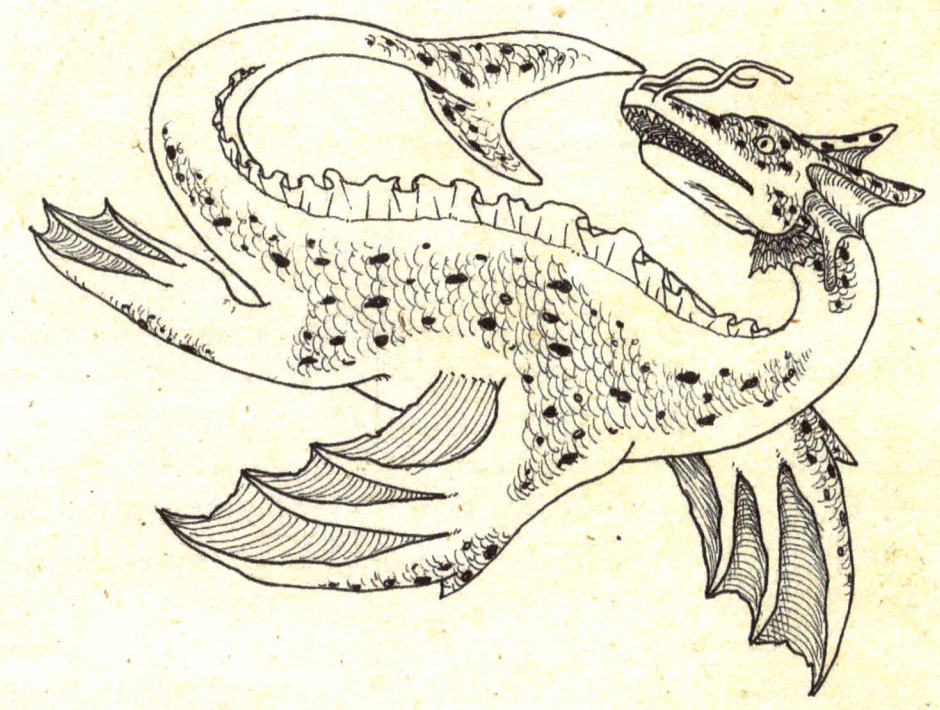

INTRODUCTION

A Fantasy Tale

Once upon a time in the Land of Enchantment, a rather middle-aged lady found herself at a crossroads. She had finished a long career in the Halls of Academia and felt her potential for employment was limited. Instead, she embarked on a creative project. Utilizing the works of a beloved author, she created a cookery book—the recipes followed the story and built on the characters. It was a loving homage to that author.

After two and a half years, her quest was completed. She found representatives for the work and chefs eager to purchase it. The rumor of the charming cookbook spread to all the corners of the knowable world. Not all were pleased, however, and the guardians of the original author's world swooped down upon the naïve lady, shouting, "You shall not publish!" The lady spent a moment cowering in a corner eating cookies. Hundreds, nay, thousands of hungry people occupied the guardian's stronghold, clamoring to have the recipes. The intoxicating scent of cinnamon broke through the guardian's protections and the cookbook was allowed to exist. The lady wrote other cookbooks and lived, as you would hope, happily ever after.

A Few Personal & Realistic Details

Good fantasy literature must have various elements rooted in reality, and the ridiculous preceding story indeed does. I do live in the Land of Enchantment, or New Mexico, a rather obscure state filled with mythology and magic and green chile. I am currently middle-aged and did spend lots of time in college, especially as a returning student. In 1998, at the age of 36, I returned to the University of New Mexico (UNM) after a 16-year absence to complete my BA. I majored in English and minored in Latin. In December 2002, I finally completed the BA after a total of seven and a half years. In December 2008, I completed an MA in Comparative Literature and Cultural Studies after a total of six years.

Why did I feel my employment prospects were slim and why did I decide to write a cookbook instead? There were some personal reasons, of course, but it was mainly the fact that the United States economy was (and unfortunately still is) in a rather sorry and complicated state. My potential employers, meaning specifically UNM and the Albuquerque school system, were in a hiring freeze. I had taught Latin at UNM for four years (and you can imagine there were not dozens of jobs available for teachers in that subject…), but I really did not relish the thought of a full-time teaching job anyway and, fortunately for me, I was married to someone who was still gainfully employed and liked to eat comfort food. So if I did not take the opportunity now, when would I? I decided to try.

The author mentioned above happened to be J. R. R. Tolkien. Perhaps you've heard of him; he is usually considered the grandfather of modern fantasy literature. For most of my life, I have been in love with the works of Tolkien and, while at UNM, I tried to find any sort of courses I could that concentrated on his works. I was fortunate enough to discover a professor in the Honors Department (now the UNM Honors College) who was offering a course on Tolkien. Dr. Leslie Donovan encountered a class brimming with enthusiastic Tolkien fans who sometimes acted more like elementary school students—and I mean this in a very positive sense. Each student had a final semester project to complete and since I loved to cook and bake, I wrote up a small cookbook with about 15 recipes and commentary. We all presented these projects to the class, and I seem to recall I brought cookies. One student built a model of Minas Tirith; another wrote and illustrated a story about a lonely orc who found love. Lest you think it was all fun and games, we also wrote papers, had highly animated class discussions, and read massive amounts of literature.

Eventually, I had finally completed my 13½ years at UNM and at the informal defense of my thesis, my graduate committee (with Dr. Donovan as chair) and I ate nachos and drank margaritas as we discussed university politics (gossip) and my future now that I was finally done at the age of 46½. As she had occasionally suggested before, Leslie wistfully brought up my old cookbook project from years before, saying she wished I could expand it and try to have it published. I suddenly realized I was truly in a position to work on the project at this particular time.

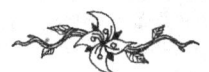

Academics

At UNM, I always tried to write papers on Tolkien as much as possible. As an undergraduate, I examined Tolkien's female characters three times and his whimsical novella, *Roverandom*. I wrote a miniature version of this cookbook in 2000. As a graduate student, I examined canine themes in Tolkien's works more extensively and also turned toward Nationalist and Orientalist themes. My master's thesis was entitled "Why Does 'Frodo Live?': Examining the Character of Frodo Baggins as a Cultural Indicator of Change in J. R. R. Tolkien's Text *The Lord of the Rings* and Peter Jackson's Film Trilogy *The Lord of the Rings*." If you are in the mood for some fairly dry scholarly writing, you may read the Orientalism paper in its entirety at this website:

http://www.tolkienlibrary.com/booksabouttolkien/shoresofme/description.htm

This was actually not a bad output, considering that Tolkien studies were not encouraged at my university. I'm not sure if Tolkien studies are encouraged at *any* university, to be honest.[1] I also wrote what seemed like millions of other papers on other subjects as diverse as Shakespeare, Milton, mythology (Greek, Roman, Celtic, Russian, and Norse), Tolstoy, Dostoevsky, and witchcraft in Roman literature, to name a few. I toyed with the idea of pursuing a Ph.D. in Medieval Studies, but after taking a course on Bede, I decided there was way too much obsession with religion and plague, and since I can generate enough angst in my normal everyday life, the last thing I needed was another decade (or in my case, more like two decades…) of stressed-out academia with its dull conferences and endless writing of papers.

My Brief & Sketchy Biography

I was born in 1962 on Long Island, New York, but my family moved to Albuquerque, New Mexico in 1968 mainly for the weather (my father was a surveyor). My mother was a homemaker and also an aide in the public school system. I have one sister who is three and a half years younger than I am. I graduated from high school in 1979 and attended UNM for two and a half years until I quit for what became a 16-year gap.

For 20 years I was a professional dressmaker (specializing in bridal) while I married, had two daughters, did lots of volunteer work in my children's schools, and attended school myself. As a typical older returning student, I worked extra hard to do well at UNM while still being a homemaker/mother/wife/Latin teacher. So, this is an

---

[1] Since my time in college, however, I have heard of a new program at the Mythgard Institute in New Hampshire (https://mythgard.org). This would have been right up my alley.

incredibly brief biography just for context. Inevitably, other biographical facts will be divulged throughout this book; maybe more than you might want to know...

Cooking Experience

I started basic cooking in elementary school. In high school, my mother let me take a few classes at a cooking school run by a chef. These were fun and exposed me to various regional cuisines, from China to Morocco. Then I decided to cook very extensively, favoring ethnic cuisines. I also took the full-length professional baking course at our community college, but decided against this as a career (probably because early mornings are a better time for baking and I'm a night owl). I catered occasionally. After my wedding (which I catered—talk about crazy), my cooking and baking skills were constantly in use for my husband Bob, our daughters Chloë and Callista, family functions, parties, and school functions. Thus, I have no elite, formal training from any sort of culinary institute, nor have I worked in any sort of restaurant as a chef (though I have waitressed, bartended, and delivered pizzas—worst job ever!). I am also not a trained nutritionist, though I think you will find my proportions to be moderate. This cookbook is based on lots of real-life cooking for real-life people. If you need professional or celebrity credentials in your cookbook authors, you'll need to look elsewhere.

My Geography & Family

My daughters are young adults who have completed their undergraduate college careers (how did that happen so fast?!) and are generally open to many different foods and drinks. My husband Bob, however, is another story. He would describe himself as a "meat and potatoes kind of guy," but he has certainly been exposed to lots of strange foods since we've been married (30 years now). I expressly asked him if I could make fun of him in my cookbook and he said okay, with my daughters as witnesses (he might regret that). I did tell him I was grateful that he gave me a (metaphorical) "room of my own" (which is actually the couch in my living room, so it is not really my *own* room...). He said, "What do you mean, a room? You have the whole house!" And unfortunately, this sounds like an episode from *Everybody Loves Raymond*.

At first, I did not include too many recipes that involved fish, but after dealing with the troublesome character of Gollum, I came up with a few that turned out well. I will justify this by saying that Tolkien did not discuss fish much at all and I've lived in the land-locked city of Albuquerque since I was six years old, so I'm just not that into fish (though I have now acquired more taste for seafood, maybe because of working on this project). The preferred basic New Mexican food groups are:

Vegetables: Red and/or Green Chile (bell peppers and jalapeños are NEVER a substitute for chile!)
Proteins: Cheese and Pork
Carbohydrates: Tortillas and Sopaipillas
Liquids: Margaritas and Beer

Okay—this is not really true... completely. I have heard of people moving to the state just for the green chile and sopaipillas, and people truly miss those particular food items when they leave (at least according to absent friends on Facebook).

As I just mentioned, Bob is more of a meat and potatoes guy whose usual comment on the occasional times I serve fish is something like, "... what is this... ? Fish... ?" This signifies to me only that Bob knows that the protein *du jour* is, indeed, fish, but he would really prefer to have a slab of beef, pork, or chicken on his plate. With potatoes on the side. He doesn't care about the suggestion that people should consume fish (besides canned tuna and deep-fried shrimp) two or three times a week. He's concerned he might come off as rather picky in this cookbook, but I assured him I was not making anything up about him.

Nevertheless, I cook a salmon fillet once in a while, and my experiments have led even Bob to have more appreciation for different types of seafood. When I need sushi, I go out with my daughters. Bob is usually on board for deep-fried seafood, but I do not like to deep-fry too much—the mess! the danger! the wonderfully, non-nutritious calories! Hence, the paucity of deep-fried recipes in this cookbook (there is actually only one—and it's fish and chips).

NOTES ABOUT OPTIONAL GREEN CHILE ADDITIONS

As you know by now, I live in New Mexico. My family and I thrive on green chile and plenty of other spicy foods. I have a feeling that lots of New Mexicans live for green chile, so I've included special notes not only for them, but also for anybody who wants to add some heat to these recipes for variety's sake. Most of the foods included in the cookbook are not particularly spicy, since they were designed to reflect Middle-earth. However, many of the recipes are conducive to an addition of heat. Around Albuquerque, we know autumn is coming when the fragrance of chiles roasting in large, black metal bins starts to permeate the air all over the city. Purists might buy them fresh and roast them at home like you would bell peppers, or have them roasted right where they've bought them. But then you have to bring home a large sack of chiles that require immediate attention—they need to be peeled, seeded, and cut up according to your particular needs. You can leave them whole for one of our local specialties, *chiles rellenos*, cut them into strips, or chop them up. Then you end up freezing them. The chiles will exude some moisture when you thaw them out; sometimes you'll want to use the juice; sometimes you won't.

But even if you live far away from the Land of Enchantment, you probably have access to green chile; all you really have to do is decide whether you like it mild, medium, or hot. You can use canned green chiles in a pinch, though they might add a tinny quality to your recipe (though this might be better than no chile at all). Lazy, busy people (like myself—yes, I'll freely admit it) always keep 4-ounce packages of hot, roasted, and chopped green chile (I use the Hatch, New Mexico variety straight out of the freezer from my favorite store, Costco) in the freezer for emergencies.

I'm just going to include notes about adding green chile—don't get me started on red chile or salsa. I'm also not going to discuss or suggest other types of chiles, such as serranos, jalapeños, or poblanos. Any of these items will undoubtedly work out fine, but salsa, in particular, comes in too many varieties for me to recommend specific ones. How about various other hot sauces or relishes from other regional cuisines? You are free to experiment, and I bet you'll find many new condiments that will complement your favorite recipes.

At the end of appropriate recipes, check out the green chile ICON, as represented to the side, and I'll offer you suggestions for how much green chile you might want to add.

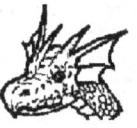

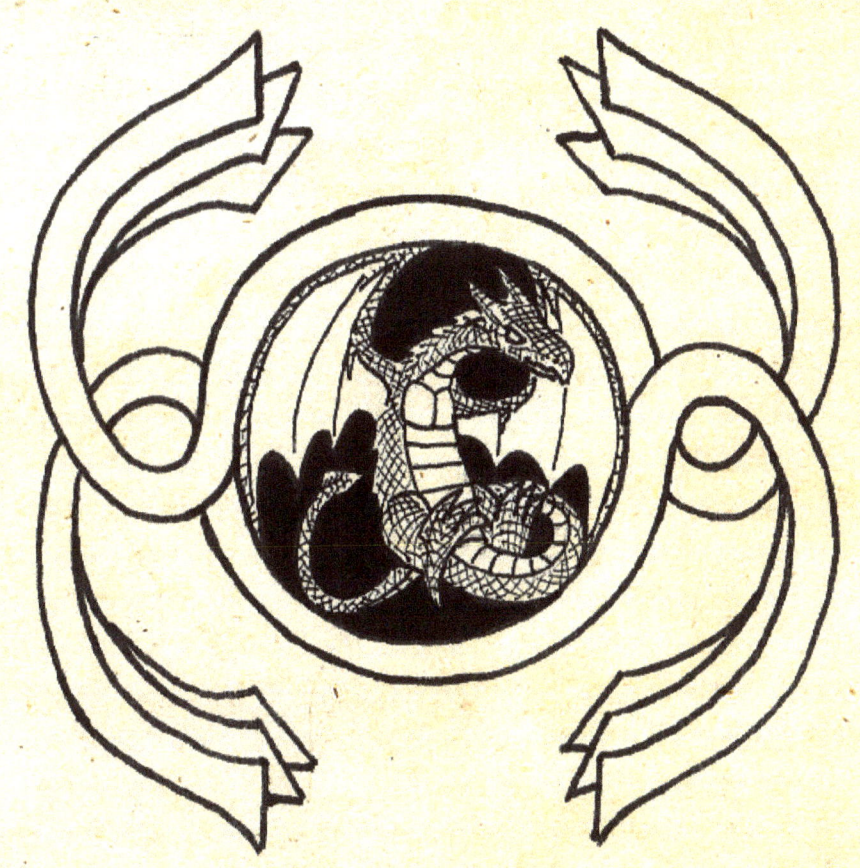

A Few Notes on Methodology

What Drives the Cookbook

As I said above, I combined my love for cooking and my love for the works of Tolkien in a quirky cookbook. It was designed to follow the plot of *The Hobbit* and *The Lord of the Rings*. I freely (and naïvely) used anything Tolkien mentioned about food and drink within my recipes; items were named after specific characters, a character might mention a dish so I created one, or an event in the story might be the catalyst for a dish. Since Tolkien's world of Middle-earth is rather British and rather medieval, I did some research into those cuisines and incorporated those elements into my recipes. Yet I intended everything to be completely modern.

The cookbook was announced in the publishing world and the Internet was abuzz. The Tolkien estate immediately sent an email to my publisher stating that legal action would occur if we went ahead with the project. They did not swoop down on me and they were extremely polite. I could not quote from the texts, name recipes after anything or anyone, and could not attach any sort of marketing to the project. I could, however, write *about* Tolkien and his created land of Middle-earth, and other aspects of that world or his works. I had originally made a point of citing all of this information just as I would in an academic treatise and we felt we had grasped the "fair use" concepts, but the Land of Copyright Law is a dangerous place and few should venture there. To finish with the details in my fantasy tale at the beginning of the introduction, nobody occupied the estate, but that would have been amusing. I also did not eat cookies in a corner, and as for living happily ever after, well, does anyone of us know this until later on?

In the end, I resigned myself to the situation and realized it was an incredibly quixotic journey I had enjoyed over the past three years. And I did enjoy it; even now, I enjoy developing a recipe and seeing people enjoy eating or drinking it. When I was in my early twenties, I wanted to write fiction (fantasy, what else?), but I quickly realized I did not have the proper mindset for it. Writing cookbooks, however, seemed like a good career for me to pursue at this stage in my life. How could I salvage the existing cookbook?

Around the winter holidays of 2011, all of this legal stuff was happening and also not happening, since holidays tend to put many things (including myself) into a state of hibernation. I was desperately thinking about how I could save the cookbook. In the shower one day, I was thinking about removing all the Tolkien references and wondering whether the cookbook still had potential: I could only utilize Middle-earth as an essence, a hint of flavor. It could no longer be an ingredient. Then I was left with 111 sort of British, sort of medieval, comfy, cozy recipes specifically designed for Middle-earth, but which were still perfectly good recipes for any cook.

Well, I could have redesigned the book in a medieval way with more research and more authenticity to the time, but I almost nodded off just thinking about that idea. Then I fiddled with the idea of devoting the whole thing to many different types of fantasy literature, but that did not flow easily; certainly not as easily as the original concept did. I was reluctant to leave Middle-earth; it is such a lovely place. I was bereft of Tolkien's characters, settings, and situations; I was now as alone as Frodo standing at the precipice in Mordor with that damned precious ring, tormented by indecision. Okay, it wasn't that dramatic, but I really thought I had no hope of finding myself able to transform the cookbook.

During another shower, I was thinking about my original chapters and how the only one that seemed cohesive now was my chapter that took place specifically at Tolkien's Prancing Pony Pub. Lo and behold, an idea for a halfling bistro hit me, then a dwarf café. Once the restaurant concept started, the book drastically changed from its original form and flowed with a new ease (just as the original one had).

So, when you want to write, you have to resign yourself to rewriting, but much of what I originally wrote was still valid. If you are a Tolkien fanatic, you'll still be able to recognize elements of his work within mine. However, this cookbook is now my own created fantasy work and evokes more than just Middle-earth—it can evoke your own favorite fantasy atmosphere, even if your version of fantasy only involves eating lots of good food without caloric consequences. Now, there's a fantasy. Archetypes now common in our cultural psyche are all reflected within this cookbook: hero, monster, dwarf, elf, and halfling.

Recipes

All of the recipes within this cookbook are of my own invention. They are informed by lots of experience in the kitchen and lots of experience manipulating (and improving) other people's recipes with an occasional glimpse at my basic edition of *The Better Homes and Gardens Cookbook* to gain a sense of proportion (just how many cups of flour do I really want in this loaf of bread?). Although I did some research into the history of food, I purposely did not consult historical cookbooks because my recipes are meant for a "modern" cook—I do not want or need to use techniques from the medieval, Elizabethan, or Victorian kitchen. I have a stove, a refrigerator, and a KitchenAid stand mixer and I intend to use them.

Also, ultimately the recipes are things I would mostly like to eat: as author, that is my prerogative, though I will admit I have some recipes that I favor over others. As a family, we generally tend to eat Italian, Chinese, and Mexican cuisines, and lately we have been experimenting more with Mediterranean and Indian foods, but none of that is in this book. Bell peppers, olives, bananas, avocados, and peanuts never appear as essential ingredients, yet I have taken liberties with various other ingredients. This cookbook is not meant to be specifically a British cookbook; it is filled with recipes that I imagined the characters of Middle-earth would like to eat, which means people in general—for don't we see ourselves in the monsters, heroes, and dwarves of the fantasy world, and isn't that why the stories resonate so well with so many of us?

Back to reality—the recipes are homemade and do not utilize any overly processed convenience foods, such as cake mixes or canned soups. In my own life, I am certainly not vegan or vegetarian; I'm also not too interested in trendy foods. I am so tired of modern cuisine's impulse to attach fancy names to basic foods. On a recent shopping trip, I saw three types of smoked bacon in a woman's cart—applewood, cherrywood, and pecanwood. And this was Walmart. It seemed pretentious to me, for some reason. It's just bacon—perhaps a higher quality, but come on now. There are plenty of vegetarian recipes included here, as well as some recipes that can be modified either way. Some canned or frozen foods are used occasionally, but these are generally certain vegetables. Of course, you are welcome to shell peas if you like; however, I think frozen peas are acceptable to use. This cookbook is for a modern cook and I expect you will take advantage of modern technology, even though you might have an attraction to the medieval worlds of fantasy.

For completely non-fantastic, nuts and bolts information on the practical aspects of this cookbook, please consult the "Practical Matters" section, following the recipes. Here, you can read about altitude, ingredient substitutions, measuring, baking, salt, butter, herbs, spices, mushrooms, and pie crusts. You will also find a listing of necessary kitchen utensils and their dimensions and/or capacities, as well as some handy Conversion Charts.

Skill Levels

Hobbits (otherwise known as halflings) might be small, but their story is epic. Therefore, do not be fooled into thinking this cookbook is geared toward young, inexperienced children—certainly some of the easier recipes might appeal to kids who are curious about cooking, but I'm assuming a basic knowledge of cooking skills here and you would definitely want to supervise youngsters. I'm assuming you know how to wash vegetables and boil eggs; I'm also assuming you have some knowledge of cooking vocabulary.

This book has many items for beginning to intermediate cooks, yet there are some advanced concepts within some recipes. The teacher buried deep in my heart would be pleased if you are a beginning cook but you have picked up a more advanced skill because of one of my recipes. However, the cookbook never intends to put on *Top Chef* or Cordon Bleu or CIA airs (meaning the Culinary Institute of America, of course). None of these recipes are intended to win any sort of *Top Chef* contest. If, however, the producers of that show ever decided to have an elimination challenge involving cooking for dwarves, I would whip up a recipe such as "Hild's Mushroom Bacon Dish of Might." This would win because it thoroughly represents what dwarves would like to eat and it has a large amount of bacon. Everybody loves bacon… right?

I don't include any aspics (does anyone really want to eat aspic anymore?), nor do I work with offal (which is kind of ironic, since characters such as orcs and trolls and other assorted monsters would definitely appreciate some good offal, preferably raw). I know offal is all the rage in the cooking world today, but do most people really want to eat it? Not around my house. Nothing is made with the *sous vide* technique, nor do I use any sort of molecular gastronomy, but a few more advanced recipes are in Chapter Five, the wizard's restaurant.

Environmental

In keeping with environmental ideals that are quite apparent in Middle-earth and should be apparent in our modern world, this cookbook strives to be relatively green. This means that I try not to use disposable items overly much, such as plastic wrap and bags, and I try to conserve water, energy, and time whenever and wherever possible. So if you don't need to wash out a pot or bowl, I'll let you know this. I always strive to dirty as few dishes as possible so I don't have to deal with them later.

Ingredients

All items required in this cookbook are fairly common and should be readily available in many of your local grocery stores. I get annoyed at recipes that require you to order rather bizarre ingredients online, especially when you end up with a large amount of an item that ends up sitting in your fridge or pantry for months, or even years. Except for seasonal availability depending on the reader's geographical location, I don't use ingredients that must be ordered from any source, nor do I choose high-end merchandise over a perfectly good common ingredient; i.e., plain old water is fine; you certainly don't need to use spring water or distilled water. Recipes sometimes require higher quality ingredients, such as saffron or pork tenderloin, but none of the recipes should break you financially. A high quality cut of meat saves money in the long run, since you will not have to trim it as much as a cheaper cut. I sometimes had trouble getting some ingredients that seemed like they should have been rather common, such as pearl onions and currants. I think these items must have been considered seasonal in my neighborhood stores—when this happens, I try to give you options to substitute.

Why 111?

Perhaps you have wondered—why 111 recipes? Why not just 100? Believe me when I say that early on I did not think I could ever come up with 111, but finally I did. I figure a cookbook needs around 100 recipes to seem substantial. The real reason, however, is a link to Tolkien. In the first chapter of *The Fellowship of the Ring*, the first section of *The Lord of the Rings*, the character of Bilbo Baggins is about to celebrate his one hundred and eleventh birthday. I also just like the number eleven. I haven't numbered the recipes in this edition, since I thought it looked cluttered—but the primary recipes number 111, with additional smaller recipes.

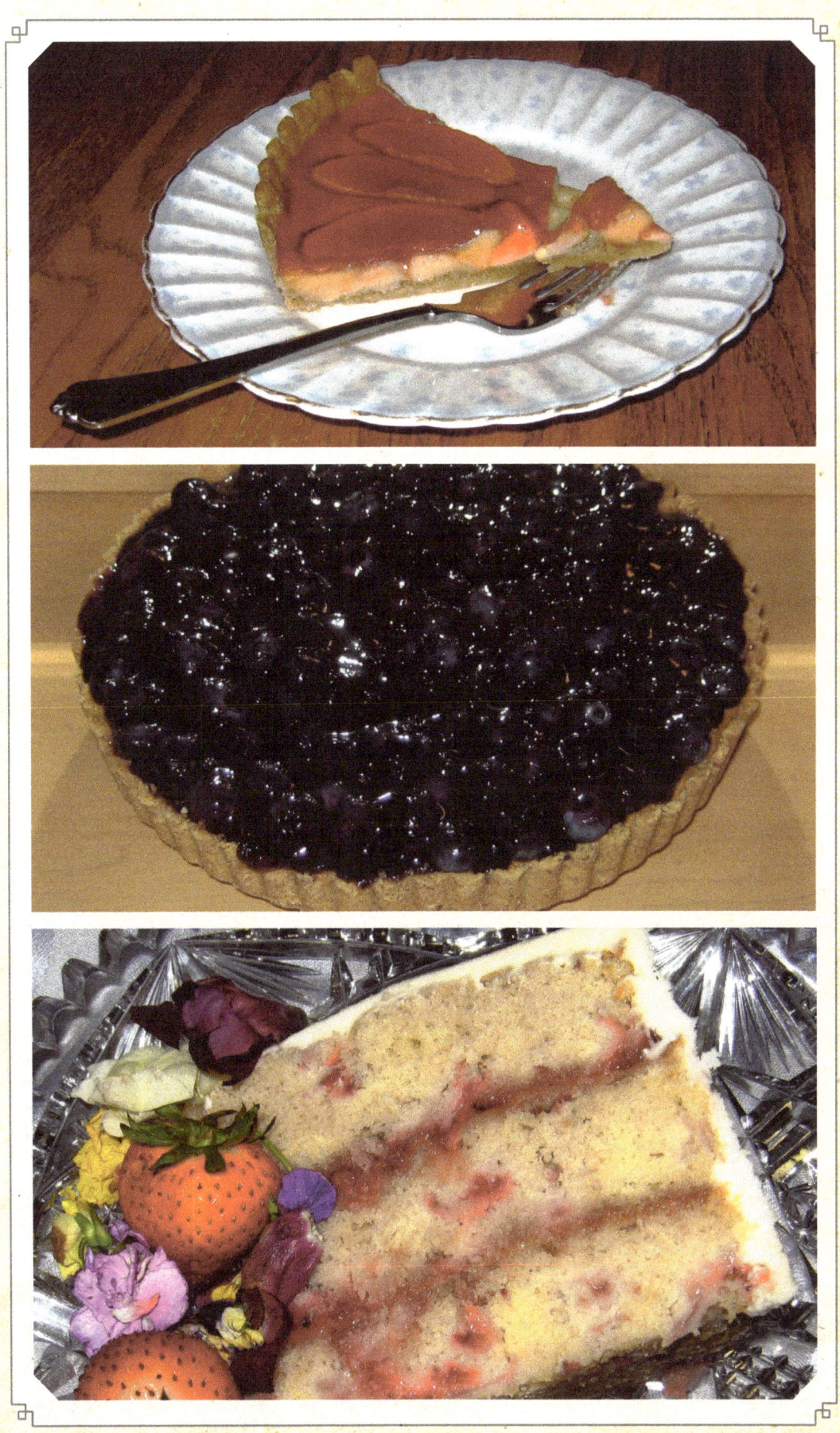

Musings About Dieting & Water

Is this cookbook good for you and your diet? Well… I am not a nutritionist or a doctor and I cannot claim any responsibility for your weight problems (especially since I have had troubles managing my own). We Americans are constantly bombarded with conflicting messages about food and drink. Women's magazines advertise their new miracle diets on one side of their covers; on the other side, they post gorgeous photographs of the fattening recipes within. We must be thin, yet restaurant portions are gigantic. We are more sedentary. Our children get fatter as they rely on juice drinks, soda, and junk food; their recesses have disappeared from their school days. As I said before, this is not a cookbook geared toward children. I've rejected the idea of inventing whimsical recipes, or recipes designed specifically for children who, I firmly believe, should be encouraged to eat real foods that adults should also be eating. It is condescending and unhealthy for children to be fed fake food full of processing, chemicals, and dyes. We eat on the run and in our cars; we consume foods with ingredient names that can hardly be pronounced.

But I am not trying to depress you; I'm just waxing a bit philosophical. This cookbook is full not only of butter and cream, but also of cheeses, meats, breads, fruits, and vegetables—these ingredients are certainly mentioned frequently in Tolkien's texts and they all seem appropriate when dealing with comfort food. I have tried to be sensible in my proportions, however. The cookbook is not vegan nor do I care if you want to buy into the organic trend—currently, all food trends seem to be under fire in one way or another. I want you to think about real ingredients and enjoy them. Though plenty of beer and wine are consumed in Middle-earth, the primary beverage mentioned is water. Eating and drinking in moderation is so important, but is too often forgotten. So make my butter-filled cookies—whether you eat one or seven is really up to you. Try to eat one (okay, eat two…).

A Summation

For me, the concept of "Halflings & Monsters" has come to represent all of my significant others, both the endearing ones and the exasperating ones. It especially represents the loved ones who embody both qualities at various times. You might think of the word "halfling" as a child who is dear to you, but you also know that child can sometimes be a "monster." You might consider your spouse or partner as another part of your own life, a better half perhaps, one who can help you to tame your own personal monsters.

In the end, I have made a sincere effort to be consistent in sharing my recipes, regarding presentation and directions. I suppose that deep down, I'm a teacher, so if you're a beginning cook, you might find my directions helpful, and before you know it, you'll be an intermediate cook. My primary goal has always been to help you bring a warm atmosphere of community and comfort to your kitchen, whether you are cooking for a crowd or even just for yourself (most recipes can easily be increased or decreased accordingly—and many are excellent as leftovers, or can be frozen for later consumption). Although this cookbook is all about the fantasy world of Middle-earth, it's really a metaphor for reality. So, crank up some Led Zeppelin (preferably from their salad days, when they, too, were obsessed with Middle-earth), cook something real, and enjoy a real beverage with it—sometimes we forget just how refreshing a simple glass of water can be.

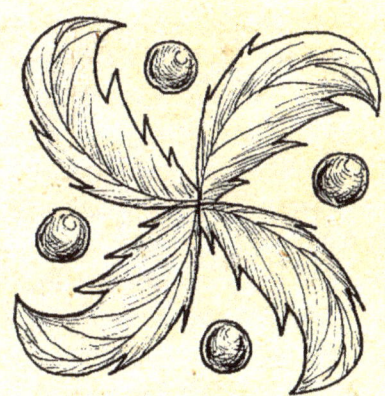

Essential Seasoning Mixes

 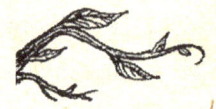

If you really want to cook and bake every item in this cookbook, please prepare the first three recipes ahead of time (Savory Seasoning, Easy Herbes de Provence, and Simple Cinnamon Sugar). All are easy to make and will save you some time (and money) in the long run! If you only have time for one, however, be sure to make up a batch of Savory Seasoning—it is the MOST important ingredient to have on hand.

The other recipes included in this section have been provided for your convenience; the salad dressings in larger quantities and the herb/garlic cheese just because you might want to make it on its own, without its bread accompaniment.

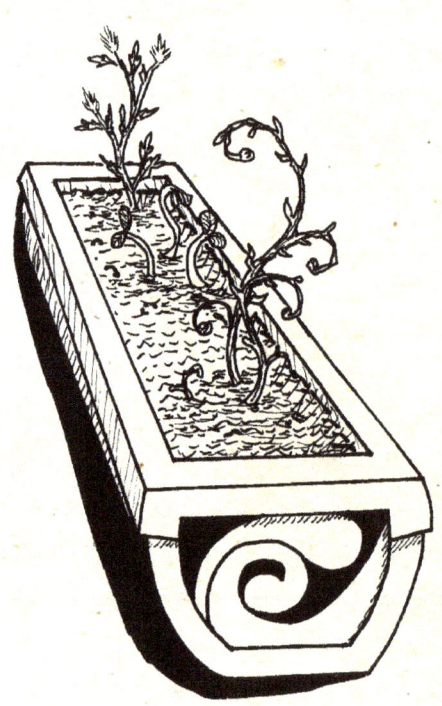

Savory Seasoning

Sometimes one needs more complex flavors than just salt and pepper and sometimes one doesn't have access to different varieties of fresh herbs growing in the garden. This convenient dry seasoning mix is used throughout the restaurants in this cookbook.

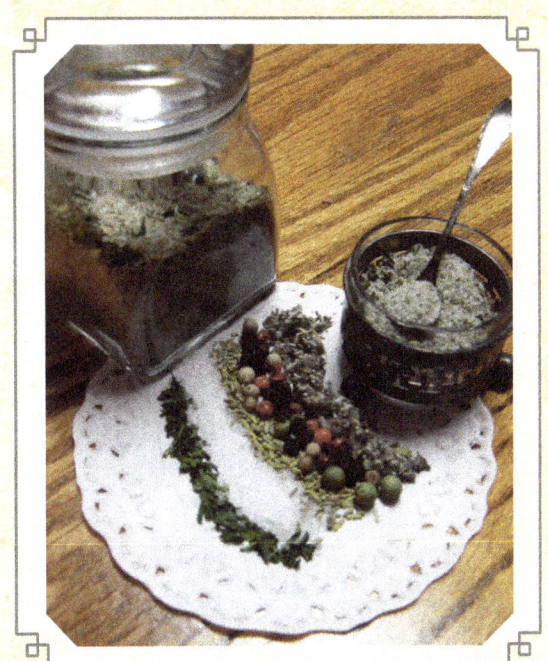

2 tablespoons coarse sea salt
1 tablespoon each:
　whole peppercorns (all black or
　　a mix of colors)
　dry parsley
　sugar
1 teaspoon each:
　onion powder
　garlic powder
½ teaspoon each:
　dry thyme
　dry marjoram
　dry sage
　dry rosemary
　celery seed

Combine the salt and peppercorns in a blender or a small food processor. Pulse until the peppercorns are mostly broken; this will take about a minute. Add the remaining ingredients and pulse another 20 seconds or so. Keep in a tightly covered container in your pantry. Shake or stir before using. Makes about ⅓ cup and retains pungency for about three to four months.

 *I like to leave some of the peppercorns almost whole for a zesty flavor. I use this in many other recipes as well as sprinkling it on various foods, such as steaks or pork chops, eggs or vegetables, and even an occasional sandwich.*

Essential Seasoning Mixes

Easy Herbes de Provence

This dry herb mix is readily available in many grocery stores. However, you can easily mix this up on the spot with herbs you probably already have in your pantry. Often, dried lavender is part of the mix—this ingredient might be harder to obtain, though I found some at Whole Foods. It is optional; some people don't like the flavor, others do. I'm starting my version with a cue from Simon and Garfunkel:

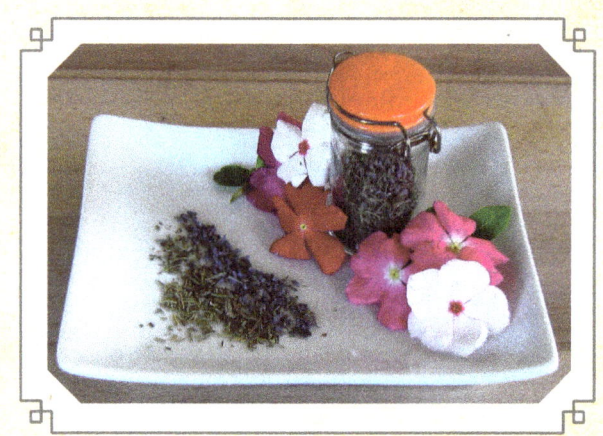

You'll need 1 teaspoon each;
   all in dried form:

Parsley flakes
Rubbed sage
Crushed rosemary
Thyme
Summer Savory
Marjoram
Lavender (optional)

Combine all in a small bowl. You may use a mortar and pestle if you want a finer consistency, but I just use my fingers to crush it all together. Keep in an airtight container in your pantry. Makes about 2 tablespoons.

 Since this is a dry mix, it will keep in your pantry for a few months and still smell herby. Use it on many different foods— eggs, meats, fish, salads, and vegetables. The lavender adds an oddly delightful flavor dimension to the mix! You might experiment with adding lavender to various baked goods, if you have some left. Lavender grows so well in Albuquerque that we have an annual Lavender Festival, where you can buy all sorts of locally produced products, from foods and drinks to soaps and lotions.

Simple Cinnamon Sugar

A few recipes require cinnamon sugar. Whip this up and you'll have easy access to it whenever you need it!

1 cup sugar
2 tablespoons cinnamon

Mix well in a medium bowl. Store in an airtight container in your pantry. Makes 1 cup and keeps for a long time.

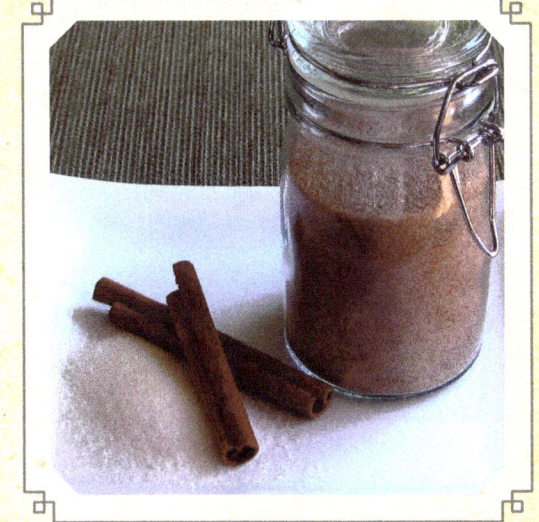

 *Now if you only want a small amount of cinnamon sugar, use these proportions: combine ¾ teaspoon sugar with ¼ teaspoon cinnamon. You can increase these measurements accordingly. To the whole recipe above, however, try adding a teaspoon or even two of spices such as nutmeg, cardamom, mace, or cloves for added flavors, especially around the winter holiday season. Try just adding one or a couple at a time to see which combination appeals to you the most.*

Aradosa's Cheese

Here's another recipe you'll see mentioned a few times within the cookbook. This herby cheese spread accompanies a rustic bread (see page 109 for the full recipe), but perhaps you'll find it helpful to be listed here on its own. There are times when you might not want to commit to baking a loaf of bread, but you feel the need for some garlic/herb cheese and something crispy/carby, such as pita chips or something like baby carrots, if you need a more healthful option.

1 rather large head of fresh garlic
½ teaspoon walnut oil
8 ounces light cream cheese (Neufchâtel), softened
1 cup Ricotta cheese
1 ounce Parmesan or Romano cheese, finely shredded
¼ cup fresh chives, minced
2 tablespoons fresh sage, minced
½ teaspoon salt
½ teaspoon pepper

Preheat oven to 450°. Cut off the top ¾" of the garlic and place it root-side down on a 12" square of aluminum foil. Drizzle with the oil and enclose loosely. Set on a medium baking sheet and bake 35 minutes. Let cool in the foil 30 minutes. Squeeze out the cloves onto the foil and mash coarsely with a fork or chop into small pieces. Set aside.

Meanwhile, in a large bowl, beat the cream cheese with a hand mixer until smooth. Add the remaining ingredients. Mix well, then add the garlic and mix. Season, as desired. Cover and refrigerate leftovers. Makes about 2 cups.

Salad Dressings

Sometimes I get fed up with certain bottled salad dressings. I figured I'd increase the proportions of all the dressings included in the cookbook mainly so I could whip one up whenever I wanted. All four recipes will keep for quite a long while, without any of the strange preservatives you see listed on ready-made dressings. They can be served on any salad you might create. And if you can't obtain (or don't want to bother purchasing) the nut oils listed, feel free to substitute your more basic vegetable oils, such as olive or avocado.

Cress Dress

1 cup walnut oil
¼ cup cider vinegar
2 tablespoons honey
2 tablespoons Dijon mustard
2 teaspoons Herbes de Provence
½ teaspoon pepper
½ teaspoon salt

Combine all ingredients in a 16-ounce jar with a tight-fitting lid. Shake very well; season, as desired. Store covered in the refrigerator. Makes approximately 1½ cups.

Ellen's Dressing

¾ cup almond oil
3 tablespoons white vinegar
3 tablespoons honey mustard
1 tablespoon sugar
1 tablespoon mayonnaise
1½ teaspoons Savory Seasoning
¾ teaspoon salt

Combine all ingredients in a 16-ounce jar with a tight-fitting lid. Shake very well; season, as desired. Store covered in the refrigerator. Makes approximately 1¼ cups.

Lise's Tangy Vinaigrette

¾ cup hazelnut oil
¾ cup red wine vinegar
3 tablespoons lemon juice
3 tablespoons sugar
1 tablespoon salt
1 tablespoon minced garlic
1½ teaspoons pepper

Combine all ingredients in a 16-ounce jar with a tight-fitting lid. Shake very well; season, as desired. Store covered in the refrigerator. Makes approximately 1½ cups.

Ted's Dressing

¾ cup walnut oil
3 tablespoons sugar
3 tablespoons malt vinegar
3 tablespoons sesame seeds, lightly toasted
2 tablespoons soy sauce
1 tablespoon Dijon mustard
1 tablespoon lemon juice
1½ teaspoons Savory Seasoning

Combine all ingredients in a 16-ounce jar with a tight-fitting lid. Shake very well; season, as desired. Store covered in the refrigerator. Makes approximately 1½ cups.

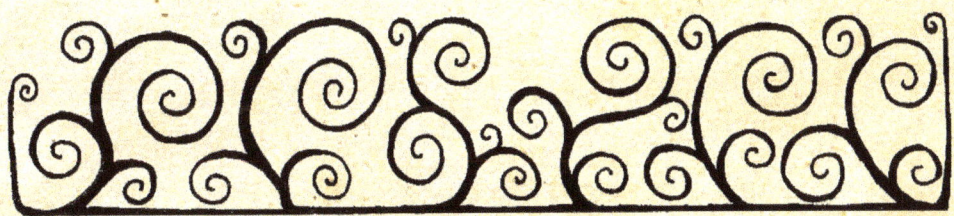

Chapter One

Halfling Hideaway

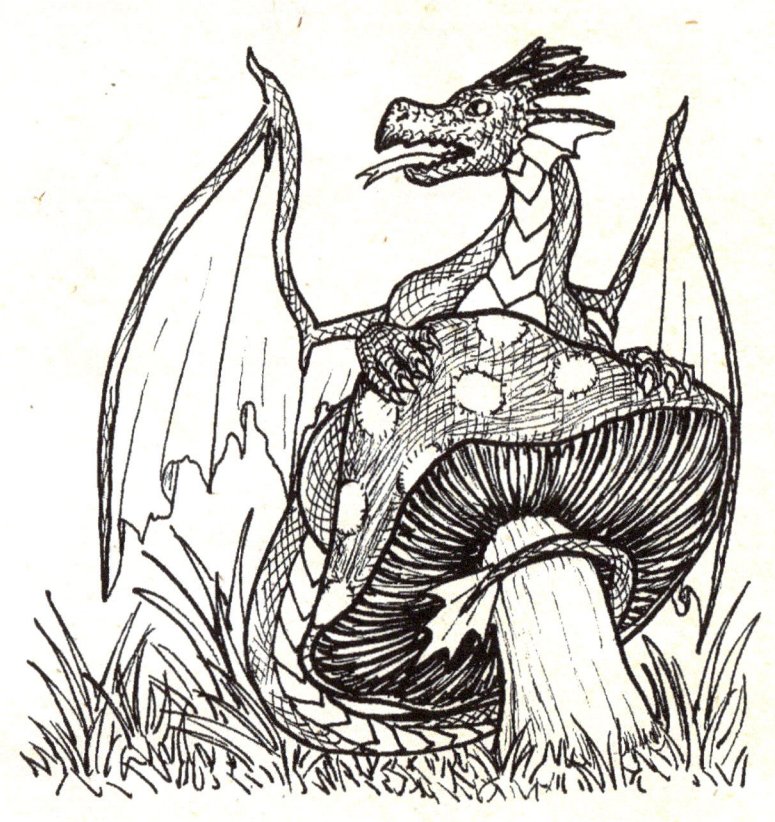

The perfect cozy spot for characters small of stature, yet big of heart.

Six of One Half a Dozen Soup

Ellen's Favorite Salad

Grape & Chicken Cups

Cheddar Sage Scones

Hideaway Sandwich

Halfling Home-Style Fish

Hearty Lunch Pie

Chloë's Macrows and Chese

Stout & Sturdy Chicken & Dumplings

Mushroom Steaks

Nutty Honey Bars

Marcella's Cherries

Apple & Raspberry Jam Tart

Comforting Chai

HALFLING HIDEAWAY

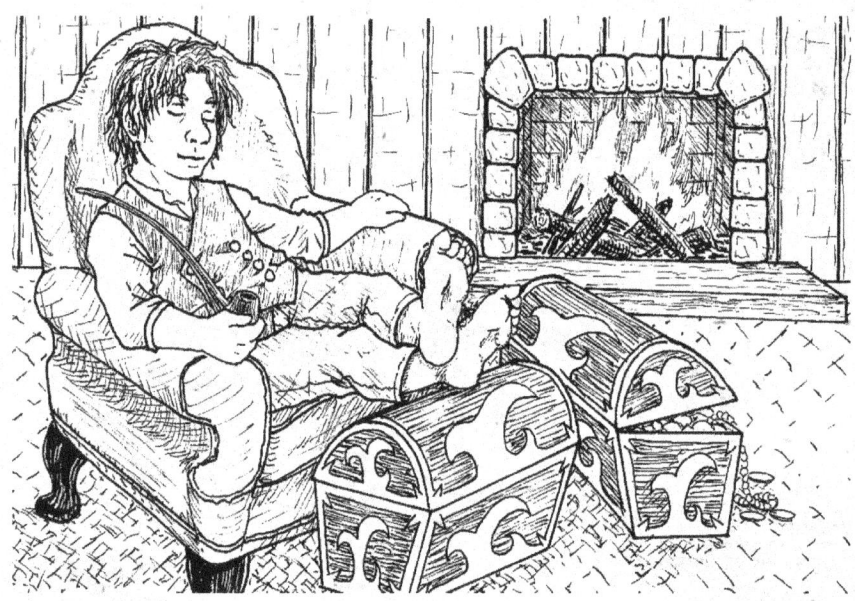

A typical halfling likes to stay at home. He or she feels most comfortable there, whether it be a modest cottage or a more sumptuous dwelling. Some work, some hobbies, some laughter; camaraderie and/or solitude—plus some good food and drink, of course—all these pleasures combine to help make home a halfling's favorite place.

But sometimes a halfling just needs to get away from it all, so he or she might occasionally visit a cozy hideaway spot, where he or she can still have comfort food and then avoid doing the dishes. Sometimes leaving your favorite place for a while makes you appreciate it all the more when you return.

Six of One Half a Dozen Soup

Six cups of liquid and half a dozen cups of vegetables produce a delicious soup no matter what you call it. It feeds about six people, as well. Be sure to check out all of the options listed below and you might even think up a few of your own, depending on what's around in your pantries, gardens, or local marketplaces.

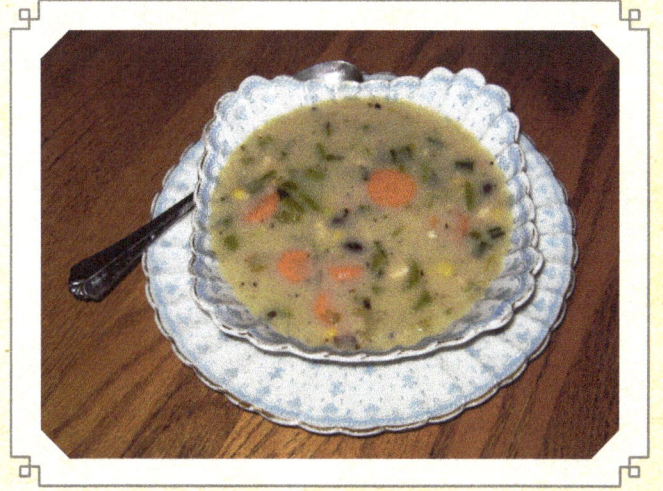

2 tablespoons salted butter
1 cup each (diced or sliced):
   celery
   onion
   carrot, peeled[1]
3 cups assorted vegetables[2]
1 teaspoon dry marjoram (or 2 tablespoons fresh marjoram, minced)
½ teaspoon salt
½ teaspoon pepper
5½ cups low-sodium chicken broth
½ pound cooked chicken, diced[3]
½ cup heavy cream
½ cup all-purpose flour or Wondra

Use a 4-cup glass measuring cup for preparing this recipe and don't bother washing it out. In a 4-quart saucepan, melt the butter over rather high heat. Add the celery, onion, and carrots and sauté 5 minutes. Add the 3 cups additional assorted (see Sidebar) vegetables and seasonings; sauté another 5 minutes. Add the broth and chicken. Bring to a boil; lower heat to a medium simmer and cook 15-20 minutes, uncovered,

[1] A trick to making a good soup is to keep your raw vegetables a rather uniform size. You don't want to have diced celery along with potatoes that are in 2" chunks. So decide on dicing or slicing and try to keep everything harmoniously similar.

[2] Use fresh or frozen vegetables. You can use 3 cups of one vegetable, or 1½ cups of 2 different vegetables. This soup is completely versatile, depending on your whim. Here are some good suggestions: potatoes, sweet potatoes, leeks, spinach, cabbage, mushrooms, asparagus, peas, corn, lima beans, bell peppers, turnips, cauliflower, broccoli, beets, and squash (winter or summer). Drain and rinse a 14½-ounce can of any sort of bean and add near the end of cooking.

[3] I usually just use some grilled chicken strips in a rotisserie-style flavor. Other cooked meats work well, such as ham, sausage, bacon (add at the end), or leftover roasted meats.

Chapter One: Halfling Hideaway

until the vegetables are tender, stirring occasionally. If you use some vegetables that are already cooked or if you use canned (drained) vegetables, just add them in the final 5 minutes of cooking time, before you thicken the soup.

In the 4-cup glass measuring cup, whisk together the cream and about 1 cup of hot soup, then whisk in the flour until smooth. Add this to the soup and bring to a boil again; cook 5 minutes over a medium heat until soup has thickened. Adjust seasonings, if desired. Cover and refrigerate leftovers. Serves 4-6.

 **Vegetarian Option**—Replace the chicken broth with vegetable broth. Replace the chicken with 2 additional cups of vegetables.

Add about 4 to 8 ounces of roasted, chopped green chile to the soup near the end of cooking. You can drain the chile or not; some chile juice will make your soup spicier.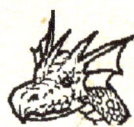

 *Sometimes I might seem to go nuts with options (you'll get used to it), but I think it's important to have the occasional recipe that you can change quite a lot, depending on what's around, while knowing that your base is reliable.*

Ellen's Favorite Salad

This is a lovely salad to accompany just about any sort of main dish. Dried cranberries or even blueberries would work well; and feel free to ramp up your Bleu cheese, if you like stronger flavors (Feta would also be a nice substitute).

5-6 cups light green lettuce, torn into large pieces (such as Bibb, Boston, Butter, or living lettuce)
2 ounces sliced almonds, lightly toasted
½ cup dried cherries
2 ounces Gorgonzola cheese, crumbled into small bits
1 cup celery, cut diagonally into ¼" slices
¼ cup almond oil
1 tablespoon white vinegar
1 tablespoon honey mustard
1 teaspoon sugar
1 teaspoon mayonnaise
½ teaspoon Savory Seasoning[1]
¼ teaspoon salt

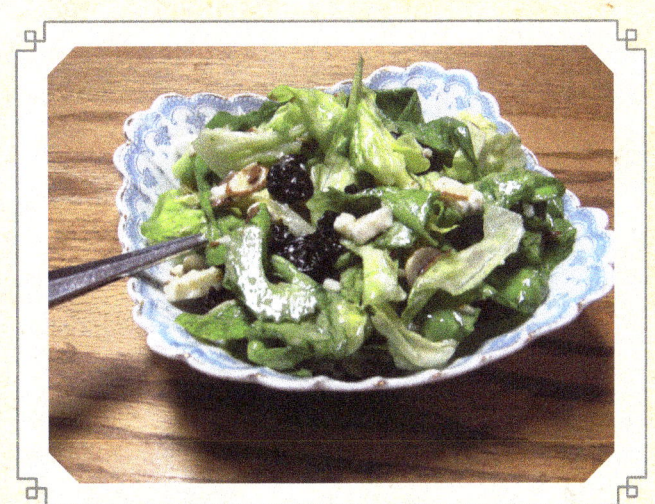

In a very large bowl, combine the lettuce, almonds, cherries, cheese, and celery. In a shaker jar with a tight-fitting lid, combine the remaining ingredients and shake well. Adjust seasonings, if desired. Pour over the greens and toss. Serve immediately. You can make the dressing in advance and mix your greens, but don't toss together until right before serving because these types of lettuces are rather fragile. Not recommended as leftovers. Serves 4.

---

[1] For all recipes that call for Savory Seasoning, see Essential Seasoning Mixes on page xxi for recipe.

Grape & Chicken Cups

You could easily use turkey instead of chicken in this refreshing salad. I often use the packaged, grilled chicken strips because they are super-convenient. If you can't find puff pastry shells, or don't want to bother with them, good carbohydrate substitutes are toasted cocktail bread slices, bagels, or multi-grain crackers.

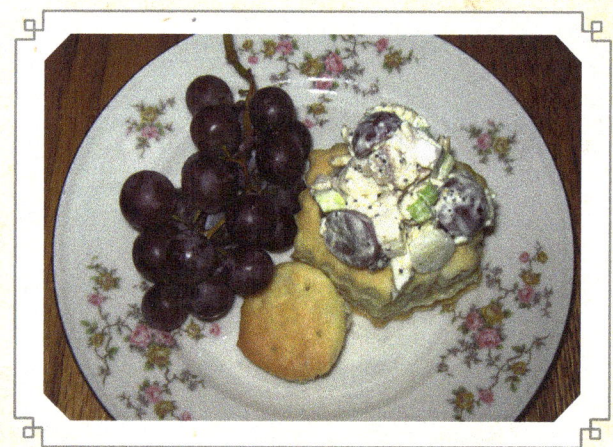

6 puff pastry shells, baked and cooled according to package directions (take off the lids and let stand on the baking sheet—such as Pepperidge Farm)
3 tablespoons mayonnaise
2 tablespoons light sour cream
2 teaspoons lemon juice
1 teaspoon poppy seeds
½ teaspoon hot Madras curry powder
½ teaspoon Savory Seasoning
½ pound cooked chicken, cut into ½" bits
½ cup red seedless grapes, halved or quartered
¼ cup scallions, thinly sliced
¼ cup raisins (or currants)
1 ounce slivered almonds, lightly toasted

In a medium bowl, whisk together the mayonnaise, sour cream, lemon juice, and the 3 seasonings. Add the remaining ingredients and combine well. Season, as desired. Use a teaspoon to fill each shell all the way to the bottom and mound on top (you will probably have some salad leftover—cover and refrigerate). Set the lids next to each shell. Serves 6.

I have a real weakness for bread products. When I really want to be decadent, I'll put this on some naan (mmm, naan). But usually I'm on some sort of diet. So sometimes I'll skip the carbs completely and serve a scoop of this salad over some mixed field greens, spinach, or arugula; and thus, it will serve as one of those low-carb recipes, which are extremely rare in this cookbook...

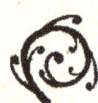

Cheddar Sage Scones

A substantial companion to any hearty soup or stew. You can certainly substitute different herbs for the sage.

1¼ cups all-purpose flour
1 cup cake flour
1 teaspoon baking powder
½ teaspoon baking soda
¾ teaspoon salt
1 teaspoon dry sage (or 2-3 tablespoons fresh sage, minced)
½ cup soft salted butter
4 ounces sharp Cheddar cheese, shredded
½ cup 1% milk, room temperature
1 extra large egg, room temperature

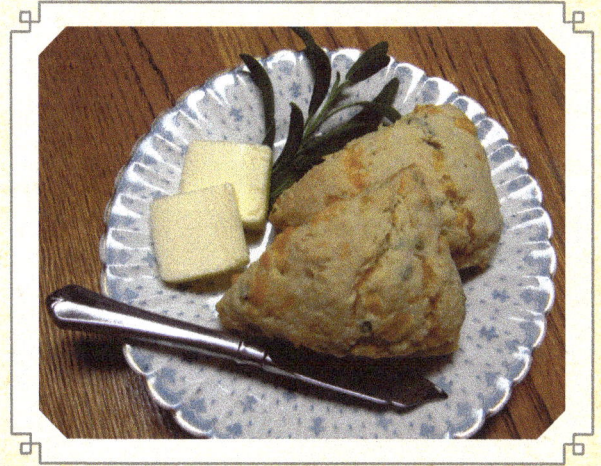

Preheat oven to 400°. Coat a large baking sheet with cooking spray or grease lightly. In a large bowl, combine the first 6 ingredients. Add the butter and cheese and combine. In a 1-cup glass measuring cup, whisk together the milk and egg, then add to flour mixture and combine just until incorporated. Turn out onto a floured surface. With floured hands, knead dough a few times, then pat into a 1" thick circle, about 8" in diameter. Cut into 8 wedges. Place on prepared sheet 1" apart. Bake 12-16 minutes, until light golden brown on bottom. Let stand 5 minutes on pan. Keep leftovers covered at room temperature. Makes 8.

Mix 4 ounces of well-drained green chile in when you add the milk and egg mixture.

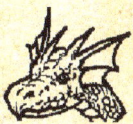

Chapter One: Halfling Hideaway

Hideaway Sandwich

Here's a quick and easy boiled egg sandwich with a salty bacon crumble mixed in for extra oomph. Excellent for a second breakfast when you're feeling a bit peckish at mid-morning, or an afternoon snack when your little halfling brings a few monsters over.

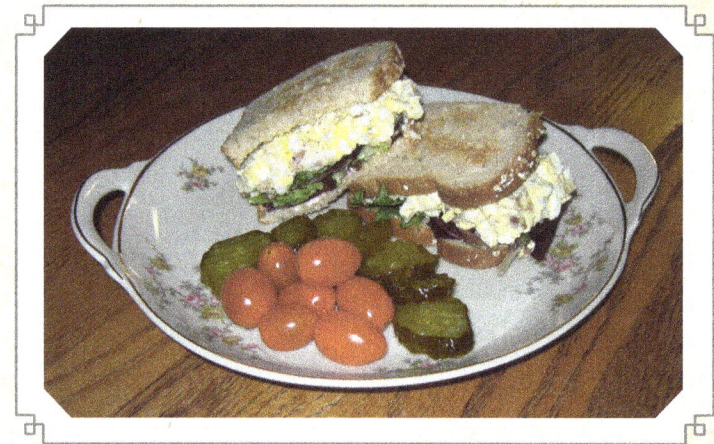

- 6 extra large eggs, hard boiled and peeled
- 2 ounces good quality precooked bacon (cook until crispy, set on paper towels to blot the fat, then crumble or chop into ¼" bits)
- ½ teaspoon Savory Seasoning
- ½ cup plus about 3 tablespoons mayonnaise
- 6 slices whole grain bread, toasted lightly
- 6 leaves of red leaf lettuce (torn or cut to fit your bread)

Place an egg in an egg slicer and slice once horizontally. Turn egg once and slice vertically. Repeat with all the eggs and place in a medium bowl. Add the bacon, Savory Seasoning, and ½ cup mayonnaise and combine. Adjust seasonings, if desired. Spread about 1 tablespoon mayonnaise on 3 slices of toast. Arrange 2 lettuce leaves on each of these slices. Divide the egg salad evenly on top of the lettuce, then top with the remaining slices of toast. Slice in half. Cover and refrigerate leftovers. Serves 3 or 6.

 *I made this up when I was first testing Troy's Springtime Pie (see page 91). At the time, I just didn't want to face making a whole pie, but then I had six hard boiled eggs hanging around. Actually, this happened twice... This sandwich also led to the creation of Savory Seasoning, so my laziness ended up being serendipitous all around.*

Halfling Home-style Fish

I'm of Norwegian descent, so here's a Scandinavian-influenced dish for you. You'll see a few items that are inspired by that cuisine in the cookbook. Remember, I live in a land-locked area and I often don't have access to fresh fish, or at least fresh fish that I can afford to buy. I've used frozen salmon, cod, and tilapia for this recipe; all are fine. If you use frozen fillets, thaw according to package directions. Nice accompaniments for this recipe are green vegetables and beets.

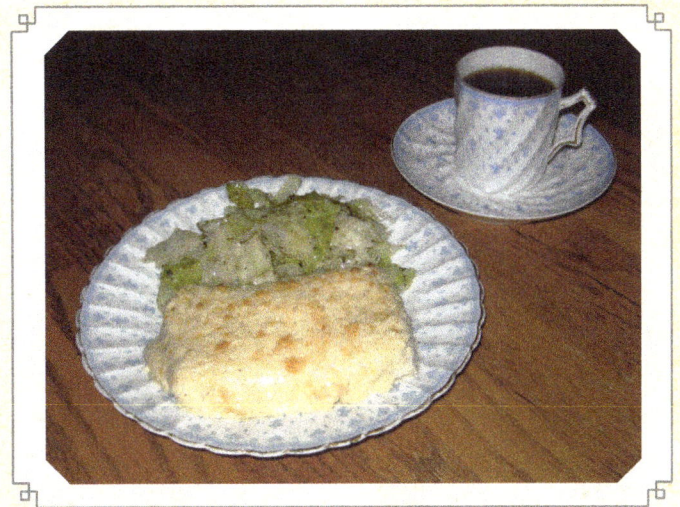

- 4 boneless, skinless fish fillets (your choice, between 1½ and 2 pounds total)
- ¼ teaspoon plus ½ teaspoon salt
- ¾ teaspoon pepper, divided
- 3 tablespoons lemon juice
- 1 tablespoon plus 1 tablespoon salted butter
- 1 tablespoon all-purpose flour
- 1 teaspoon ground coriander seed
- 1 cup half-and-half
- 1 extra large egg yolk
- 2 ounces Parmesan or Romano cheese, finely shredded

Preheat oven to 400°. Coat a 13" by 9" baking dish with cooking spray. Sprinkle the pan with ¼ teaspoon each of salt and pepper. Place fish in pan. Pour lemon juice all over fish. Sprinkle fish evenly with ½ teaspoon salt and ¼ teaspoon pepper. Cut 1 tablespoon butter into 4 pieces and place 1 on each fillet. Bake 15-25 minutes, until flaky in the center (test with a fork), yet still moist (cooking time will depend on the thickness of your fillets).

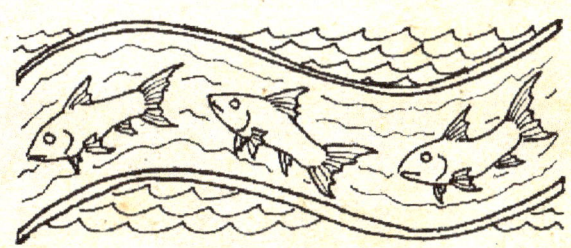

Meanwhile, melt the remaining butter in a 1½-quart saucepan over moderately high heat. Whisk in the flour until well-combined. Add the remaining pepper and the coriander. In a 2-cup glass measuring cup, whisk together the half-and-half and egg yolk. Add this to the butter mixture, whisking over moderate heat just until thicker. Season, as desired. Cover and let stand.

Remove fish from oven and set broiler to high. Coat a broiler-proof 11" by 7" baking dish with cooking spray and place fish here; discard any cooking liquids. Whisk the cream sauce and spread this all over the fish, then sprinkle the cheese evenly over all. Broil about 5-7 minutes, until the cheese is bubbly and golden brown. Cover and refrigerate leftovers. Serves 4.

 *Everyone in my house enjoys this recipe, even Bob. I suppose it's hard to go wrong when you top things with cream sauce and bubbly cheese.*

Hearty Lunch Pie

You know this will be a favorite dish for any halfling. Monsters will love it, too. Please prepare the Mini-Mashers first!

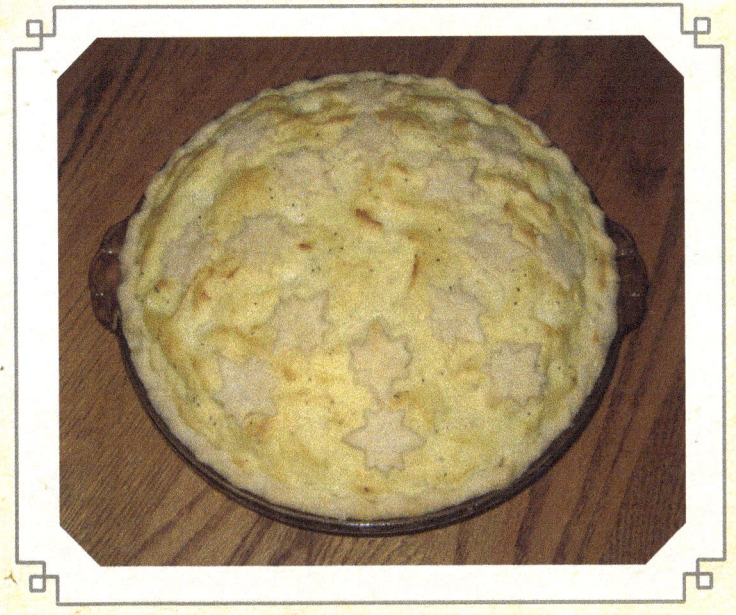

Mini-Mashers

1 pound russet potatoes, peeled and cut into 1" chunks
3 cups water
2 tablespoons salted butter
½ teaspoon salt
½ teaspoon pepper
⅓ cup half-and-half
1 extra large egg

Combine the potatoes and water in a 2-quart pot. Bring to a boil; lower heat a bit and cook, uncovered, for about 15 minutes or until fork-tender. Using the lid for the pot, drain potatoes well and put back in the pot. Add the remaining ingredients and mash until smooth, either by hand or with a hand mixer. Combine well, cover, and set aside. Season, as desired. Makes a smidge over 3 cups.[1]

---

[1] If you don't want to make these, you can use 3 cups leftover, seasoned mashed potatoes mixed well with 1 extra large egg. Or, purchase a 24-ounce container of ready-made potatoes and add the egg.

 *These are only called "mini" because the recipe only makes about three cups, which is just enough to cover the Hearty Lunch Pie which follows. It's also just enough to feed 3-4 people for dinner if you don't want any leftovers.*

Hearty Lunch Pie (Proper)

Mini-Mashers, (see preceding recipe)
1½ cups plus 2 tablespoons all-purpose flour
1 teaspoon salt, divided
3 ounces chilled lard, cut into ¼" bits (or other shortening)
6-8 tablespoons ice water
1 pound lean ground beef
1 cup onion, coarsely chopped
4 ounces fresh mushrooms, coarsely chopped
14½-ounce can petite diced tomatoes, drained well
1 cup low-sodium beef broth
1½ teaspoons Worcestershire sauce
½ teaspoon Savory Seasoning
½ teaspoon Kitchen Bouquet[2]
½ teaspoon plus ¼ teaspoon pepper
2 tablespoons plus 1 tablespoon salted butter
10-12 ounces fresh baby spinach

[2] This concentrated browning sauce is widely available in America. It is definitely worth purchasing a small bottle, rather than attempting to make your own. If you have trouble obtaining this, you may substitute sauces such as soy or Worcestershire, depending on the other seasonings in a particular recipe. Check out online sources if you can't locate some; it keeps for years on your pantry shelf.

Be sure to have your Mini-Mashers ready and waiting. Meanwhile, combine the 1½ cups flour, ½ teaspoon salt, and lard in a large bowl with a pastry blender. Add the water one tablespoon at a time and mix well to form a dough. Flatten into a disk, wrap with plastic wrap or set in a covered container, and refrigerate while preparing the filling.

Coat a 5-quart deep skillet with cooking spray. Over rather high heat, cook the ground beef, onion, and mushrooms until almost dry. Add the tomatoes. In a 2-cup glass measuring cup, combine the broth, Worcestershire sauce, 2 tablespoons flour, Savory Seasoning, Kitchen Bouquet, ½ teaspoon pepper, and ¼ teaspoon salt with a whisk. Add to the meat and bring to a boil. Lower heat a bit and cook, uncovered, for 5-10 minutes until saucy. Adjust seasonings, if desired. Let stand.

Preheat oven to 375°. On a floured surface, roll out dough to a 13" circle and lay in a 9½" glass pie dish. Trim edge, fold and flute edge generously. Reserve scraps for decorations, if desired. Pour meat mixture into dish. Wash out skillet. In skillet, melt 2 tablespoons butter over very high heat. Add the remaining ¼ teaspoon salt and pepper. Add the spinach and cook over rather high heat just until wilted, about 2-3 minutes, covered. Uncover and cook over very high heat until fairly dry, stirring frequently, about 2-3 minutes (dry, but don't let it burn). Cover meat with spinach mixture.

Mix the potatoes and carefully spread to cover the spinach; seal at the crust edge. Decorate, if desired. Cut the 1 tablespoon butter into 16 bits and evenly dot the potatoes. Bake 46-50 minutes. Let stand 15 minutes before slicing. Cover and refrigerate leftovers. Serves 6-8.

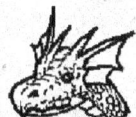

Drain 4 ounces roasted and chopped green chile and add into the meat mixture at the end of cooking.

Because of a number glitch (I decided to combine two smaller recipes into one and then forgot to change the numbers, duh…), I realized I was one recipe short in June, 2010. So, Callista and I were standing around the kitchen thinking of something else to finish the book—111 was the goal! Luxurious hot chocolate? Fancy coffee? Too Starbucky. Mead? It takes too long and you need space for storage. Fancy oatmeal? I felt I had enough dried fruit going on. At first, I had thought of a Shepherd's Pie and I actually did have a version in my original college cookbook project from 2000. But I figured it's been done to death—it was even deconstructed on a Top Chef *episode. We went to bed and I said something will come to me eventually.*

I actually woke the next morning after dreaming about this particular recipe. It had to have spinach. Then it had to go in what used to be the Farmer Maggot section. This was really odd to dream about something so specific and, even odder, to remember it. I unfortunately didn't remember exact proportions, however, so I still had to work on it a few times. So, this is the one hundred and eleventh recipe I developed—a Shepherd's Pie, yet different and delicious enough to include. What's wrong with revisiting old classics, anyway? I guess that's why they're called classics and that's why they often stay in style.

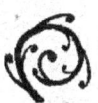

Chloë's Macrows and Chese
(a.k.a. Chloë's Macaroni and Cheese)

I would find it hard to imagine that any halfling would be dissatisfied with this recipe as a meatless supper.

2 quarts water
8 ounces elbow macaroni (or other small-shaped pasta)
½ teaspoon salt
1¼ cups heavy cream
¼ cup salted butter
½ cup seasoned dry bread crumbs
4 ounces Gouda cheese, shredded
2 ounces Parmesan or Romano cheese, finely shredded

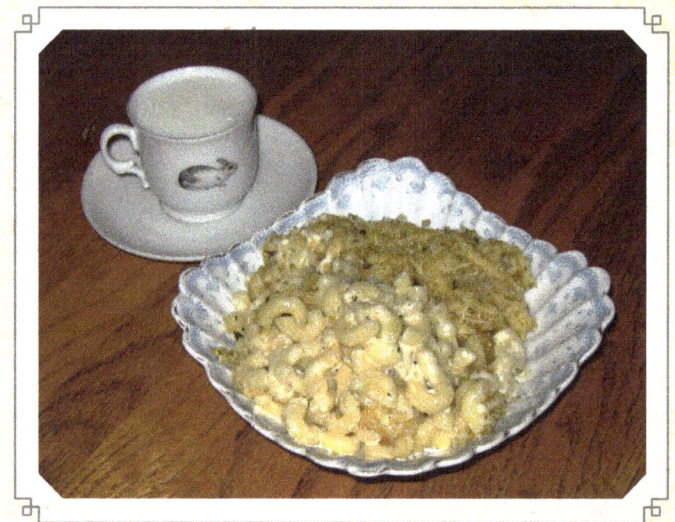

Preheat oven to 400°. Coat a 2" deep, 11" by 7" baking dish with cooking spray or grease lightly. Bring the water to boil in a 4-quart saucepan. Add the macaroni and cook as directed on the package. Drain and put back in the saucepan. Add the salt and cream and combine. Pour this into the prepared dish (it will be soupy).

Meanwhile, microwave the butter on HIGH in a medium glass bowl in 20-second intervals until fully melted. Add the remaining ingredients and combine. Sprinkle this evenly over the macaroni. Bake for 16-18 minutes, until golden brown on top. Let stand 5 minutes before serving. Cover and refrigerate leftovers (the macaroni will completely absorb the cream and you will be left with buttery, bready, cheesy noodles—if you have any leftovers; don't count on it). Serves 4-6.

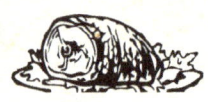 **Meat Lover's Option**—Add between 1-2 cups of any kind of diced, cooked meat to the pasta—this is a good place to use up some leftovers (you can cut up 2 or 3 hot dogs and watch this disappear extra fast!).

Drain 4 ounces of roasted and chopped green chile and mix in with the cooked pasta and cream.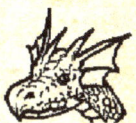

 *I consider this "mac & cheese" in its purest essence and as far removed from a box as possible. Callista disagrees since the cheese is not mixed in with the macaroni; yet I've noticed this recipe is quite popular around my house. It is one of Chloë's absolute favorites, and the two of them sometimes argue about this dish (in a friendly way…).*

I came up with this recipe after doing some research into food history. According to Reay Tannahill, "macrows" makes an English appearance in the 14th Century: it is served with butter and grated cheese on the side (236). C. Anne Wilson discusses more of an 18th Century concept, whereby macaroni would be cooked and combined with cream; cheese would cover the pasta and it would be broiled till it became golden brown (180). And thus, you can see where I came up with this particular macaroni treatment.

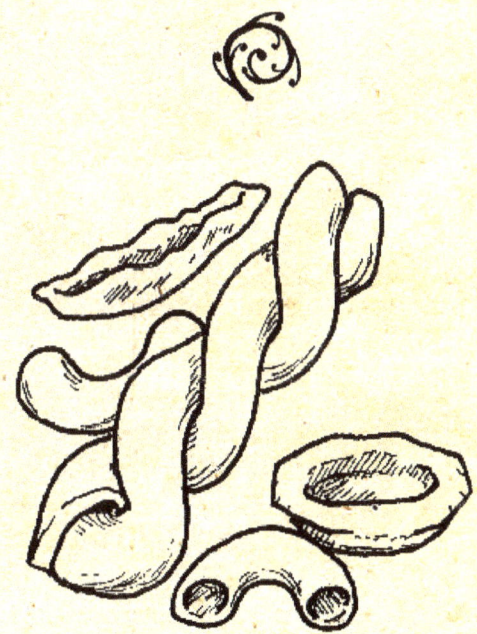

Stout & Sturdy Chicken & Dumplings

I love the smell of cumin, and it really complements the chicken in this dish. Feel free to substitute regular onions for the leeks, if you prefer.

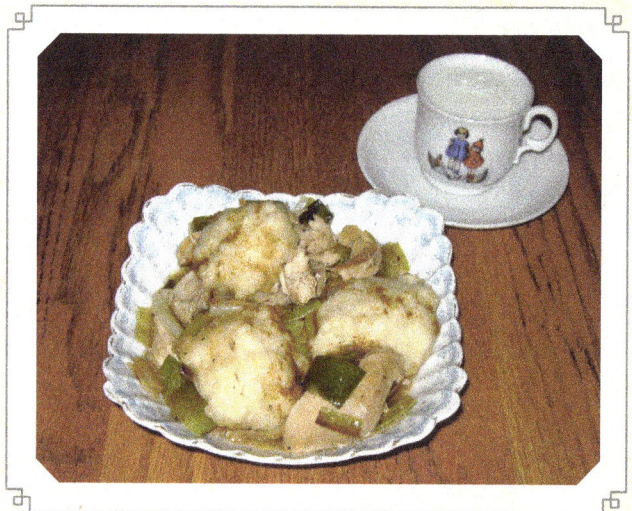

- 2 pounds boneless, skinless chicken breasts
- 24 ounces stout beer, room temperature (or use a porter or brown ale)
- 1 cup water
- ¼ cup salted butter
- 4-5 cups leeks, cut into ½" slices (clean well; use white and light green parts)
- 14½-ounce can low-sodium chicken broth
- 2 tablespoons plus 1½ cups all-purpose flour
- 1 teaspoon plus ½ teaspoon cumin
- 1 teaspoon pepper
- ½ teaspoon plus 1 teaspoon salt
- ½ teaspoon poultry seasoning
- ½ teaspoon baking powder
- 2 ounces softened lard (or other shortening)
- ½ cup 1% milk

Pour 1 cup beer into a 4-cup glass measuring cup and set aside. Place chicken, remaining beer, and water into a 5-quart deep skillet. Bring to a boil, then simmer over low heat, covered, 15 minutes. Turn meat over and simmer over low heat, covered, another 15-20 minutes. Place chicken on a plate or cutting board; discard all cooking liquid and rinse out the skillet. When chicken is cooler, shred it into 1-2" pieces; set aside.

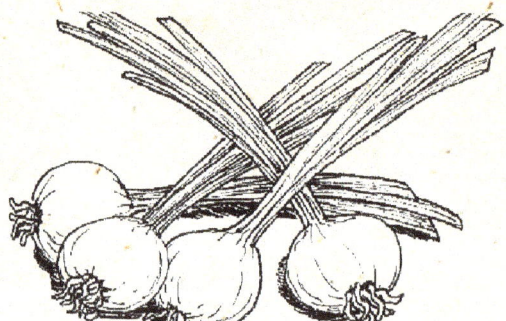

In the skillet, melt the butter over high heat. Add the leeks and sauté 5 minutes, stirring frequently. Add the broth, 2 tablespoons flour, 1 teaspoon cumin, pepper, ½ teaspoon salt, and poultry seasoning to the reserved beer and whisk well to combine. Add to the skillet and bring to a boil. Cook over medium heat until the sauce thickens, about 5-10 minutes. Add the chicken and bring to a gentle simmer. Season sauce as desired.

Meanwhile in a medium bowl, combine the 1½ cups flour, 1 teaspoon salt, and the baking powder. With a pastry blender, cut in the lard until the mixture resembles coarse crumbs. Add the milk and combine well. With a spoon, divide the dough into 1½" rather rough portions; you should end up with about 16. Place on top of the simmering chicken/leek mixture 1" apart. Sprinkle mainly the dumplings with the ½ teaspoon cumin. Cover and simmer over a very low heat for 15 minutes. Cover and refrigerate leftovers. Serves 4-6.

You know, about 4 ounces of roasted and chopped green chile wouldn't hurt, if you mix it in with the broth and stout mixture. You are probably getting tired of hearing me make these suggestions, but I can't help it; 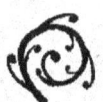 New Mexicans really do live for chiles, both red and green—they are good for you; they are full of Vitamin C and will help to clear out your nasal passages. My son-in-law's great-grandmother just turned 103. She attributes her longevity to green chile… and cigarettes (while it's probably not a great idea to start smoking, perhaps adding more spicy food to your daily diet wouldn't hurt!).

Mushroom Steaks

These are a bit like miniature meatloaves and are sure to make halflings happy. Serve with mashed potatoes and a green vegetable, such as peas.

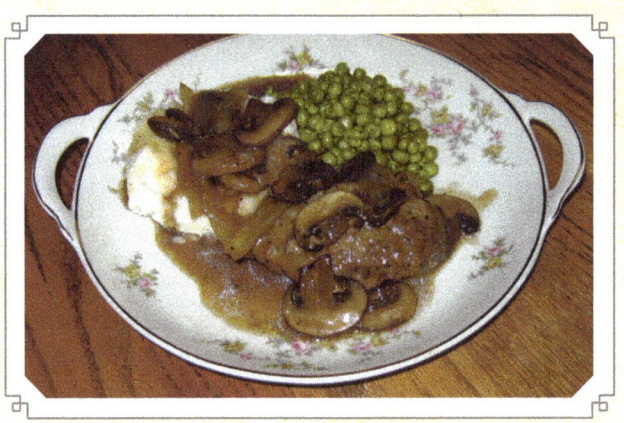

1 tablespoon salted butter
¾ pound fresh mushrooms, cut into ¼" slices
2 cups onion, cut into ½" slivers
14½-ounce can low-sodium beef broth
1 tablespoon Worcestershire sauce
½ teaspoon Kitchen Bouquet
½ teaspoon plus ½ teaspoon salt
½ teaspoon plus ½ teaspoon pepper
½ cup water
2 tablespoons cornstarch
1½ pounds lean ground beef
2 extra large eggs
½ cup seasoned dry bread crumbs
2 tablespoons dry parsley (or ½ cup fresh parsley, minced)
1 teaspoon crushed rosemary (or 2 tablespoons fresh rosemary, minced)

In a 5-quart deep skillet, melt the butter over high heat. Add the mushrooms and onion. Cook on medium/high heat, covered, for 5 minutes. In a 4-cup glass measuring cup, combine the broth, Worcestershire sauce, Kitchen Bouquet, ½ teaspoon salt, ½ teaspoon pepper, water, and cornstarch with a whisk. Add to skillet and bring to a boil. Boil, uncovered, for 3 minutes until sauce thickens. Adjust seasonings, if desired.

Meanwhile in a large bowl, combine the beef, eggs, bread crumbs, and all remaining seasonings with your hands until thoroughly mixed. Divide into 8 equal oval-shaped patties and place each on top of the mushroom gravy. Cover and simmer on low heat for 10 minutes. Turn patties over, spoon some gravy over the top of each, and cook over medium heat for 15 minutes, uncovered. Cover and refrigerate leftovers. Serves 6-8.

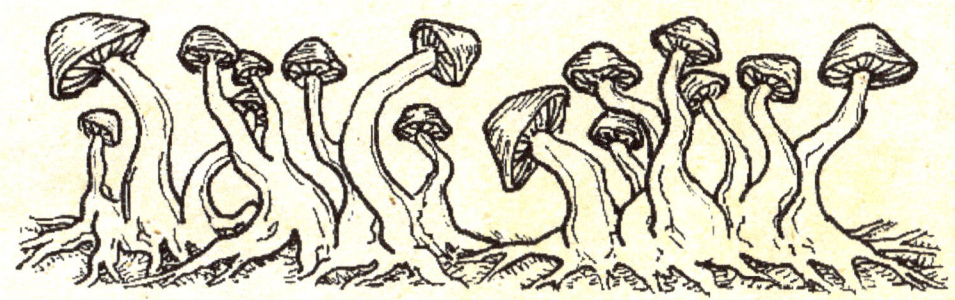

Well, I thought I could restrain myself, but 4 ounces of roasted and chopped green chile (drained or not) would certainly be nice in the gravy here; just mix it in with the broth. Or mix 4 ounces into the gravy and 4 ounces (drained) into the meat for a really intense experience. Good thing desserts are next, so I'll shut up about green chile for the moment.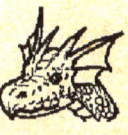

 *One of Callista's favorites, and you can imagine it's one of Bob's as well!*

Nutty Honey Bars

Almonds have a long history in British cuisine and are a natural companion for honey.

1 cup plus 1 tablespoon all-purpose flour
½ cup powdered sugar
½ teaspoon plus ½ teaspoon cinnamon
½ cup soft salted butter
1 tablespoon half-and-half
½ cup almond butter, room temperature
½ cup honey
2 ounces sliced almonds; toast lightly; cool, then grind finely
2 extra large eggs, room temperature
¼ teaspoon salt
¼ teaspoon baking powder
Extra powdered sugar

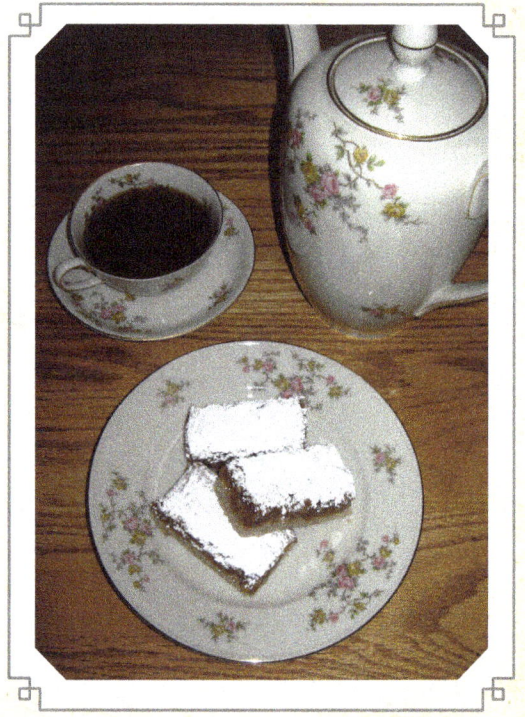

Preheat oven to 350°. Line a heavy 9" square pan with regular aluminum foil; extend about 2" of foil on two sides. Liberally coat the foil and sides of the pan with cooking spray. In a large bowl, combine the 1 cup flour, ½ cup powdered sugar, ½ teaspoon cinnamon, butter, and half-and-half until well blended. Press evenly into prepared pan (don't bother washing the bowl). Bake 10 minutes.

Meanwhile in the bowl, whisk together the almond butter, honey, almonds, eggs, 1 tablespoon flour, salt, baking powder, and ½ teaspoon cinnamon. Pour over baked crust and bake another 22-24 minutes, until the center is set. Cool completely on a rack, about 2 hours. Lift out by the foil extensions, using a sharp knife along the edges, if necessary. Cut into 24 pieces. Sprinkle liberally with powdered sugar. Store covered at room temperature. Makes 24.

 *I think cashews and cashew butter would also work well here—you could also try macadamias/macadamia butter, or even a chocolate and hazelnut butter with hazelnuts (NOT Nutella, however—it's too sweet for this purpose). You can sprinkle more sugar on top after it soaks in, if you like.*

Marcella's Cherries

Perhaps you have a cherry tree in your yard—this is a simple, but quite delicious, crisp; it also works with other fruits, such as apricots, peaches, or nectarines (pit and cut into 1" pieces).

1½ pounds fresh or frozen cherries[1]
1 cup sugar
1 cup all-purpose flour
2 teaspoons cinnamon
¼ teaspoon salt
½ cup soft salted butter

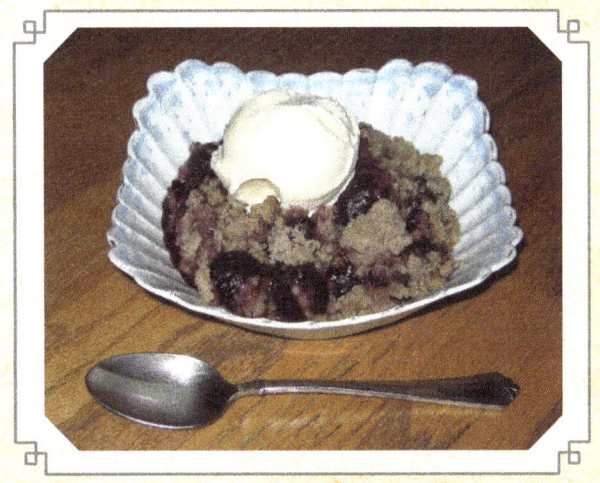

Preheat oven to 400°. Coat an 11" by 7" baking pan with cooking spray or grease lightly. Put all the cherries in the prepared pan. In a medium bowl, combine the sugar, flour, cinnamon, and salt. Mix in the butter until crumbly, while leaving small bits of butter throughout. Sprinkle all over the cherries and spread to cover. Bake 30 minutes. Place on a rack for 30 minutes before serving. Serve warm with whipped cream or ice cream. Store covered at room temperature or refrigerate. Serves 4-6.

This is a slight modification of a dessert my mother-in-law used to make. I was blessed with a sweet and kind mother-in-law. She was thrilled to learn, at the age of 79, that she would finally have a grandchild. Both of my girls usually spent a few hours every Saturday at "choo-choo baba's"—named so because Grandpa Bill and Grandma Marcella lived right next to the railroad tracks—exploring nature, eating lots of good food, doing projects, and basically being loved like crazy by two people who never thought they would ever be grandparents. They had a small house, but a huge yard and garden in Albuquerque's North Valley. When the cherry tree was ready, everyone went out to pick the tart fruit, then came the washing and the pitting. The best part was when Marcella made her tart cherry cobbler and you could eat it warm with vanilla ice cream. My in-laws are both gone now, but I hope that making this recipe will remind my daughters of those times. It may remind you of more carefree days, as well.

[1] Any variety is fine. If using fresh cherries, stem and pit them. Cut in half if they are large, or use whole small ones. If using frozen cherries (I prefer to do this, since frozen cherries are available year-round and they're already pitted), use unsweetened, pitted ones and let them stand in a strainer for a couple of hours before using. Do NOT use canned cherries or cherry pie filling.

Chapter One: Halfling Hideaway

Apple & Raspberry Jam Tart

Sweet jam, apples, and nuts—sort of a perfect halfling dessert. My own favorite apples are varieties such as Fuji, Honey Crisp, Pink Lady, and Gala—all are appropriate for any of the apple recipes in the cookbook; use whichever is your own favorite!

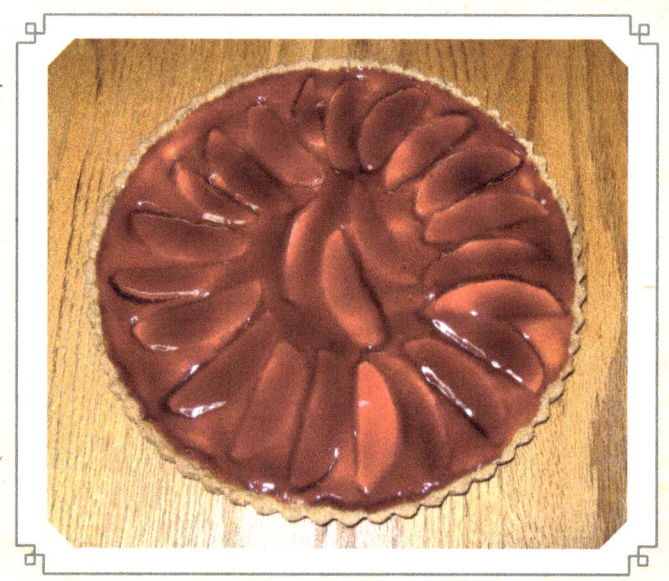

4 ounces walnut halves, lightly toasted and cooled
½ cup all-purpose flour
2 tablespoons plus ½ cup sugar
¼ teaspoon salt
¼ cup soft salted butter
4 ounces light cream cheese (Neufchâtel), softened
1 tablespoon packed golden brown sugar
2 extra large eggs
1 teaspoon vanilla extract
1 large apple, peeled and cored, then cut into ¼" slices
½ cup seedless raspberry jam

Preheat oven to 350°. In a large food processor, pulse the walnuts, flour, 2 tablespoons sugar, and salt until the nuts are ground. Add and pulse the butter until thoroughly mixed. Liberally coat a 9½" tart pan (1" deep) with removable sides with cooking spray or grease well. Scrape nut mixture into pan (don't bother washing bowl and blade); press evenly up the sides, then press evenly onto the bottom of the pan.

Bake 15 minutes. Put on a rack; maintain oven temperature. Be sure to handle pan on the sides only, so you don't shift the bottom.

Meanwhile, process the ½ cup sugar, cream cheese, brown sugar, eggs, and vanilla. Spread evenly over shell. Decoratively arrange the apple slices over the egg mixture, but don't overload. Bake 36-40 minutes. While tart is baking, melt jam in a 1-quart saucepan over medium heat, whisking just until smooth. Remove from heat and let stand, uncovered.

When done, carefully place the tart on a rack and spread the jam over all, using a spoon or bent spatula. Cool on rack for one hour. Refrigerate at least one hour before serving. Remove pan sides and place on a serving plate. After cutting, store covered in refrigerator—you can bring it to room temperature before serving again or enjoy cold. Serves 6-8.

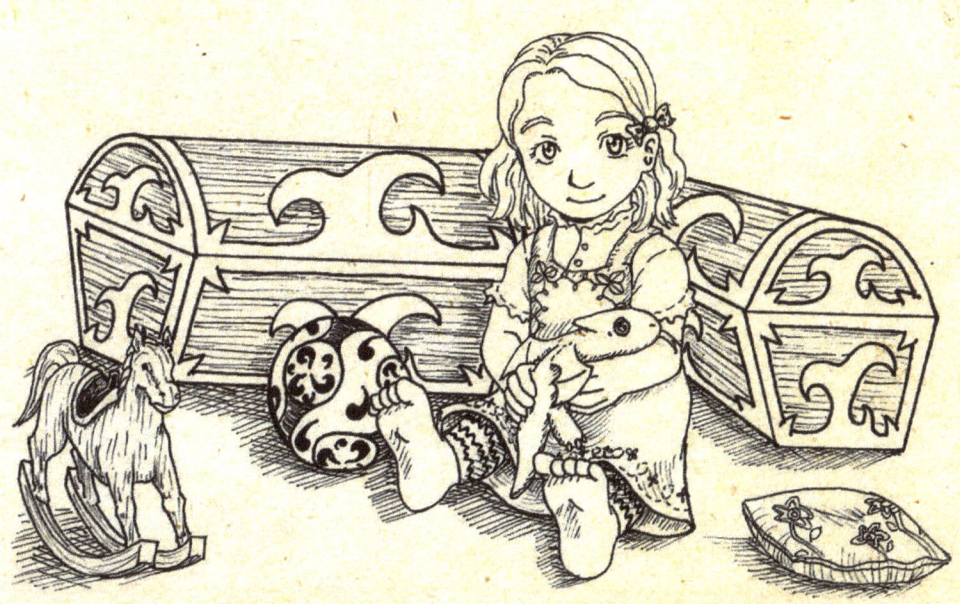

Comforting Chai

Mmm, all of these lovely spices will smell so good simmering in your kitchen.

- 1 large cinnamon stick, broken into 3 pieces
- 2 star anise
- 6 cardamom pods
- 8 whole cloves
- 20 whole peppercorns (any colors)
- 1" piece of fresh ginger, washed, unpeeled, and cut into ¼" slices
- 3 cups water
- 3 regular-sized tea bags (use any fruity variety, such as Constant Comment or Orange Zinger)
- 3-4 tablespoons honey, or more to taste
- 1 cup 1% milk

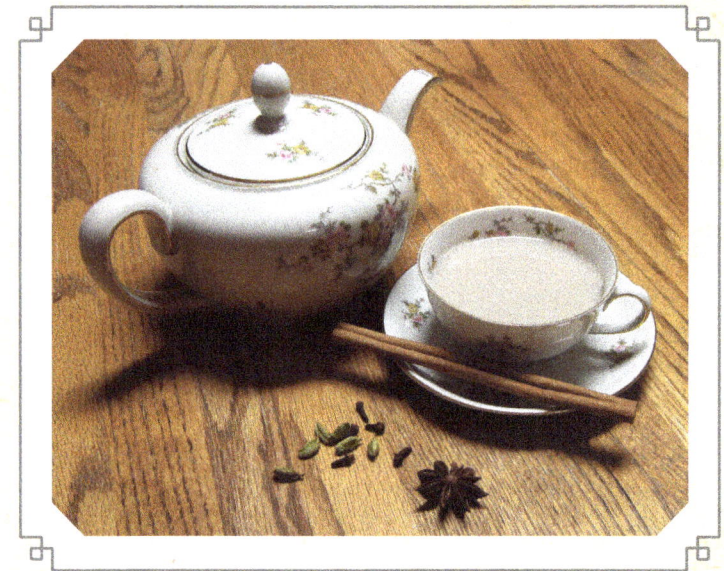

Use a 4-cup glass measuring cup to prepare this recipe. In a 2-quart saucepan, combine the first seven ingredients. Bring to a boil, then simmer over medium heat, uncovered, for 10 minutes. Turn off the heat, add the tea bags, then cover. Let it steep 5 minutes. Put a small fine-mesh strainer over the 4-cup glass measuring cup. Pour the liquid into this and squeeze out the liquid from the tea bags. Discard all solids. You'll have about 2½-2¾ cups left. Pour this back into the saucepan. Add the honey and milk. Stir over low heat just until the honey dissolves. Carefully pour into 2-3 mugs, or pour this back into the 4-cup glass measuring cup so you can pour it more carefully. Cover and refrigerate leftovers; microwave to desired temperature. Serves 2-3, depending on how much comfort you need.

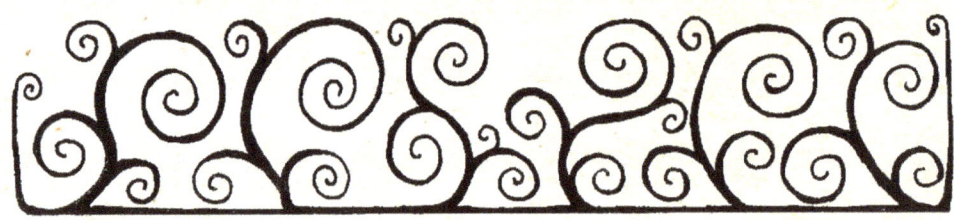

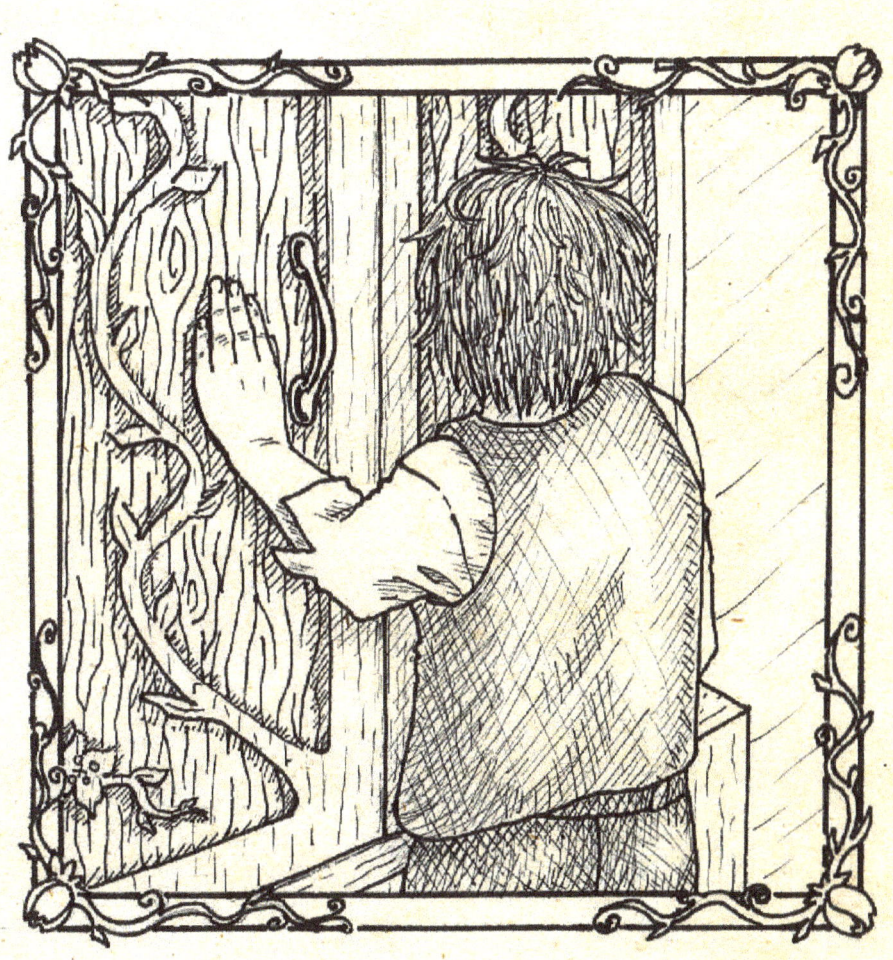

Chapter Two

The Inn of the Doughty Hero

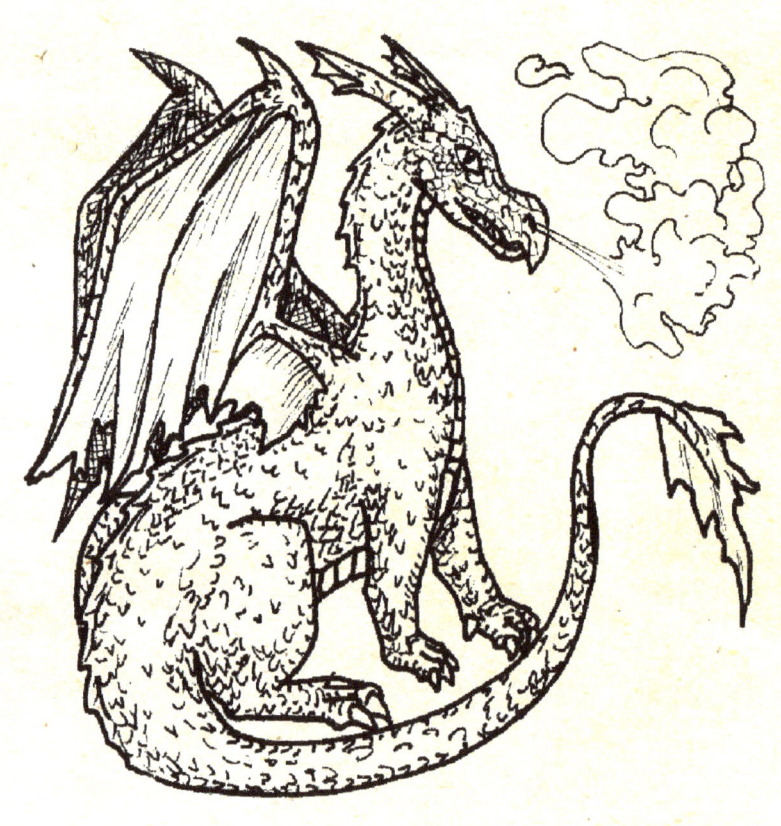

Hearty food for the hero on the move.

Golden Barley Beef Soup

Roast Beef Toasties

Cress Composition

Dilly Bread & Butter

Lise's Lentils

Courageous Low-Carb Chicken

Doughty Hero Casserole

Beery Beef Stew

Rabbit Braised with Herbs

Jan's Baked Apples

Brave Blackberry Tart

Busy Day Rice Pudding

Elfryda's Apple Crisp

Healing Chocolate Chai

The Inn of the Doughty Hero

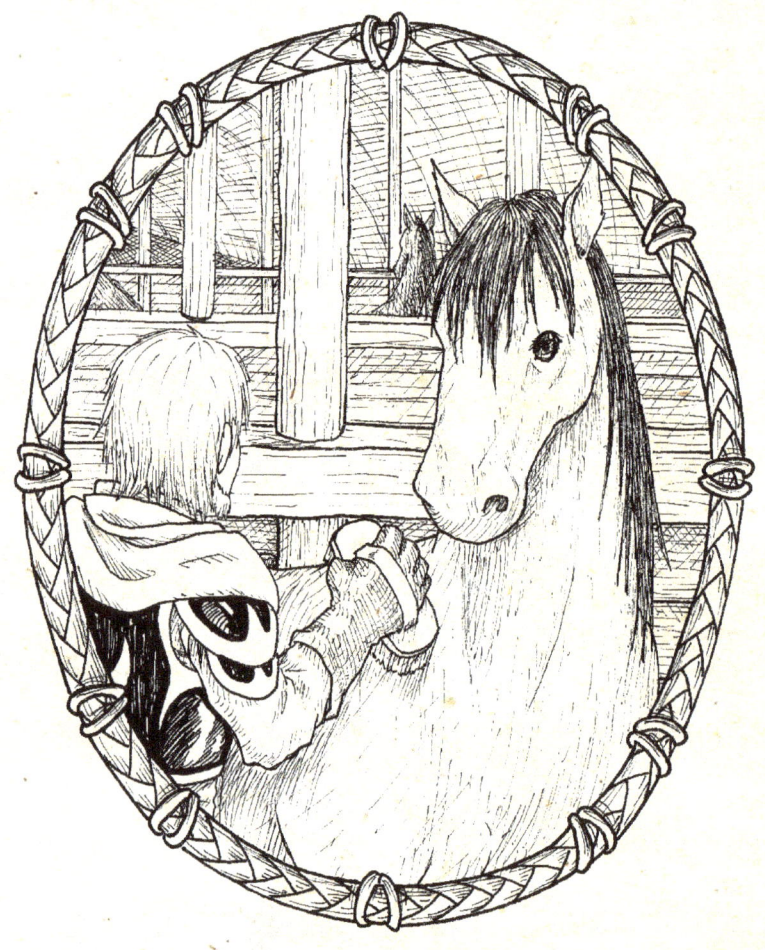

Here's a warm and casual restaurant/inn where wandering ranger-type heroes could bring items they have picked up along their travels and have them prepared in a gentler atmosphere; things such as watercress, apples, roots, and rabbits will all be prepared for the tired champion. So, stay and wash your hands and hair for a change, hero (heroine), and sit back to enjoy some quiet time before you have to tackle the wilderness again.

Golden Barley Beef Soup

A hearty, savory soup—perfect for the hero who has come in from the cold. If you use quick barley, you can reduce your cooking time by about 15 minutes.

1 tablespoon salted butter
1 tablespoon minced garlic
1 cup each, coarsely chopped:
    celery
    onion
    carrot, peeled
½ pound fresh mushrooms, sliced thinly
½ pound sirloin steak, cut into ½" bits
1 quart low-sodium beef broth
½ cup dry red wine, such as Cabernet Sauvignon or Merlot
1 teaspoon saffron threads, crushed
½ teaspoon salt
½ teaspoon pepper
⅓ cup regular pearl barley

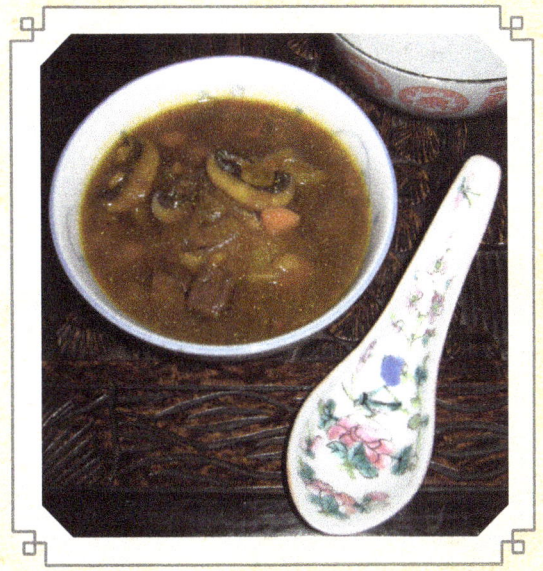

In a 4-quart saucepan, melt the butter over rather high heat. Add the garlic, celery, onion, and carrot and sauté 5 minutes. Add the mushrooms and steak; sauté 5 minutes until the beef loses its red/pink color. Add the remaining ingredients and bring to a boil. Lower heat to a low simmer, cover, and cook 40-45 minutes or until the barley is tender. Stir occasionally. Adjust seasonings, if desired. Cover and refrigerate leftovers; do not store in a plastic container because the saffron will most likely stain it. Serves 4.

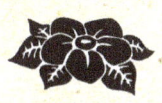 **Vegetarian Option**—Replace the beef broth with vegetable broth. Replace the beef with another ½ pound of fresh mushrooms, or other desired vegetables.

 *I know you might be thinking saffron is expensive, and it certainly can be. I found it cheapest at a local Middle Eastern grocery. Saffron has always been expensive, even in the Middle Ages; however, its relative expense did not prevent its popularity. If you've never tried it before, here's a tasty way to do so.*

Chapter Two: The Inn of the Doughty Hero

Why is saffron expensive? Saffron is made from the stigmas of the crocus plant. If you look at a picture of your basic crocus flower, you'll see two or three red filaments within the flower. You pull these out, dry them, and you now have saffron. You can see that one flower yields about 1/100 of a teaspoon of saffron. In the spring in my garden, I probably have about 100 crocus flowers blooming (if I'm lucky). I could spend a few back-breaking days harvesting crocus stigmas and end up with a teaspoon of saffron. Now I can make some soup. Or I can go ahead and treat myself to a small bottle of it, which won't break the budget much more than lots of other dried spices.

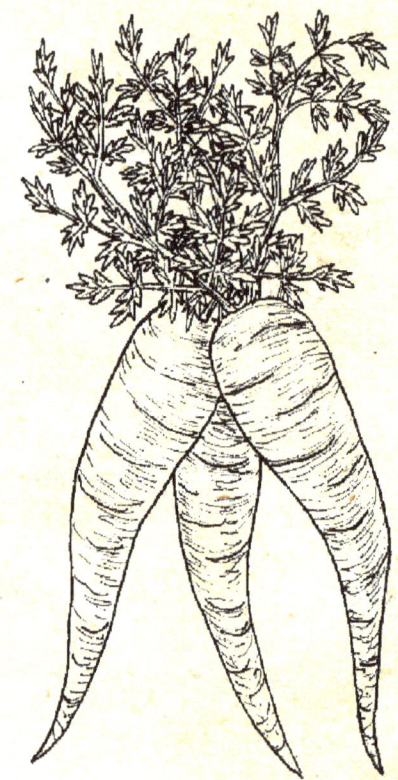

Roast Beef Toasties

These would make a substantial snack at a halfling/monster smörgåsbord, or serve a few as an open-face sandwich for lunch.

- 18 slices of rye or pumpernickel cocktail bread (such as Pepperidge Farm)
- ½ cup mayonnaise
- 4 ounces Gorgonzola cheese, crumbled into small bits[1]
- ½ teaspoon plus ½ teaspoon Savory Seasoning
- 1 tablespoon heavy cream
- 18 slices of shaved roast beef deli meat (from ½ pound)
- 1 unpeeled English (seedless) cucumber, scored, then cut into 18 diagonal slices, each ¼" thick
- 3-4 large radishes, cut into ⅛" slices
- ¼ cup white wine vinegar
- 2 teaspoons sugar
- Salt
- 2 tablespoons fresh parsley or dill, minced (or 1 teaspoon dry parsley or dill weed)

[1] You can use any type of Bleu cheese, depending on your taste, such as Gorgonzola, Bleu, Stilton, or Roquefort.

Preheat oven to 400°. Place the bread slices on a large baking sheet and bake for 8 minutes. Leave on the sheet and set aside to cool. In a medium bowl, whisk together the mayonnaise, cheese, ½ teaspoon Savory Seasoning, and cream. Spread equally onto the toasts, about 1½ teaspoons on each. Fold the beef in halves or quarters to fit on each toast. In a medium bowl, whisk together the vinegar, sugar, and ½ teaspoon Savory Seasoning. Place the cucumber in this to coat, then place a slice on each toast. Place the radishes in the same mixture, then place 2 or 3 slices on top of each cucumber slice (discard the vinegar or chop up any remaining vegetables and toss together for a tiny salad). Lightly sprinkle all with salt. Sprinkle with the parsley or dill. Cover and refrigerate leftovers. Makes 18.

Vegetarian Option—Omit the beef and increase the cheese to 6 ounces.

 Bob *likes about four or five of these for lunch, along with a small can of something like Campbell's tomato soup.*

Chapter Two: The Inn of the Doughty Hero

Cress Composition

If you have difficulties obtaining watercress (or you feel daunted by all the trimming involved), feel free to substitute spinach, arugula, or other mixtures of field greens. You can use one or a combination.

4-5 cups trimmed watercress
¼ cup walnut oil
1 tablespoon cider vinegar
½ tablespoon honey
½ tablespoon Dijon mustard
½ teaspoon Herbes de Provence[1]
⅛ teaspoon salt
⅛ teaspoon pepper
½ cup each:
    radishes, sliced very thinly
    English (seedless) cucumber, sliced very thinly (peeled or not)
    peas (thawed, if using frozen)
¼ cup fresh chives, minced
1 ounce walnut halves, lightly toasted and chopped coarsely

Place the watercress in a large bowl. In a shaker jar with a tight-fitting lid, combine the oil, vinegar, honey, mustard, and the 3 seasonings. Shake until well combined. Season, as desired. Pour 2 tablespoons dressing over the watercress, toss, and arrange on a platter. Arrange the radishes, cucumber slices, and peas in rows or some other artistic fashion. Sprinkle the chives and nuts all over, then pour the remaining dressing over all. Serve immediately. Not recommended as leftovers. Serves 4.

This will serve two (or maybe even three, depending) as a main dish—add about 6 ounces of proteins (any variety of cooked and sliced or chopped meats and/or shredded or diced cheeses) and serve some bread or crackers on the side.

[1] If you don't have access to ready-made Herbes de Provence, see the recipe in the Essential Seasoning Mixes section on page xxii for a homemade version.

Dilly Bread & Butter

There's nothing like a loaf of this hearty, multi-grain bread with its savory, dill-flavored butter to round out your meal. It's good with any soup in the cookbook, or serve it with a substantial salad. This bread combines lots of flavors into a harmonious blend; herby, slightly sweet, yet with a tang of rye in the background. It is also great with other spreads, cheeses, and even jams.

½ cup water
½ cup honey
1 cup buttermilk
2 packets regular active dry yeast
1½ cups plus 2-2½ cups bread flour
½ cup wheat flour
¼ cup dark rye flour
1 tablespoon dill seed
1½ teaspoons salt
1½ teaspoons onion powder
Dilly Butter, recipe below

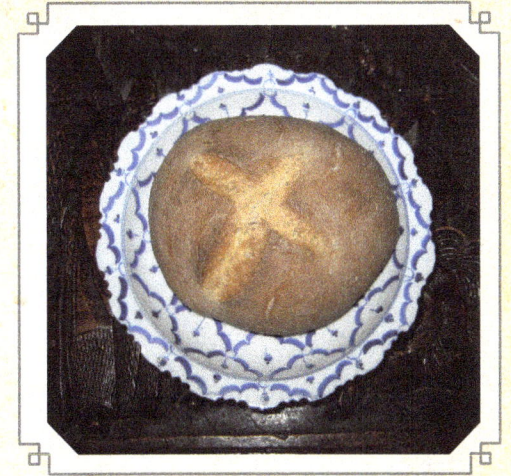

In a 1½-quart saucepan, combine the water, honey, and buttermilk. Whisk and cook over medium heat to 120°, then remove from heat and whisk in the yeast (if you exceed this temperature, let the liquid stand until it is back down to 120°—you don't want to kill your yeast). Let this stand.

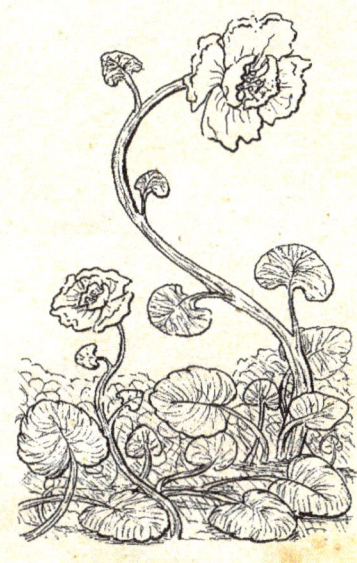

In a very large mixing bowl, combine the 1½ cups bread flour, wheat, rye, and the 3 seasonings. Add the liquid and mix on a low speed for 1 minute. Add the remaining bread flour, starting with 2 cups. If the dough seems very sticky, add the remaining ½ cup, or maybe just a few tablespoons. Mix for another minute on low speed. Change to a dough hook and mix at the lowest speed for 5 minutes. Place dough in a lightly oiled large bowl; turn dough to coat all over. Cover with a towel and let rise 1 hour in a relatively warm, draft-free place.

Chapter Two: The Inn of the Doughty Hero

Coat a large baking sheet with cooking spray or grease lightly. Press down dough and divide into 4 portions. Form each into a ball by rolling on a counter until smooth. Place on sheet, 2" apart. Cover with the same towel and let rise another 45 minutes.

Preheat oven to 375°. With a very sharp knife, cut a deep X on top of each loaf. Bake for 30-34 minutes. Cool on pan 10 minutes, then cool on a rack for at least 15 minutes before cutting. Serve with Dilly Butter. Cover and store at room temperature. Makes 4 small, round loaves; serves 8-12.

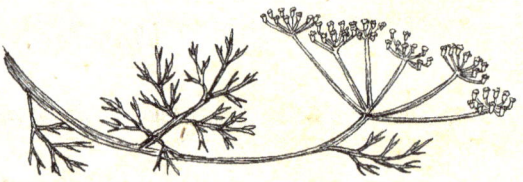

Dilly Butter

¾ cup soft salted butter
¾ teaspoon onion powder
¾ teaspoon dry dill weed (or about 2 tablespoons fresh dill, minced)

Combine all in a medium bowl. Cover and refrigerate leftovers; bring to room temperature to serve. Makes ¾ cup.

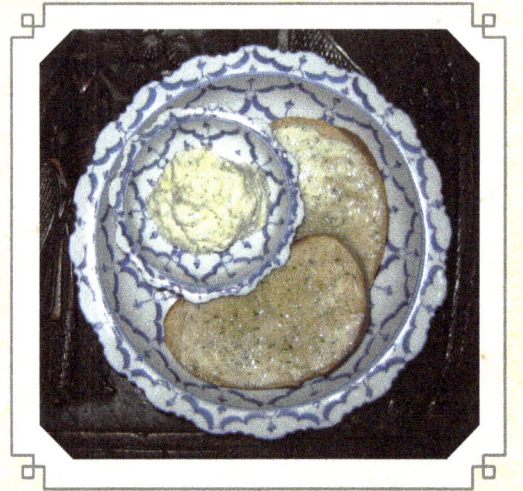

 *This bread and butter combination is oddly addictive. It's all I can do to prevent myself from cutting another slice... oh well, diet tomorrow, right?*

Lise's Lentils

This salad would make a unique addition to a potluck; it is very hearty.

8 ounces lentils
1 quart water
14-ounce can quartered artichoke hearts or bottoms (cut these into ½" bits), drained well[1]
2 hard boiled extra large eggs, peeled and cut into ½" pieces
2 tablespoons small capers, drained well
½ cup red onion, diced
½ cup fresh parsley, chopped coarsely
10 grape tomatoes, halved
¼ cup hazelnut oil
¼ cup red wine vinegar
1 tablespoon lemon juice
1 tablespoon sugar
1 teaspoon salt
1 teaspoon minced garlic
½ teaspoon pepper

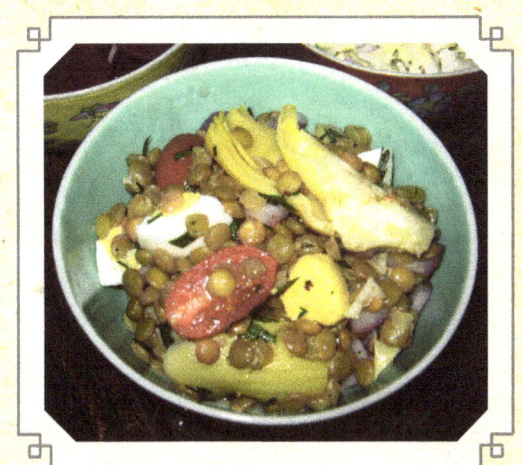

In a fine-mesh strainer, rinse and sort the lentils. Combine the lentils and water in a 2-quart saucepan and bring to a boil. Reduce heat to medium and cook 16-20 minutes, until tender. Pour into strainer, rinse with cold water, and drain well. In a large bowl, combine the lentils, artichokes, eggs, capers, onion, parsley, and tomatoes. Combine the remaining ingredients in a jar with a tight-fitting lid; shake well, then mix with the lentils. Adjust seasonings, if desired. Place in a 7-cup container, cover, and chill at least 1 hour before serving; stir a couple of times. Cover and refrigerate leftovers. Serve with a slotted spoon. Serves 6-8.

[1] You can use fresh artichokes that you have cooked, but you'd need quite a few to equal the amount in a can; besides, I know I'm too busy to mess with all of that preparation, aren't you?

Courageous Low-Carb Chicken

This is one of the few low-carbohydrate recipes included in the cookbook. You can use chicken (or leftover Thanksgiving turkey) from your own roast or use prepared grilled chicken strips. If you have made Sine Qua Non Chicken (see page 121), you might have some meat leftover.

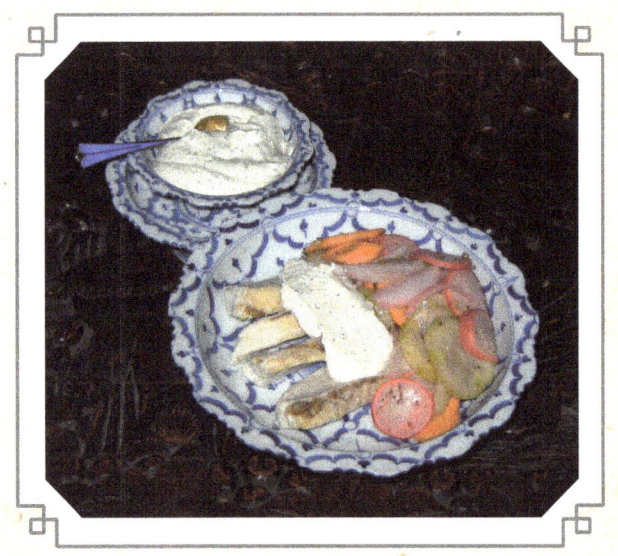

½ cup cider vinegar
2 tablespoons sugar
½ teaspoon mustard seed
¼ teaspoon celery seed
A pinch of salt
½ cup each, all sliced thinly:
    English (seedless) cucumber, peeled or not
    radishes
    celery
    carrot, peeled
¼ cup red onion, cut into ¼" slivers
½ pound cold cooked chicken
¼ cup light sour cream
1 tablespoon heavy cream
1 tablespoon coarse ground mustard
¼ teaspoon pepper
⅛ teaspoon salt

In a 1½-quart saucepan, combine the first 5 ingredients. Bring to a boil and stir just to dissolve the sugar. Turn off heat and add the 5 vegetables. Cool ½ hour. Put in a covered 3-cup container and refrigerate for 1 hour; stir a couple of times. Drain to serve.

Shred, slice, or dice the chicken. In a small bowl, whisk together the remaining ingredients. Adjust seasonings, if desired. Dollop sour cream sauce on chicken or combine as a salad. You may serve this plain with the pickles on the side or, if you want some carbs, serve as a sandwich with the pickles as a relish. Cover and refrigerate leftovers separately. Vegetables look best the first day; the color fades afterwards. Both keep about 3 days. Serves 2-4.

 *I believe you do have to be courageous to give up carbs completely. Come to think of it, if you're following that kind of diet, you should probably just put this cookbook away now to avoid temptation. Then you can just fantasize about the carbs within these pages…*

Doughty Hero Casserole

A convenient and rib-sticking casserole, you could assemble it early in the day (or even the night before); cover, then refrigerate. Let stand at room temperature for 30 minutes before you do the final baking later on (bake about 25 minutes if you make this in advance). A half recipe will easily fit in an 8-inch square baking dish.

- 3 pounds assorted root vegetables, peeled and cut into rather uniform 1" chunks[1]
- 1 tablespoon plus 2 tablespoons salted butter
- ½ teaspoon plus ½ teaspoon Savory Seasoning
- 1 pound bulk sage-flavored pork sausage
- 1½ cups onion, diced
- ¼ cup all-purpose flour
- ½ teaspoon pepper
- ½ teaspoon poultry seasoning
- 2 teaspoons dry sage (or about 3 tablespoons fresh sage, minced)
- 14½-ounce can low-sodium chicken broth
- 1 cup half-and-half
- ¼ cup heavy cream
- 1 ounce Parmesan or Romano cheese, finely shredded
- 2 tablespoons seasoned dry bread crumbs

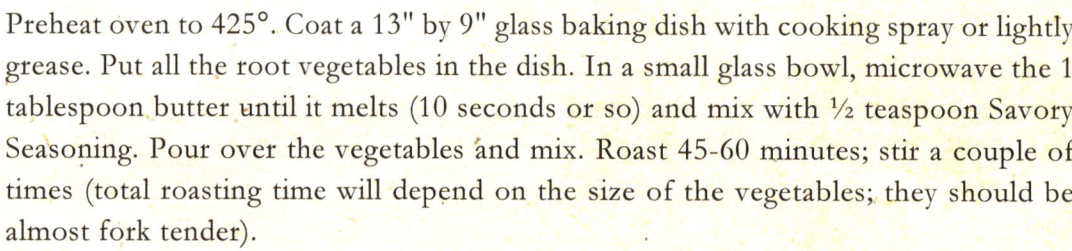

Preheat oven to 425°. Coat a 13" by 9" glass baking dish with cooking spray or lightly grease. Put all the root vegetables in the dish. In a small glass bowl, microwave the 1 tablespoon butter until it melts (10 seconds or so) and mix with ½ teaspoon Savory Seasoning. Pour over the vegetables and mix. Roast 45-60 minutes; stir a couple of times (total roasting time will depend on the size of the vegetables; they should be almost fork tender).

[1] Your best choices are potatoes, carrots, parsnips, turnips, or rutabagas—try to use at least two different varieties. If you use smaller red potatoes, you don't need to peel them.

Meanwhile, coat a 5-quart deep skillet with cooking spray and place over high heat. Fry the sausage and onion until the meat is no longer pink. Drain and set aside (don't bother washing the pan). In the same skillet, melt the 2 tablespoons butter and whisk in the flour until fully combined. Add all the remaining seasonings, broth, half-and-half, and cream. Keep heat on medium/high and whisk until sauce is thicker. Add back the meat and onions and combine well. Season, as desired. Pour this over the vegetables, covering all. Combine the cheese and bread crumbs; sprinkle this over the meat. Bake at 425° for 15 minutes, until golden brown on top. Remove and let stand 5-10 minutes. Cover and refrigerate leftovers. Serves 6-8.

Mix 4 ounces roasted and chopped green chile (undrained) into the gravy right at the end of cooking, before pouring onto the vegetables.

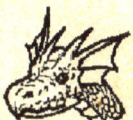

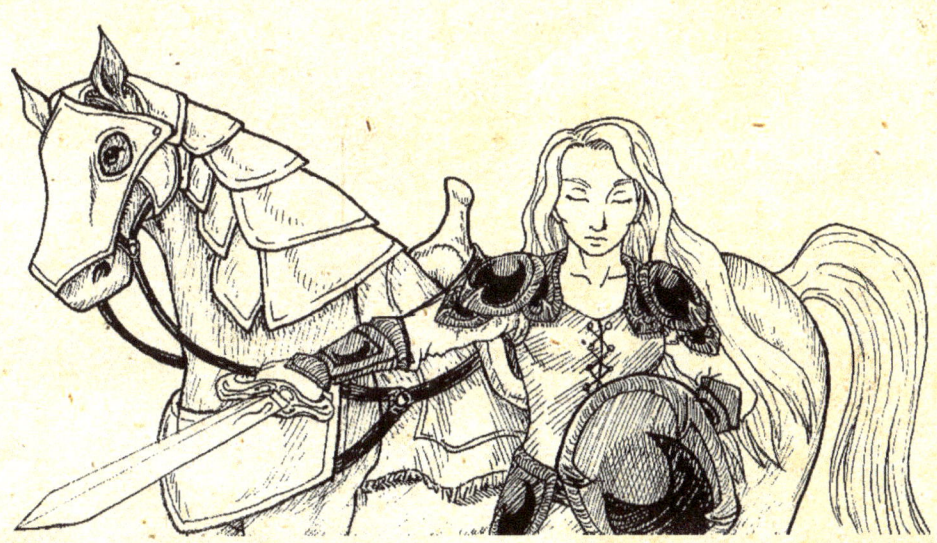

Beery Beef Stew

This hearty stew will taste slightly differently depending on your beer. Use one you wouldn't mind drinking by itself; life's too short to skimp on your spirits, don't you think? Though the recipe calls for a lager or ale type of beer, you could also go amber, dark, or stout for variety. You can use any brand you like here, foreign or domestic; even light or non-alcoholic ones will work (though this stew cooks for a while and you don't have to worry about alcoholic content).

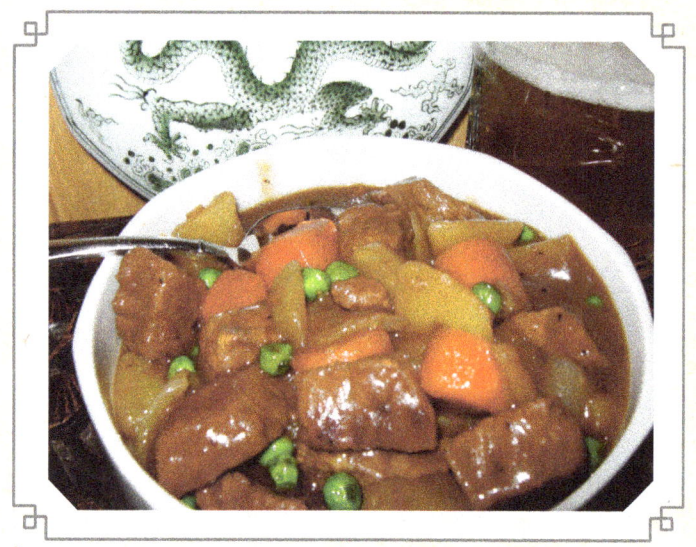

2 tablespoons salted butter
1 tablespoon minced garlic
2½ pounds beef stew meat, cut into 1" chunks (lamb or pork would work as well)
¼ cup all-purpose flour or Wondra
1 teaspoon salt
1 teaspoon pepper
3 cups beer (lager or ale, 24 ounces), room temperature
½ pound onion, cut into 1" chunks
½ pound carrots, peeled and cut into 1" chunks
1½ pounds potatoes, peeled (or not) and cut into 1" chunks
1 tablespoon Worcestershire sauce
1 tablespoon Kitchen Bouquet
1 cup frozen peas (or lima beans)

Coat a 6-quart saucepan with cooking spray. Melt the butter over rather high heat. Add the garlic and beef; sauté over medium/high heat until the beef starts to brown, about 8-10 minutes. Add the flour, salt, and pepper and mix in. Add the beer slowly and bring to a boil. Reduce heat to a very low simmer, cover, and cook 1½ hours, stirring occasionally.

Add the onions, carrots, potatoes, Worcestershire sauce, and Kitchen Bouquet. Bring to a boil again, then simmer on a low heat, covered, for 45 minutes (stir occasionally). Add the peas, raise heat a notch or two and cook, uncovered, about 10-15 more minutes, until the meat and vegetables are tender. Stir a few times. Adjust seasonings, if desired. Cover and refrigerate leftovers; don't freeze. Serves 6.

Mix anywhere from 4-8 ounces of undrained, roasted, and chopped green chile anytime during cooking.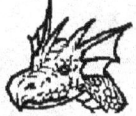

This ranks in Bob's top five recipes (surprise!). He is definitely a meat and potatoes halfling (monster). I like a lot of beers, though I sure don't drink many on a regular basis anymore. Albuquerque is one of the best locations for award-winning local breweries. But sometimes you buy a brand of beer that tastes skunky or dish-watery. Then you're stuck with it, and you really don't want to drink it. Well, here's the perfect place for it—it will mellow out and coat your meat and vegetables with rich, savory goodness.

Rabbit Braised with Herbs
(a.k.a. A Halfling Hero's Dream)

Sometimes a hero gets lucky and discovers some game along the road. Here is a savory, simple recipe for rabbit, though I usually use chicken here, for reasons I will give below. This reflects a dreamier version of a scene depicted in Middle-earth. Be sure to serve some crusty bread or rolls with this, to sop up the light sauce.

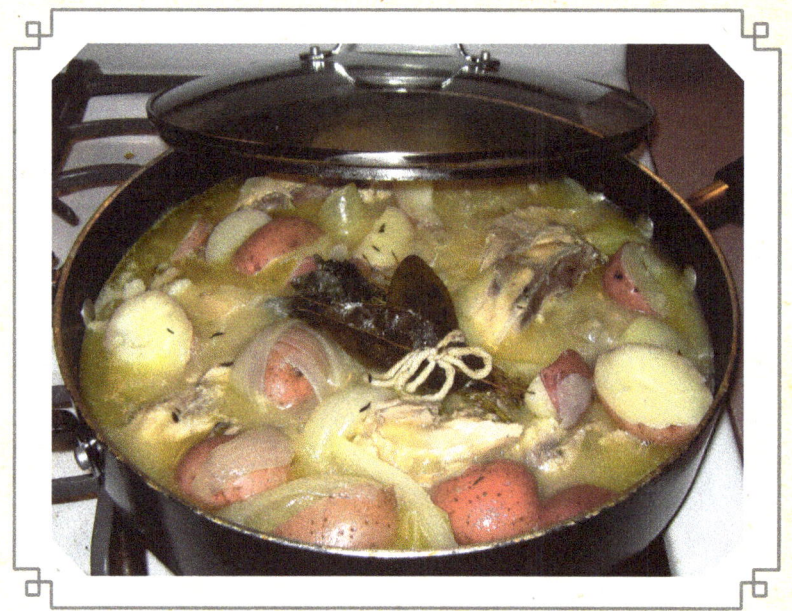

5 pounds whole, cut-up rabbit (or chicken—a little more or less is fine; remove as much skin as you can easily)

3 sprigs fresh thyme (each about 4" long—only fresh will do!)

A handful of fresh sage leaves (only fresh again)

3 large bay leaves (fresh or dry)

1 teaspoon salt

6 cups low-sodium chicken broth (if using homemade, skim off any noticeable fat before measuring)

1 pound small red potatoes, unpeeled and cut in halves or quarters

About a ½ pound onion, peeled and cut into 8 wedges

¼ cup all-purpose flour or Wondra

¼ cup water

Kitchen twine

Place the rabbit in a 5-quart deep skillet. Tie the herbs together with a 12" long piece of twine and place on top of the meat. Sprinkle the rabbit evenly with the salt, then pour the broth over all. Bring to a boil, then reduce heat to a nice simmer. Cook 30 minutes, covered.

Uncover; set the herbs aside and turn over all the pieces of meat. Add the potatoes and return the herbs, cover, and cook 15 minutes. Add the onions and raise heat to cook on a gentle boil, uncovered, 30-40 minutes or until the potatoes are tender.

Remove all meat and vegetables to a platter (use the skillet lid to cover them). Discard the herbs. Measure out 3¼ cups of the broth and discard the rest (this is most likely about what you'll have left anyway). Pour back in the pan and raise heat. In a 1-cup glass measuring cup, whisk together the flour, water, and about ½ cup of the broth, then whisk this into the skillet. Bring to a boil and cook until it thickens slightly. Adjust seasonings, if desired. Serve gravy alongside the meat and vegetables; don't forget to serve some crusty bread on the side as well. Cover and refrigerate leftovers; don't freeze. Serves 4-6.

When I was a teenager, I cooked a cut-up rabbit in a red wine sauce and it was fine. I am confident that the recipe above will work perfectly well with 5 pounds of cut-up rabbit, and a member of the Fellowship of the Recipe Testers used rabbit and said the recipe was delicious, though he thought rabbit was apparently rather expensive compared to chicken. Now, however, I have various problems with the thought of cooking a coney. Here are my reasons, proceeding from the most practical to the personal, and ending with the most tragic.

First, chicken is much more readily available, at least in my neighborhood, and you are welcome to use whatever cuts of chicken you prefer; all breast meat or all thighs or any combination—it should still be on the bone.

Second, people are probably more willing to eat chicken—ask them and you'll see. I was thinking of having a rabbit party, but people kind of shuddered at the thought of eating rabbit. I know you may be thinking that I'm copping out here, but I didn't want to spend money and time on a dish that nobody would eat.

Third, Bob ate lots of freshly caught rabbits as a boy. He hated eating them then and he still hates the thought of eating them now.

Chapter Two: The Inn of the Doughty Hero

And finally, the clincher: when Chloë was six years old, she got a brown lop-eared rabbit. He ended up with many names, from Cinnamon to simply Bunny. She was devoted to him. He grew to be quite large and had a rather annoying habit of spraying urine around to mark his territory. He was kept in a hutch outside, though she let him out frequently to run around the backyard, and he followed her around more like a puppy.

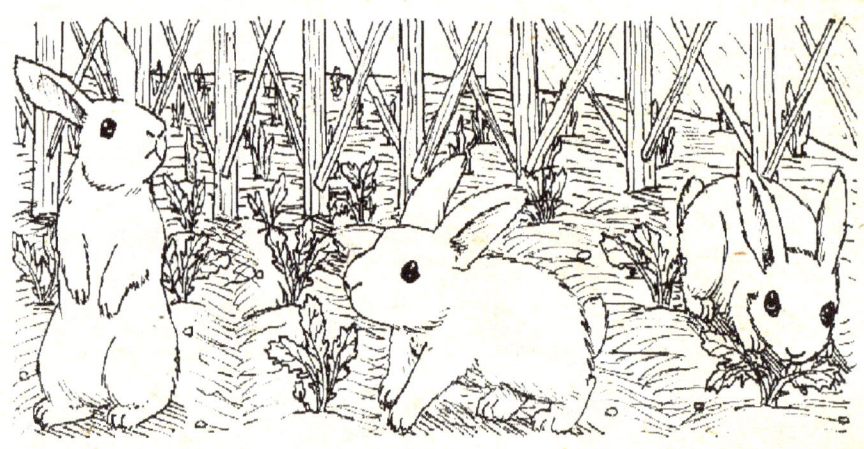

One day, when Chloë was 15, we were out in the yard with her now nine-year-old bunny right before I was going to take her to a dental appointment. The weather was beautiful and the bunny was flopping around as usual. Callista and I went inside; Chloë also came in to brush her teeth. She returned outside and discovered her bunny had suddenly died. This was actually the first pet I had ever owned who died at home. You can imagine the three of us were horribly upset, and, of course, I rescheduled the dentist. I tell you, it is a hard thing, as an overly sensitive parent, to see your children lose beloved pets. It all happened so unexpectedly.

So, I hope you can see why rabbits have a special place in our family's psyche. I suppose if we kept chickens as beloved pets, I wouldn't cook them either.

Jan's Baked Apples

The perfect recipe for those large Honey Crisp apples!

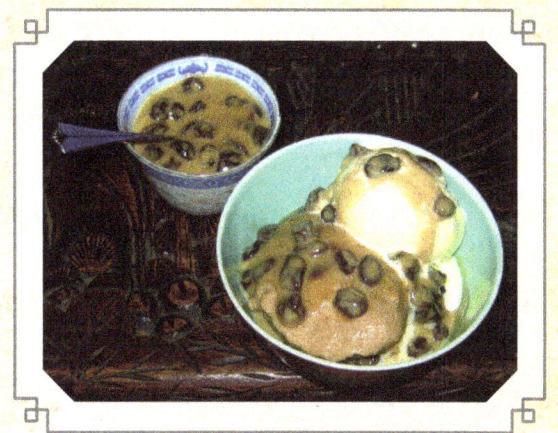

½ cup water
2 very large apples, peeled and cored; cut in half lengthwise
1 tablespoon lemon juice
1 cup raisins
1 cup hot water
4 ounces light cream cheese (Neufchâtel), softened
¼ cup plus ¼ cup packed golden brown sugar
1 tablespoon plus ¾ cup heavy cream
½ teaspoon plus ½ teaspoon cinnamon
⅛ teaspoon plus ⅛ teaspoon salt
2 tablespoons salted butter
¼ cup sugar
1 extra large egg yolk
½ teaspoon vanilla extract

Preheat oven to 375°. Coat a broiler-safe 8" square pan with cooking spray, then pour in ½ cup water. Place the apple halves rounded side down in the pan and sprinkle all over with the lemon juice. Cover with regular foil and bake 30-60 minutes until just sharp knife tender (the type and size of your apples will affect your cooking time, so be sure to check them at 30 minutes).

Meanwhile, combine the raisins and hot water in a medium bowl for 15 minutes. Strain and set aside. Dry the bowl and use next.

In the bowl, beat the cream cheese with a hand mixer until smooth. Add ¼ cup brown sugar, 1 tablespoon cream, ½ teaspoon cinnamon, and ⅛ teaspoon salt and combine well. Set aside.

In a 1½-quart saucepan, combine the butter, sugar, ¼ cup brown sugar, and the remaining cinnamon and salt. Using a whisk, cook over medium heat until the butter melts and the sugar dissolves. In a 2-cup glass measuring cup, whisk together the ¾ cup cream and the egg yolk; whisk about ¼ cup of the hot butter/sugar mixture into this, then add to the pot. Bring almost to a boil, then simmer over very low heat about 10 minutes, until it is a nice sauce consistency—whisk occasionally. Add the vanilla and the strained raisins. Turn off heat, cover, and set aside.

When the apples are done, remove and set the broiler to high. Remove foil and place apples on the foil. Pour out the cooking liquid, then coat the pan with cooking spray again. Return the apples to the pan (rounded side down) and carefully smear the cream cheese mixture equally over the apples. Broil about 2-4 minutes until they are golden brown; be careful not to burn them. Stir the sauce and pour about ¼ cup of the raisin sauce into each of 4 dessert bowls. Place an apple in each, cheese side up. Drizzle a little more sauce over each apple (any remaining sauce is great on ice cream). Serve with a scoop of vanilla ice cream or a dollop of whipped cream. Serve immediately. Cover and refrigerate leftovers separately; reheat sauce slowly. Serves 4.

Brave Blackberry Tart

You could substitute fresh raspberries, blueberries, or sliced strawberries for the blackberries depending on availability (even a combination of different berries will work nicely). If you do, be sure to change the seedless jam you use, as well. Only use fresh berries!

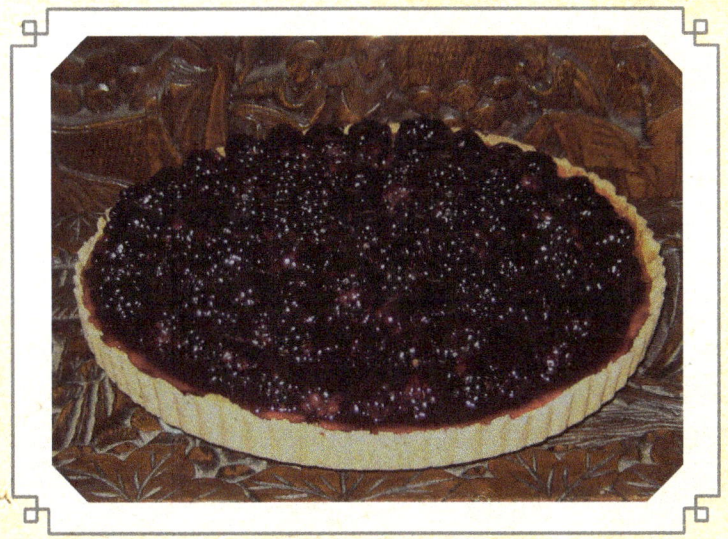

- 18 ounces fresh blackberries
- 1½ cups all-purpose flour
- 2 tablespoons plus ¾ cup sugar
- 1 ounce pecan halves, toasted lightly
- 2 whole graham crackers (8 sections)
- 1 teaspoon cinnamon
- ¼ teaspoon salt
- ½ cup salted butter, melted and cooled a bit
- 8 ounces light cream cheese (Neufchâtel), softened
- 3 extra large eggs
- 1 teaspoon vanilla extract
- 1 teaspoon cinnamon extract
- 1 cup seedless blackberry jam
- 2 tablespoons water

Wash the blackberries and let dry on a towel or a couple of paper towels while you prepare the tart.

Preheat oven to 400°. Liberally coat an 11" wide, 1" deep tart pan with removable sides with cooking spray or grease well. In a large food processor, combine the flour, 2 tablespoons sugar, pecans, graham crackers, cinnamon, and salt. Pulse until the nuts are fully ground. Add the butter and pulse until fully combined. Scrape this mixture into the tart pan (don't bother rinsing bowl or blade). Press evenly up the sides first, then press evenly onto the bottom of the pan. Bake 10 minutes. Remove; immediately lower oven temperature to 350°. Carefully place crust on a rack.

Meanwhile, combine the cream cheese, eggs, ¾ cup sugar, and extracts in the food processor and pulse until fully mixed. Scrape down sides and process again. Pour onto crust and carefully return this to the oven (it is okay if the oven has not decreased heat yet). Bake 30 minutes or until the cheese is set in the center. Place on rack for 1 hour.

Remove the pan sides and place tart on a serving dish or platter. Arrange all the berries on top. In a 1-quart saucepan, combine the jam and water. Over medium heat, whisk just until the jam has melted. Spoon jam all over the fruit and cheese—fill in empty spaces with a pastry brush. Chill at least 2 hours or overnight before serving. Cover and refrigerate leftovers. Serves 8-10.

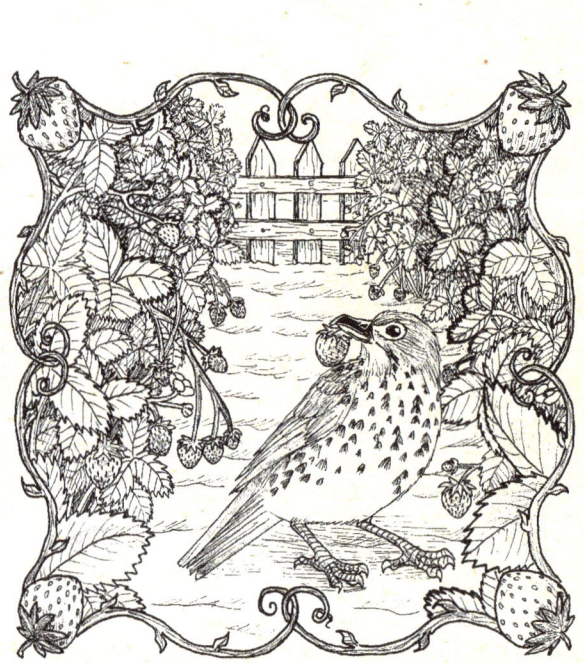

Busy Day Rice Pudding

If you are trying to recover from your "busy day" and like to imbibe, you could pour a tablespoon or so of your favorite liqueur all over your serving, if you want. I could definitely see some Amaretto or Frangelico on this.

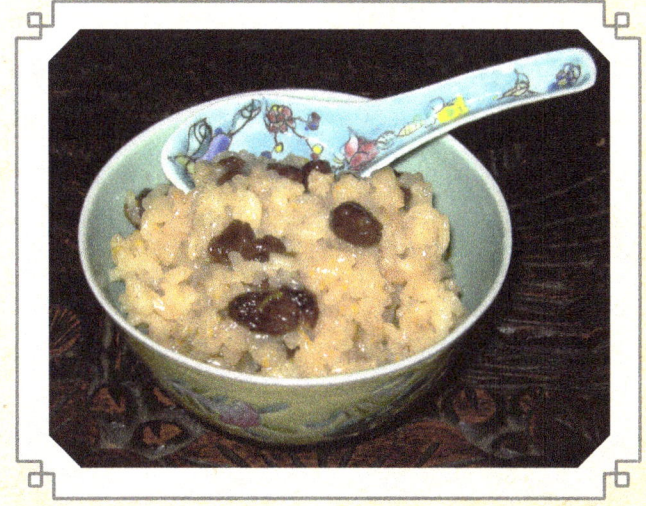

- 1 giant orange (or 2 medium oranges)
- 2¼ cups water
- 1¼ cups short grain rice[1]
- ½ cup raisins
- 2 ounces crystallized ginger, coarsely chopped
- 2 tablespoons salted butter
- ½ teaspoon salt
- ½ cup heavy cream
- ½ cup sugar
- 1 teaspoon cinnamon
- 1 teaspoon vanilla extract

With a box shredder or microplaner, zest the orange. You should end up with 1-2 tablespoons zest; set aside. Cut orange in half, juice and strain it—you should end up with 3-4 tablespoons juice. Place in a 2-quart saucepan. Add the water, rice, raisins, ginger, butter, and salt. Bring to a boil and stir once. Set heat to lowest setting, cover, and cook 20 minutes. Turn heat off; leave saucepan covered and let it stand undisturbed for 15-20 minutes.

Meanwhile in a 2-cup glass measuring cup, combine the zest and the remaining ingredients with a whisk. Combine this with the rice and serve immediately, or cover and let stand. Serve warm. You may pour some extra heavy cream over the top, or dollop with whipped cream. Cover and refrigerate leftovers. Serves 6-8.

[1] To rinse or not to rinse? That is sometimes the question regarding rice. All the recipes in the cookbook are designed to use non-washed rice, with one exception (see Treasured Tidbits, page 125). Many varieties of rice are coated with various additives and you might object to this. I usually don't bother to rinse rice because I'm lazy and I live in a desert, so I tend to be conservative with water usage in certain circumstances. You are welcome to rinse your rice, if you prefer.

My mother's mother occasionally made a delicious rice pudding with raisins, cinnamon, and milk. She would cook it in an old, battered double boiler for what seemed like hours. And she would spend lots of time stirring it. I love a warm rice pudding and she never did impart her particular recipe secrets to me before she died. So this is my tribute to Mama, though it has some extra flavors and is much easier to prepare—perfect for a 'busy day.' You may omit the ginger if you find it to be too strong for yourself or your family.

Elfryda's Apple Crisp

This is one of those recipes where people will come along and pick at it, and you'll be slapping at hands to stop them. This is a lovely fall recipe, celebrating the apple harvest.

¼ cup plus ⅔ cup water
½ cup sugar
¼ teaspoon plus ½ teaspoon salt
1 tablespoon lemon juice
1 cup dried blueberries[1]
6-7 cups apples, peeled, cored, and cut into ¼" slices (around 2¼ pounds)
¼ cup cornstarch
2 ounces plus 2 ounces nuts, coarsely chopped[2]
1 cup all-purpose flour
1 cup old-fashioned oats
1 cup packed golden brown sugar
1 teaspoon cinnamon
½ teaspoon nutmeg
½ teaspoon allspice
½ cup soft salted butter

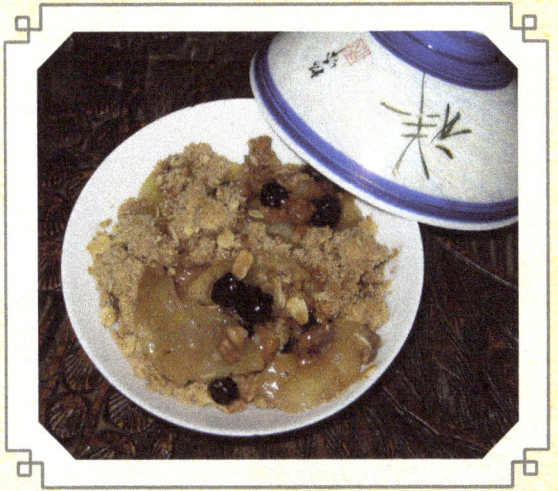

[1] Raisins, cranberries, cherries, or any combination of any small, dried fruits will also work fine.
[2] Use nuts such as pecans, walnuts, hazelnuts, or almonds, or any combination you like.

Preheat oven to 400°. Coat a 13" by 9" glass baking dish with cooking spray or grease lightly. In a 6-quart saucepan, combine the ¼ cup water, sugar, ¼ teaspoon salt, lemon juice, blueberries, and apples. Bring to a boil; lower heat to medium/high, cover, and cook 5 minutes. Stir a couple of times. In a 2-cup glass measuring cup, combine the ⅔ cup water and the cornstarch with a whisk until smooth. Bring the fruit to a boil again, add the cornstarch mixture, and cook a few minutes until the sauce thickens. Add 2 ounces chopped nuts and combine. Pour into the prepared dish. Rinse the saucepan and dry it.

In the saucepan, combine the flour, oats, brown sugar, remaining nuts, salt, and spices. Add the butter and combine until mostly incorporated. Sprinkle evenly on top of the fruit. Bake for 30 minutes. Let stand 10 minutes before serving. Serve warm, either plain or with cream, whipped cream, or vanilla ice cream. Store covered at room temperature or refrigerate. Serves about 8.

Healing Chocolate Chai

Heroes definitely need time to recover from their adventures. Tea and dark chocolate supposedly promote good health; here, they are joined in a pleasing combination, a variation on Comforting Chai (see recipe page 24)—sure to soothe a weary wanderer.

20 whole peppercorns (any colors)
4 cardamom pods
8 whole cloves
1 large cinnamon stick, broken into 3 pieces
1" piece of fresh ginger, washed, unpeeled, and cut into ¼" slices
3 cups water
3 regular-sized bags of Earl Grey tea
1 tablespoon unsweetened cocoa powder
3-4 tablespoons sugar, or more to taste
1 cup 1% milk
1 teaspoon vanilla extract

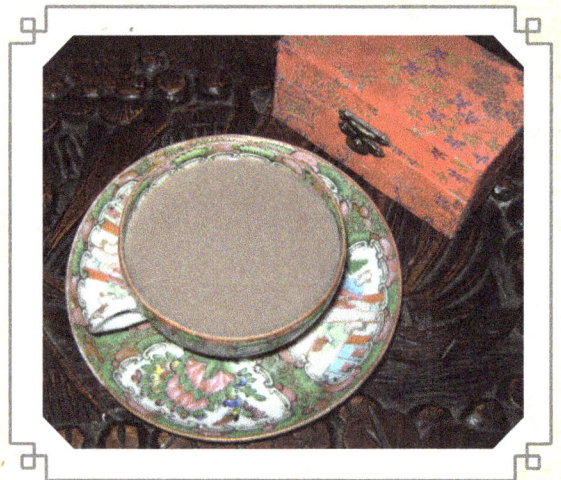

Use a 4-cup glass measuring cup for this recipe. In a 2-quart saucepan, combine the first 6 ingredients. Bring to a boil, then simmer over a medium heat, uncovered, for 10 minutes. Turn off the heat, add the tea bags, cover, and let them steep 5 minutes. Put a small, fine-mesh strainer over the 4-cup glass measuring cup. Pour the liquid into this and squeeze out the liquid from the tea bags. Discard all solids. You'll have about 2½-2¾ cups left; set aside. In the saucepan, whisk together the cocoa, sugar, and milk over medium heat until the cocoa and sugar dissolve. Pour the tea mixture back into the pot and add the vanilla. Stir over low heat about 2 minutes. Carefully pour into 2-3 mugs, or pour this back into the glass measuring cup so you can pour it more carefully. Cover and refrigerate leftovers; microwave to desired temperature. Serves 2-3, depending on how unhealthy you might be feeling.

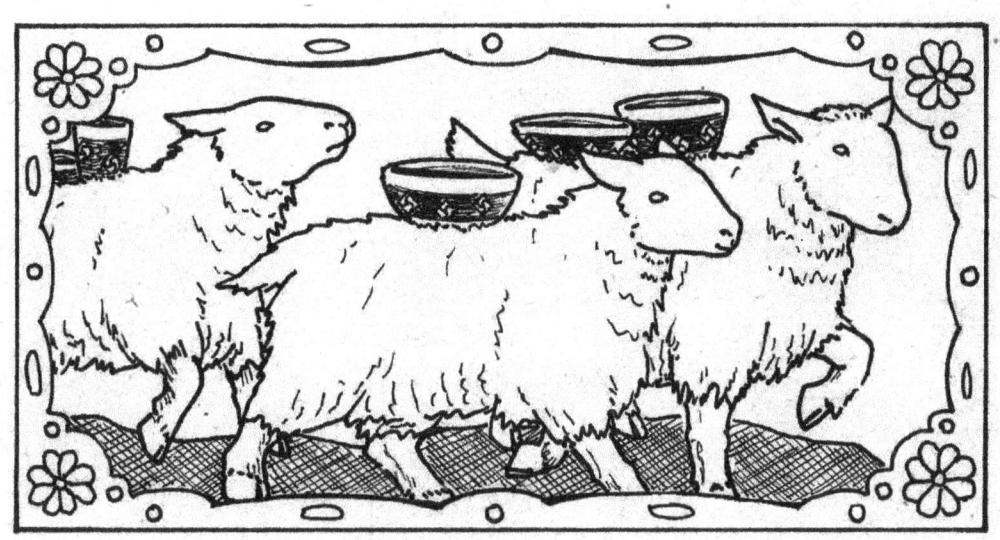

Chapter Three

Council Catering

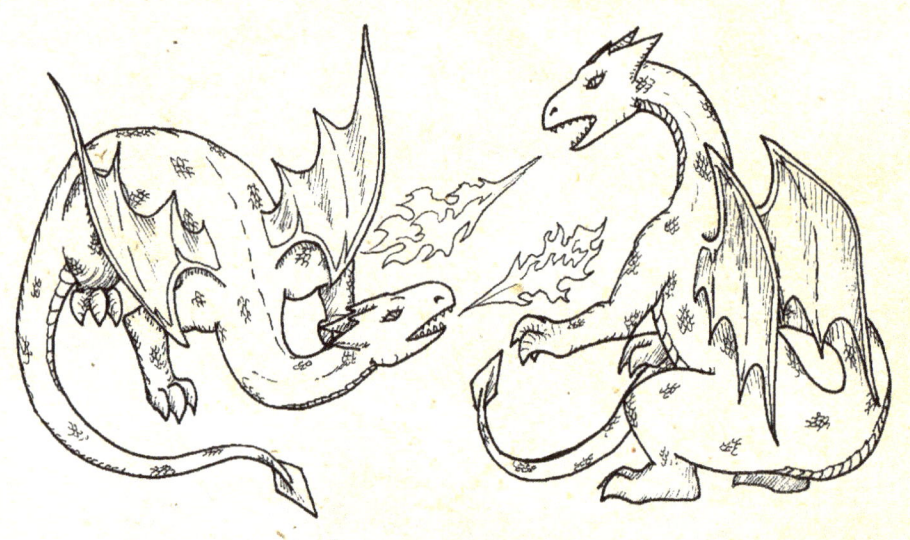

Let us help you develop a sophisticated menu to help convince your heroes to risk their lives fulfilling dangerous quests. They'll do that willingly, even eagerly, if you send them off with a good meal first…

Wisdom Chicken Soup

Ted's Spinach Mushroom Salad

Head-in-the-Clouds Biscuits

Button Pickles

Keep-You-Awake Cauliflower

Herby Cabbage Sauté

Roasted Asparagus with Mustard Sauce

Potentially Pungent Potatoes

Mellow Mushroom Meatloaf

Sweet & Savory Pork Roast

Donald's Cinnamon Sticks

Essential Mocha Tart

Council Catering Celebration Cake

Spring-in-Your-Step Punch

Council Catering

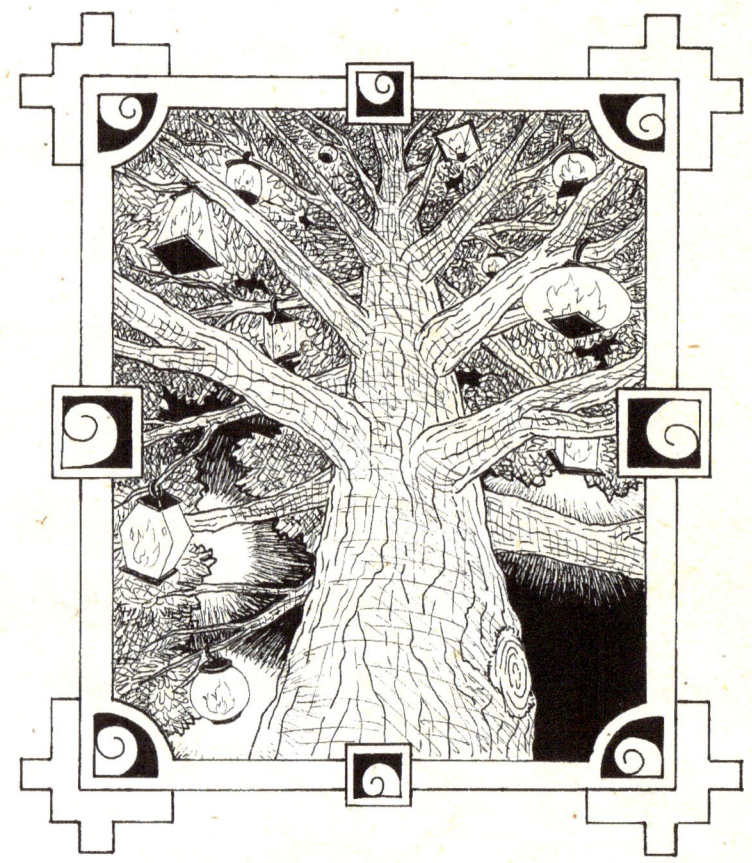

Have you ever noticed that you usually have to have some sort of meeting to convince people that the world is going to end in some horrible Ragnarökian fashion unless someone steps up and volunteers to take care of things? The least a council can do is put out some bagels and coffee, but they usually don't bother, even at some important event like the Council of Elrond. Council Catering is the place to go for help in setting up a buffet of any size, or catering a party. Some of the following recipes serve larger numbers of people, but all are easy to increase or decrease according to your needs.

Wisdom Chicken Soup

Perhaps when your heroes eat some of this soup, it will impart enough wisdom so they can get the job done efficiently (but not the kind of wisdom that makes them have second thoughts and decide to go back home and avoid doing anything that might kill or maim them…).

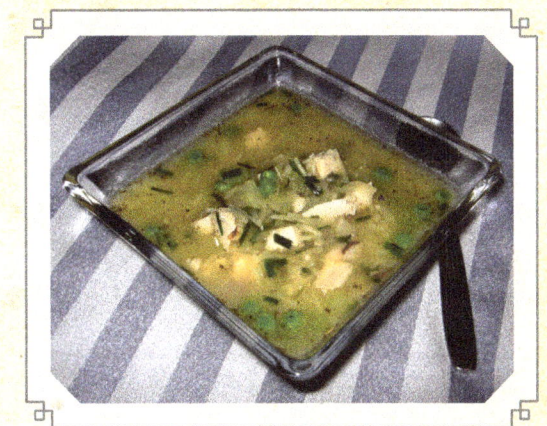

2 tablespoons salted butter
2 cups celery, cut into ¼" bits
1½ cups shallots, cut into ¼" bits
2 quarts low-sodium chicken broth
1 cup frozen peas
½ pound cooked chicken, diced or shredded
6 ounces very thin pasta (such as fideo, or break angel hair or vermicelli into 1" pieces)
½ teaspoon each:
  salt
  pepper
  garlic salt
3-4 tablespoons fresh sage, minced (or about 2 teaspoons dry sage)
½ cup fresh chives, minced

Coat a 6-quart saucepan with some cooking spray. Melt the butter over rather high heat. Add the celery and shallots and sauté about 3 minutes. Add the broth and bring to a boil. Cook over medium heat for 3 minutes, uncovered. Add the peas and chicken and cook another 3 minutes. Add the remaining ingredients and cook at a rolling simmer according to package directions, until the pasta and vegetables are tender, anywhere from 8-12 minutes or so. Stir a few times. Adjust seasonings, if desired. Cover and refrigerate leftovers. Serves 6-8.

 *Bob actually put some soy sauce in this because he thinks it's more of a Chinese soup… this works, but I prefer it the original way. You can certainly use any type of tiny pasta you like, such as stars or alphabets, though vermicelli has an older history of being added to soups (Wilson 214).*

Ted's Spinach Mushroom Salad

As with all of the salads in the cookbook, you are welcome to substitute your greenery.

¼ cup walnut oil
1 tablespoon each:
    sugar
    malt vinegar
    sesame seeds, toasted lightly
2 teaspoons soy sauce
1 teaspoon Dijon mustard
1 teaspoon lemon juice
½ teaspoon Savory Seasoning
5-6 ounces fresh baby spinach
½ cup carrots, peeled and shredded
½ cup red onion, cut into ¼" slivers
Freshly ground pepper (about 20 turns)
¼ pound fresh mushrooms, thinly sliced

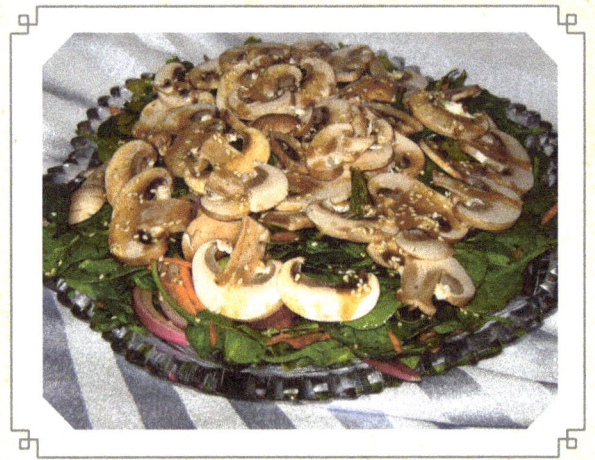

In a shaker jar with a tight-fitting lid, combine the oil, sugar, vinegar, sesame seeds, soy, mustard, lemon juice, and Savory Seasoning and shake well. Season, as desired. Place the spinach, carrots, and onion in a very large bowl. Toss ¼ cup of the dressing with this and sprinkle with the freshly ground pepper. Toss again, then arrange on a platter. Arrange the mushrooms on top of the spinach mixture. Pour remaining dressing over the mushrooms. Serve immediately. Not recommended as leftovers. Serves 4-6.

Head-in-the-Clouds Biscuits

These are moderately-sized biscuits that are delicate but will not fall apart on you—which is annoying when you are trying to spread honey or jam on them. For delicious sweet and savory variations, see below.

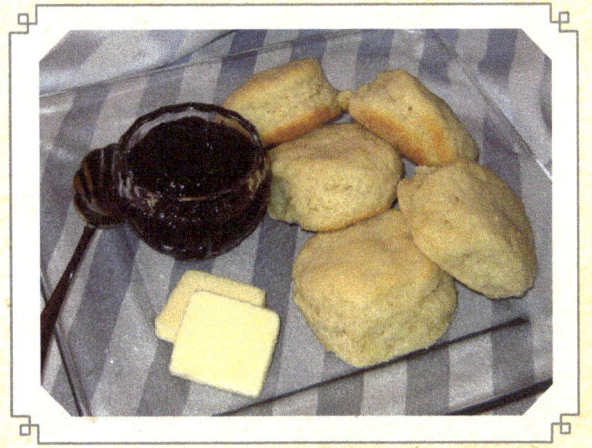

- 2 cups all-purpose flour
- ¾ cup cake flour
- 1 tablespoon baking powder
- 1 teaspoon salt
- ½ cup soft salted butter
- 1½ cups buttermilk, room temperature
- Additional all-purpose flour
- 2 tablespoons melted salted butter

Preheat oven to 450°. Coat bottom and sides of a 13" by 9" glass baking dish with cooking spray or grease lightly. In a large bowl, combine the flours, baking powder, and salt. Mix in the soft butter with a wooden spoon. Add the buttermilk and combine well. The dough might be a little sticky at first. With floured hands, turn dough out onto a heavily floured surface and knead a few times. Pat dough to about 1" thickness. Using a 2½" biscuit cutter (or an equivalent small drinking glass), cut a few biscuits and place in pan in 3 rows of 5 each (they will touch each other). Gather scraps together to cut more biscuits. For the final biscuit, gather the remaining dough and fashion a 15th biscuit (which won't be as perfect as the others; that's okay). Bake 15 minutes. Brush the tops with the melted butter and bake 3-5 more minutes, until they are barely golden brown on the bottom. Let stand in pan for 5 minutes before you tear into them. Store covered at room temperature. Makes 15.

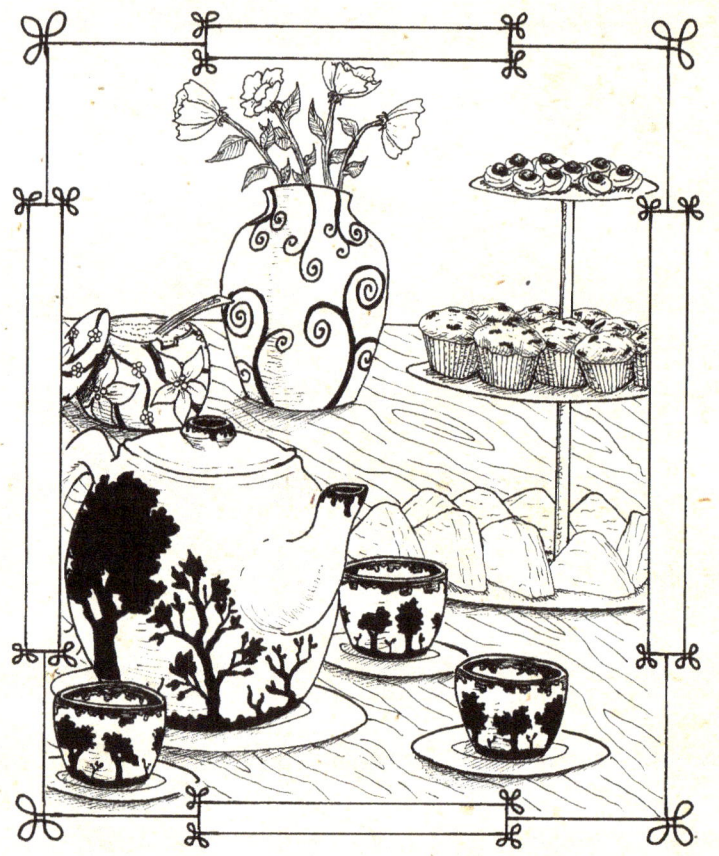

 *Here is a sweet option for you: after you brush them with butter, sprinkle 2 tablespoons of sugar all over them. After they have cooled a bit, split them, then fill with some sliced and sugared strawberries and whipped cream (a nice place to use some Cardamom Berries; see page 136).*

Or you can make them savory: mix 1-2 tablespoons fresh, minced herbs (or 1-2 teaspoons dried herbs) into the dry ingredients. Brush with butter and sprinkle 1 or 2 ounces finely shredded Parmesan or Romano cheese all over them.

Button Pickles

Button mushrooms are best here, but if you have trouble getting them (I know I certainly did, but maybe my vision of what exactly makes a mushroom a button is too harsh…), just try to find pretty small (or is that small pretty?) mushrooms and keep them whole. I'm talking about mushrooms that are 1" in diameter or even smaller. One can dream of finding the perfect mushrooms, I suppose.

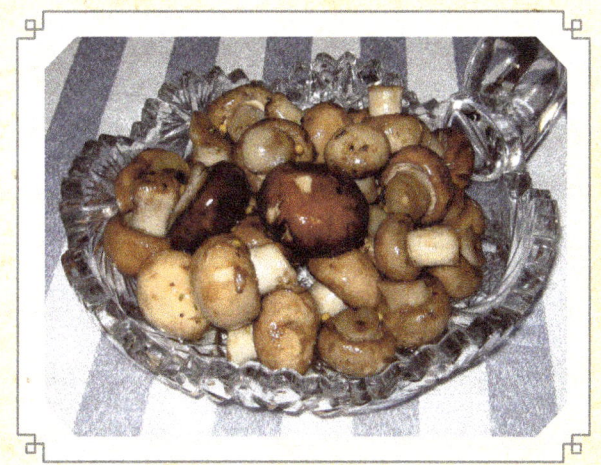

- 4 cups plus ½ cup water
- 1 pound fresh mushrooms (as small as you can get them)
- ¼ cup sugar
- ½ cup white wine vinegar
- 2 tablespoons any fresh green herb you like, minced (or 1 teaspoon dry green herb—my favorite is Herbes de Provence)
- 1 teaspoon mustard seeds
- ½ teaspoon salt
- ½ teaspoon pepper

Place 4 cups water in a 3-quart saucepan and bring to a boil. Add the mushrooms and bring to a boil again. Lower heat to medium/high and cook 3 minutes. Drain and rinse well in cold water; let stand in colander. In the same saucepan (just rinse it out), combine ½ cup water and the remaining ingredients with a whisk. Bring to a boil and cook 1 minute. Remove from heat and let stand 30 minutes, uncovered. Put mushrooms in a 1-quart container and pour the vinegar mixture over all. Cover and chill at least 1 hour before serving; stir a couple of times. Serve with a slotted spoon. Cover and refrigerate leftovers. Makes about 3 cups.

Chapter Three: Council Catering　61

Keep-You-Awake Cauliflower

Even if you don't expect a crowd, it's nice to have pickled vegetables on hand. I'll often have a few cauliflower florets, some olives, some fruit, and a little cheese and salami for a sort of Mediterranean lunch. Add some crispy, herby crackers and fantasize you're dining in Venice or Rome, perhaps… add wine… gelato… Nice substitutes for cauliflower would be fresh green beans or asparagus, cut into bite-sized portions.

5 cups plus ⅔ cup water
2 pounds cauliflower, cored and cut into 1" florets (about 4-5 cups, or an average head)
½ cup carrot, peeled and cut diagonally into ⅛" slices
½ cup celery, cut diagonally into ⅛" slices
¾ cup white wine vinegar
¼ cup sugar
½ teaspoon dill seed
¼ teaspoon each:
   Savory Seasoning
   salt
   pepper
2 tablespoons small capers, drained well

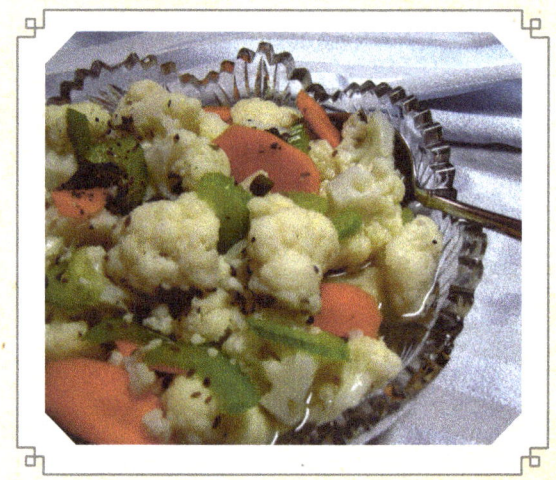

In a 4-quart saucepan, combine the 5 cups water and cauliflower. Bring to a boil; lower the heat to medium/high and cook uncovered for 2 minutes. Stir a few times. Mix in the carrot and celery and cook another 2 minutes. Drain and don't bother washing the saucepan. Place vegetables in an 8-cup container. In the saucepan, combine the ⅔ cup water, vinegar, sugar, and seasonings with a whisk. Bring to a boil and cook 1 minute. Add the capers, then pour over the vegetables. Let stand for 30 minutes. Cover and refrigerate for at least 1 hour before serving; stir a couple of times. Use a slotted spoon to serve. Cover and store in refrigerator. Makes about 7 cups.

Herby Cabbage Sauté

When you want a humble cabbage to be a little more special, break out some wine and Herbes de Provence in this delicious side dish which can be paired with many recipes in the cookbook.

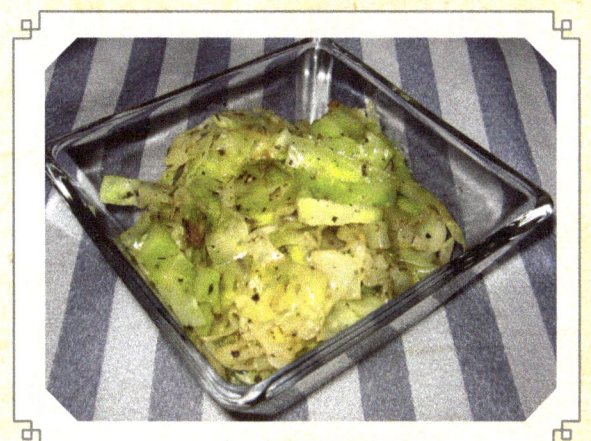

- 2 tablespoons salted butter
- 4-5 cups green cabbage, cut into slivers, 2" long by ½" wide (this is usually half of a smallish cabbage, cored)
- 2 tablespoons dry white wine, such as Chardonnay
- 2 tablespoons heavy cream
- 2 teaspoons Herbes de Provence (or any other herb you prefer; 2 tablespoons fresh, minced)
- ½ teaspoon Savory Seasoning

Melt the butter in a 3-quart deep skillet over rather high heat. Add the cabbage and sauté 2 minutes. Add the remaining ingredients; cover and cook over medium heat for 3 minutes. Uncover and raise heat to rather high. Sauté 1-2 minutes until most of the liquid evaporates, stirring frequently. Season, as desired. Cover and refrigerate leftovers. Serves 4-6.

A tablespoon or two of drained, roasted, and chopped green chile could be added right at the end of cooking.

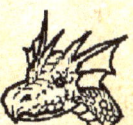

I must tell you that Bob can't stand cooked cabbage in any form (and a few other vegetables in general). However, he loves my particular recipe for coleslaw (Bob's Obsession; see page 114). So I usually end up with extra cabbage after making his favorite coleslaw, which I generally only make once a month. I have come up with a few ways to use up four or five cups of cabbage—this one is obviously showcasing the cabbage, but I usually sneak it into other dishes.

Chapter Three: Council Catering

Roasted Asparagus with Mustard Sauce

Be sure to get hefty asparagus for this dish. Skip the sauce and just roast the asparagus as a simple side dish. Be bold and use a chili-flavored sesame oil for variety.

3 pounds fresh asparagus (with ½" thick stalks)
3 tablespoons almond oil
½ teaspoon plus ½ teaspoon Savory Seasoning
3 tablespoons each:
    Dijon mustard
    heavy cream
    dry white wine, such as Chardonnay
⅓ cup light sour cream, room temperature
1 ounce sliced almonds, lightly toasted and chopped coarsely

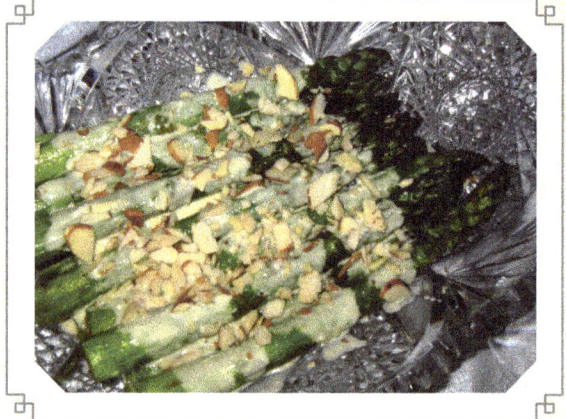

Preheat oven to 400°. Lightly coat an 11" by 7" baking dish with cooking spray. Wash asparagus, line up heads on a cutting board, and cut off the bottom 2" or so, so all the stalks are about 6½" long. Place in dish. Drizzle with almond oil and sprinkle with ½ teaspoon Savory Seasoning. Roast about 15-20 minutes until they are fork tender. Stir every 5 minutes.

Meanwhile in a 1-quart saucepan, whisk together the mustard, cream, wine, and ½ teaspoon Savory Seasoning. Bring to a boil, then reduce to a low simmer. Whisk in the sour cream and simmer 1 minute; do not boil. Right before serving, pour this over asparagus; sprinkle with sliced almonds. Cover and refrigerate leftovers. Serves 10-12.

Potentially Pungent Potatoes

When it comes to mashing, you can leave your potatoes rather chunky or mash until they are completely smooth, it is your choice. Once you've mashed them, you could simply stop there if you just want a good basic recipe for mashed potatoes. But I often like to go ahead and add the extras and bake it as a casserole, especially if I have other things going on in the kitchen.

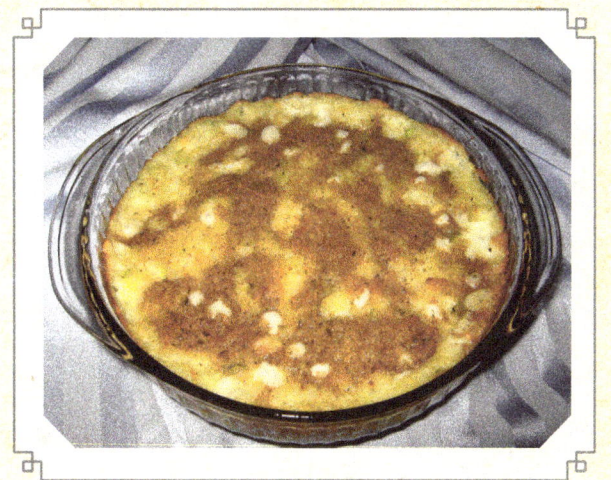

3 pounds potatoes, peeled and cut into 1" pieces
1 teaspoon plus ½ teaspoon salt
2 quarts water
½ cup soft salted butter
¾ cup heavy cream
¾ teaspoon Savory Seasoning
½ teaspoon pepper
1½ cups scallions, thinly sliced
6-7 ounces Bleu cheese (1 cup), crumbled into small bits[1]
⅓ cup salted butter
⅓ cup seasoned dry bread crumbs

Preheat oven to 400°. Coat a 3-quart baking dish with cooking spray or lightly grease. In a 6-quart saucepan, combine the potatoes, 1 teaspoon salt, and water. Bring to a boil; lower heat to medium/high and cook until the potatoes are fork tender, 15-20 minutes. Reserve ½ cup cooking liquid, then drain the potatoes well by partially covering the pot with the lid. Add the butter, cream, Savory Seasoning, ½ teaspoon salt, pepper, and reserved cooking liquid. Mash this either by hand or use a hand mixer.

Add the scallions and cheese and combine; pour into the prepared dish. Microwave the ⅓ cup butter in a small glass bowl in 20-second intervals until melted, then combine with the bread crumbs. Sprinkle over the potatoes. Bake 30 minutes, until golden and bubbly. Cover and refrigerate leftovers. Serves 10-12.

---

[1] The potential pungency comes not only from the scallions, but also from your choice of Bleu cheese—Gorgonzola is rather mild; Bleu is stronger; and a Roquefort is stronger still. Try a Stilton, or you can simply use a purchased, creamy garlic/herb cheese (such as Alouette or Boursin). If you would like to make your own, try Aradosa's Cheese, on page xxiv.

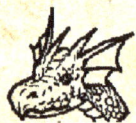 **Meat Lover's Option**—Fry up a pound of sweet or hot Italian sausage, drain, then add to the potatoes at the end. Slice up a pound of Polish sausage or use up some leftover cooked meat; cook up a quarter pound of bacon, and crumble it into bits—all would be delicious additions, though maybe not all at the same time, you know.

You can add anywhere from 4-8 ounces of well-drained chopped, roasted green chile with the cheese and scallions for a robust side dish.

Mellow Mushroom Meatloaf

Cognac adds a wonderful flavor to a classic dish.

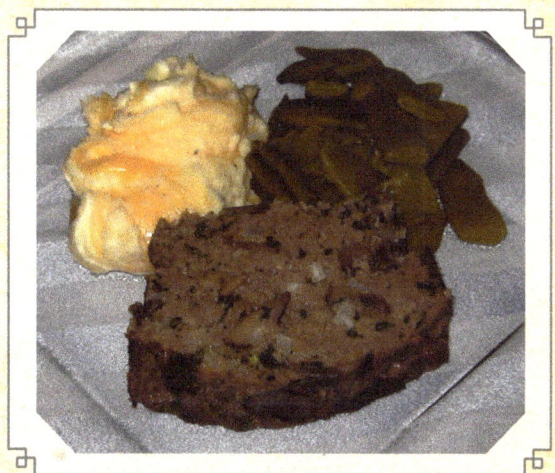

1 tablespoon salted butter
1 pound fresh mushrooms, sliced rather thinly
¼ cup cognac
½ teaspoon Savory Seasoning
1 pound ground beef sirloin
½ cup seasoned dry bread crumbs
½ cup minced onion
1 extra large egg
½ cup half-and-half
½ cup fresh parsley, minced (or 2 tablespoons dry parsley)
2 tablespoons fresh sage, minced (or 2 teaspoons dry sage)
1 tablespoon Worcestershire sauce
1 teaspoon each:
    salt
    pepper
    minced garlic

In a large skillet, melt the butter over rather high heat. Add the mushrooms and sauté 5 minutes. Add the cognac and cook over fairly high heat until most of the liquid evaporates, about 5-10 minutes. Add the Savory Seasoning; combine and set aside.

Preheat oven to 375°. Coat an 8½" by 4½" glass loaf pan with cooking spray. In a large bowl, combine the remaining ingredients with your hands until thoroughly mixed. Gently mix in the mushrooms. Put in the loaf pan and press down. Smooth top and bake 1 hour, or until a meat thermometer registers 160-165° in the center. Let stand 10 minutes before slicing. Cover and refrigerate leftovers. Serves 6-8.

Mix 4 ounces of well-drained, roasted and chopped green chile into the meat mixture.

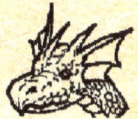

Chapter Three: Council Catering

Sweet & Savory Pork Roast

Pork and apples just seem to go together well. The idea is older than medieval times, dating back to a Roman chef, Apicius, who suggested all sorts of flavors to counterbalance the rich fattiness of various meats or to mask the tell-tale smell of a meat that might be past its prime. Hence, the reason strong flavors, such as pepper, garlic, and ginger were often used. Acidic fruits often help with the digestion of fats. Remember this when you see a ham with pineapple slices and maraschino cherries, or orange peel beef, the classic Duck a l'Orange, and even lamb prepared with mint sauce or jelly.

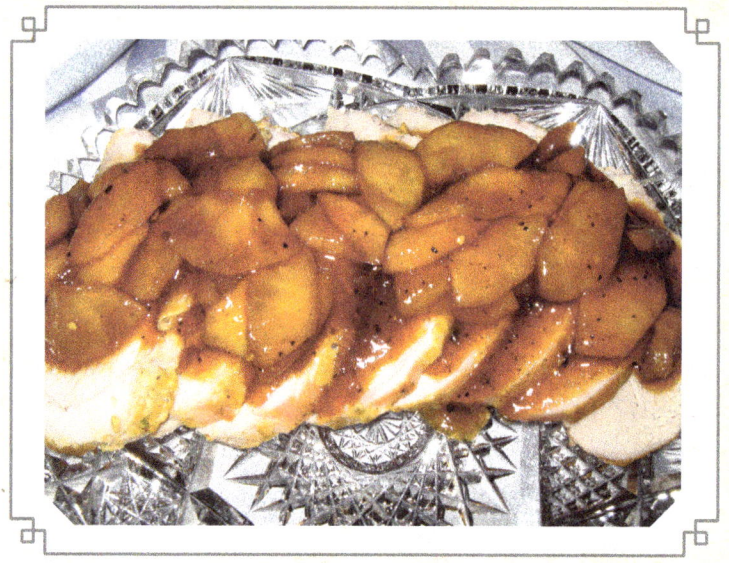

2 boneless pork sirloin tip roasts or single pork top loin roasts (you'll need a total of about 4-4½ pounds between them)

½ cup Dijon mustard

1 tablespoon plus 1 teaspoon Savory Seasoning

½ cup salted butter

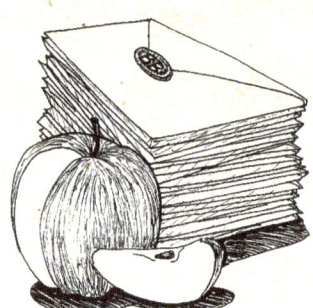

4 large apples, peeled, cored, and cut into ¼" slices

½ teaspoon pepper

12-ounce jar mango chutney (1 cup—you may cut up any large pieces of mango, if desired)

¼ cup soy sauce

14½-ounce can low-sodium chicken broth

Preheat oven to 325°. Coat a 13" by 9" glass baking dish with cooking spray or grease lightly. Place roasts in pan. In a small bowl, whisk together the mustard and 1 tablespoon Savory Seasoning. Smear this all over the tops and sides of the roasts. Bake 1 hour and 20 minutes. Insert a meat thermometer into the center of one roast and raise heat to 400°. Bake another 15-25 minutes, until the thermometer reaches 160°.

Meanwhile, melt butter in a 5-quart deep skillet over rather high heat. Add the apples and sauté about 3 minutes. Add the remaining ingredients and bring to a boil. Lower heat slightly and cook 20-30 minutes, until the sauce reduces somewhat and becomes thicker. Adjust seasonings, if desired.

Remove pork from oven; cover with foil and let it rest in the pan 15 minutes. Cut into ¼" diagonal slices and arrange on a platter. Pour the sauce over all. Cover and refrigerate leftovers. Serves 10-12.

Donald's Cinnamon Sticks

Oh, cinnamon—is there any other spice that exemplifies comfort food as much as you?

¾ cup all-purpose flour
½ cup cake flour
2 tablespoons sugar
2 tablespoons packed golden brown sugar
1 teaspoon cinnamon
¼ teaspoon salt
¾ cup soft salted butter
1½ tablespoons heavy cream
1½ tablespoons cinnamon sugar[1]

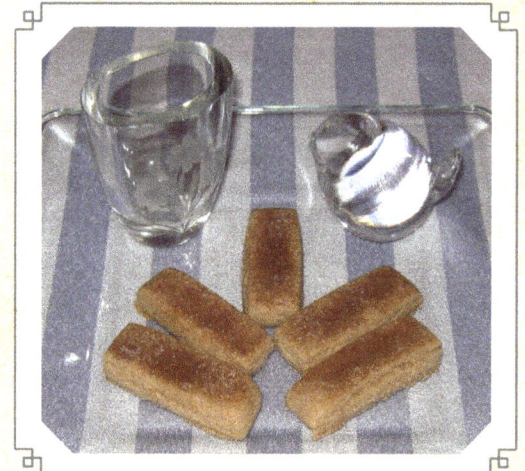

Preheat oven to 325°. Coat a large baking sheet with cooking spray or grease lightly. In a large bowl, combine the flours, sugar, brown sugar, cinnamon, and salt. Add the butter and mix until well combined. Place dough on a lightly floured surface and knead it a few times until smooth. Pat the dough out to a 4" by 10" rectangle, about ½" thick. Cut 2" by ½" strips and place on sheet ¾" apart. Bake 17 minutes. Brush cookie tops with heavy cream and liberally sprinkle the cinnamon sugar all over. Bake another 3 minutes. Cool on pan 2 minutes. Carefully remove to a rack. Store covered at room temperature. Makes around 34-36.

---

[1] For all recipes that call for Cinnamon Sugar, see Essential Seasoning Mixes on page xxiii for a recipe.

Essential Mocha Tart

Here's an intense mocha dessert—if you hate mocha, all you need to do is omit or decrease the coffee powder; everything else would remain the same.

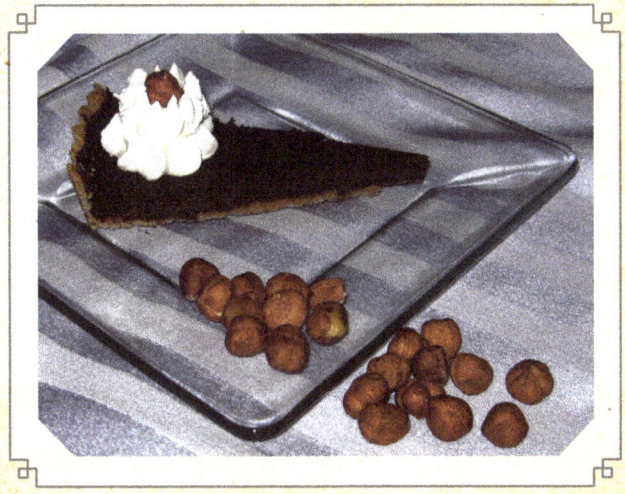

⅓ cup plus 2 tablespoons sugar
⅛ teaspoon plus ¼ teaspoon salt
1½ tablespoons instant coffee or espresso powder (regular or decaffeinated)
4 ounces semi-sweet chocolate squares, broken in half
2 ounces unsweetened chocolate squares, broken in half
¾ cup heavy cream
4 ounces hazelnuts, toasted lightly and coarsely chopped
¾ cup all-purpose flour
½ cup salted butter, melted and cooled slightly
½ cup hazelnut-flavored liqueur, such as Frangelico
3 extra large eggs, room temperature
½ teaspoon vanilla extract
½ cup heavy cream combined with 1 tablespoon sugar

Optional Garnishes (choose one or combine options, as desired):
12-16 whole hazelnuts, toasted lightly
12-16 chocolate-coated coffee beans
About 1 tablespoon cinnamon sugar
About 1 teaspoon unsweetened cocoa powder (use a fine-mesh strainer to sprinkle on the tart)
Other dessert decorations, such as sprinkles or crystallized sugars

In a 2-quart saucepan, combine the ⅓ cup sugar, ⅛ teaspoon salt, coffee powder, chocolates, and ¾ cup cream. Cook over low/medium heat just until the chocolates have melted, whisking frequently. Remove from heat and let stand uncovered.

Meanwhile, preheat oven to 350°. Liberally coat a 1" deep, 11" tart pan with removable sides with cooking spray. In a large processor, combine the hazelnuts, flour, 2 tablespoons sugar, and ¼ teaspoon salt until the nuts are finely ground. Add the butter and process thoroughly. Pour into the prepared pan and press dough up the sides first, then press evenly all over the base of the pan. Bake 10 minutes.

A couple minutes before the crust is done, whisk the liqueur, eggs, and vanilla in a 4-cup glass measuring cup. Whisk the chocolate mixture into the egg mixture well. Leaving the tart pan on the oven rack, pull the rack out partly and carefully pour the chocolate mixture onto the crust (it will be pretty full—try to keep it level). Carefully push the rack back in and bake 40 minutes, or until the center is set. Remove and place the tart pan on a rack for 1 hour. Chill at least 1 hour before garnishing. Remove sides from the pan and place tart on a serving dish.

Whip the ½ cup cream and 1 tablespoon sugar until stiff (I do this by hand in my washed and dried 4-cup glass measuring cup, but you can use a hand mixer in a medium bowl). Place in a pastry bag with a large star tip and pipe 12 or 16 rosettes equally around the tart. Place desired garnish on top of each rosette or sprinkle with the cinnamon sugar, cocoa powder, or other decorations. Or, you may simply spread the whipped cream/sugar all over the top of the tart and decorate as desired. For longer storage, cover and chill. Let it stand at room temperature about 30 minutes before serving again. Serves 12-16.

Council Catering Celebration Cake

Maybe you need a show-stopping cake to impress your potential heroes. Or maybe you just want to celebrate an elderly halfling's birthday. This can counter the effects of the previous dark chocolate dessert. **Make this impressive cake the night before you want to serve it.**

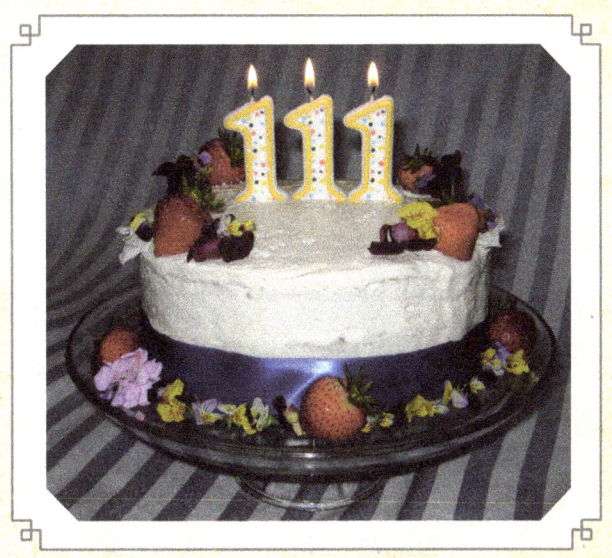

1½ pounds fresh strawberries

8 ounces plus 4 ounces white chocolate, broken into smaller pieces (chips are okay)

1 cup plus ½ cup soft salted butter

1 cup sugar

4 extra large eggs, room temperature

3 cups cake flour

1¼ cups buttermilk, room temperature

1 teaspoon baking soda

1 teaspoon plus 1 teaspoon vanilla extract

¾ cup seedless strawberry jam

1 pound powdered sugar

¼ cup 1% milk

Parchment paper

Optional Garnishes, see below

Wash, then stem all the strawberries. Cut them into ¾" pieces and lay on 2 paper towels. In a medium glass bowl, microwave the 8 ounces white chocolate in 30-second intervals until fully melted. Set aside. Cut parchment paper to line the bottoms of three 9" round, heavy aluminum baking pans. Coat each pan with a little cooking spray, place paper in each, then spray bottom and sides of each pan.

Preheat oven to 350°. In a very large bowl, beat the 1 cup butter and sugar on medium speed until fluffy. Add the eggs, one at a time, beating well especially after the last addition, scraping down the sides as needed. Place the buttermilk, baking soda, and 1 teaspoon vanilla in a 4-cup glass measuring cup and whisk until fully combined. Add 1 cup flour to the butter mixture, then half of the buttermilk mixture. Add 1 cup flour, the remaining buttermilk, then the remaining 1 cup flour; beat well on medium speed, especially after the last addition. Scrape down sides. Add the melted chocolate and combine well (don't bother rinsing the chocolate bowl—use later). By hand, gently fold in the strawberries. Divide batter into the prepared pans. Bake 36-40 minutes until all three centers test done. Cool on racks 20 minutes. If necessary, run a sharp knife around the edges and carefully turn out of the pans, but flip each cake over with the paper remaining underneath back onto the racks. Cool 1 hour.

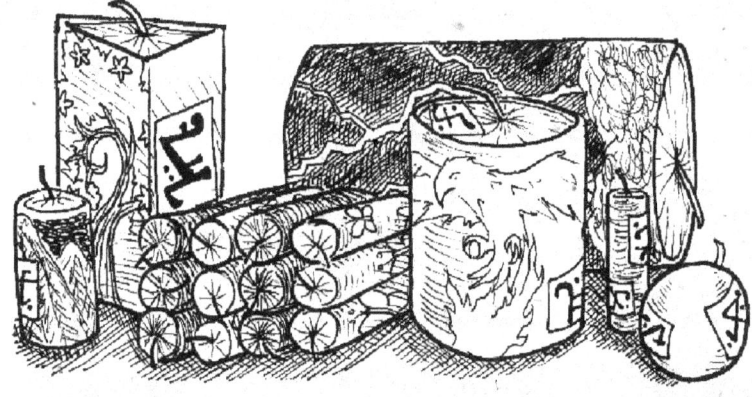

Meanwhile, heat the jam in a 1-quart saucepan just until it is melted, stirring with a whisk until smooth; set aside. Melt the remaining white chocolate in the bowl used previously and set aside to cool, but you still want it to be liquid.

For frosting: combine the powdered sugar, ½ cup butter, 1 teaspoon vanilla, milk, and cooler chocolate in a very large bowl. Beat on low speed to combine, then beat 1-2 minutes on high speed until fluffy.

Carefully remove paper from one cake layer and place the bottom side on a serving dish or cake pedestal. Using a bent (or recessed) spatula, spread a thin layer (about ⅓ cup) of frosting over the top, then spread half of the jam over the frosting. Repeat with another cake layer, ⅓ cup frosting, then the remaining jam. Place the last cake layer on top. Spread a thin layer of frosting all over the sides; refrigerate for about an hour to set it. Cover the remaining frosting with a towel and let it stand. Spread remaining frosting on sides then top of cake as evenly and smoothly as you can. Frosting should cover any cracks, so don't worry. Cover with a cake dome and chill overnight. Let stand at room temperature 1-2 hours before serving or enjoy cold. Garnish before serving, if desired (see below). If you have leftover cake, first remove all the garnishes and store it covered in the refrigerator (it actually keeps well for about a week or so; it also freezes well). Serves 12-16.

Optional Garnishes:
½ pound of medium strawberries, as nicely shaped and unblemished as possible
1½" wide ribbon, any color you choose; satin, grosgrain, or velvet. You'll need 32" or ⅞ yard.
Various fresh edible flowers and/or decorative candles, depending on the occasion.

Wash the strawberries and leave them to dry on a kitchen towel—don't remove their stems. Place ribbon around the base of the completed cake. Fold over one edge and use a few straight pins to hold in place. Cover this fold with garnishes and be sure to remove the pins before serving. Decorate top and sides with strawberries and flowers as desired and place candles on top.

Spring-in-Your-Step Punch

All that talking about danger on the road is bound to make your potential heroes quite thirsty. Use the refreshing alcoholic option if you want to make them agree to your requests more readily. **Start the night before serving.**

4 cups fresh or frozen whole strawberries (remove stems)
2 cups orange juice, no sugar added
2 cups cold water
½ cup lemon juice
11-12 ounces apricot nectar[1]
3 cups apple juice, no sugar added
750 ml. bottle of sparkling apple cider (or Asti Spumante or Prosecco)

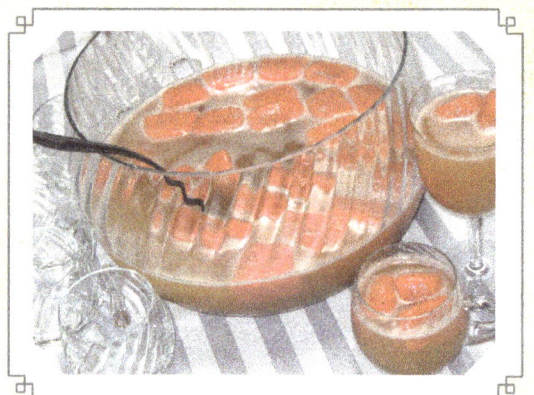

The night before serving: if using frozen strawberries, place in a 4-cup glass measuring cup and let stand for 1-2 hours. Place strawberries in a blender with orange juice. Blend until completely smooth. Pour or spoon equally into 2-3 plastic ice cube trays and freeze overnight. Be sure the lemon juice, nectar, apple juice, and sparkling cider are chilled for use the next day.

Right before serving: combine the water, lemon juice, and nectar in a 4-cup glass measuring cup; pour into a punchbowl. Add the apple juice and sparkling cider. Put all the prepared ice cubes into the punchbowl; as they melt the punch becomes slushier and is never diluted. Cover and refrigerate leftovers. Makes about 12 cups. Serves 12-16.

---

[1] Other nectars are fine, such as peach, pear, or mango.

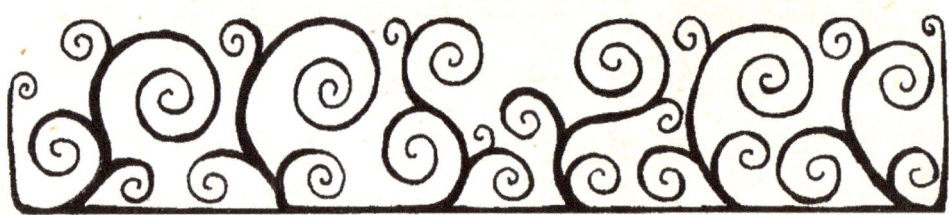

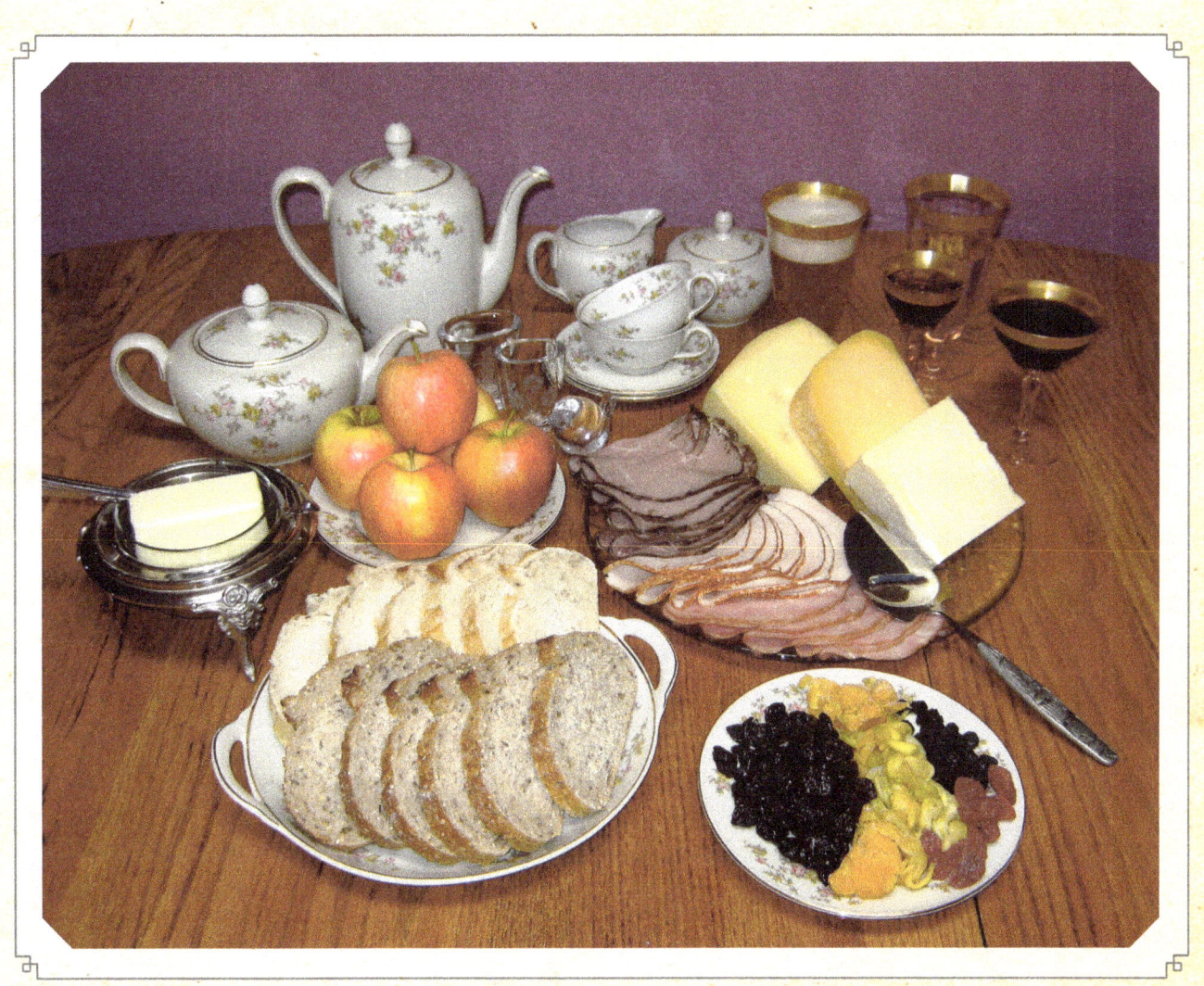

Chapter Four

Quest Depot: Supplies for the Seemingly Hopeless Enterprise

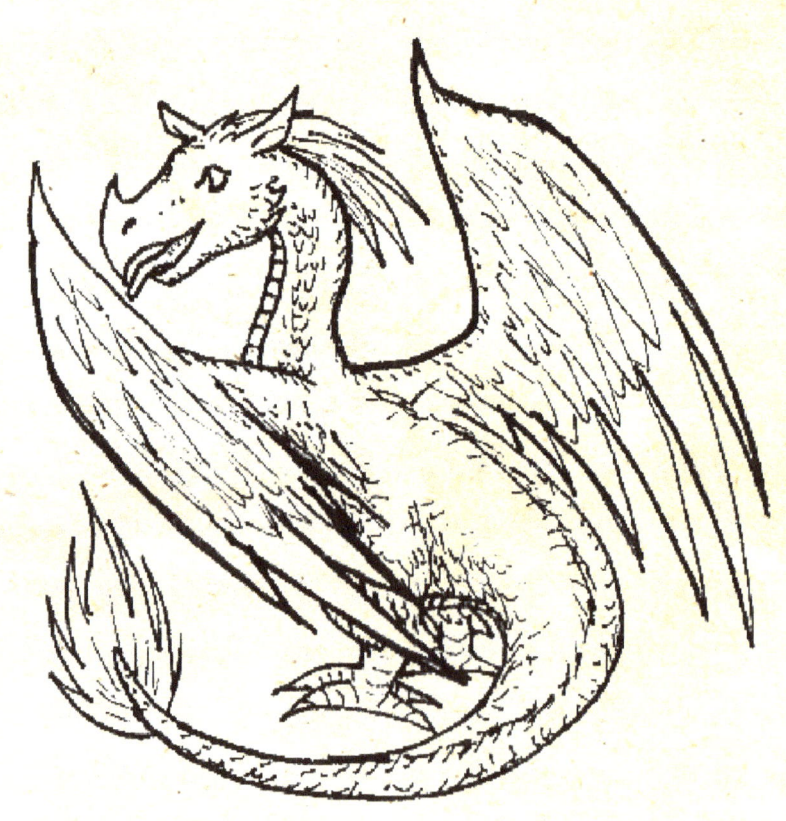

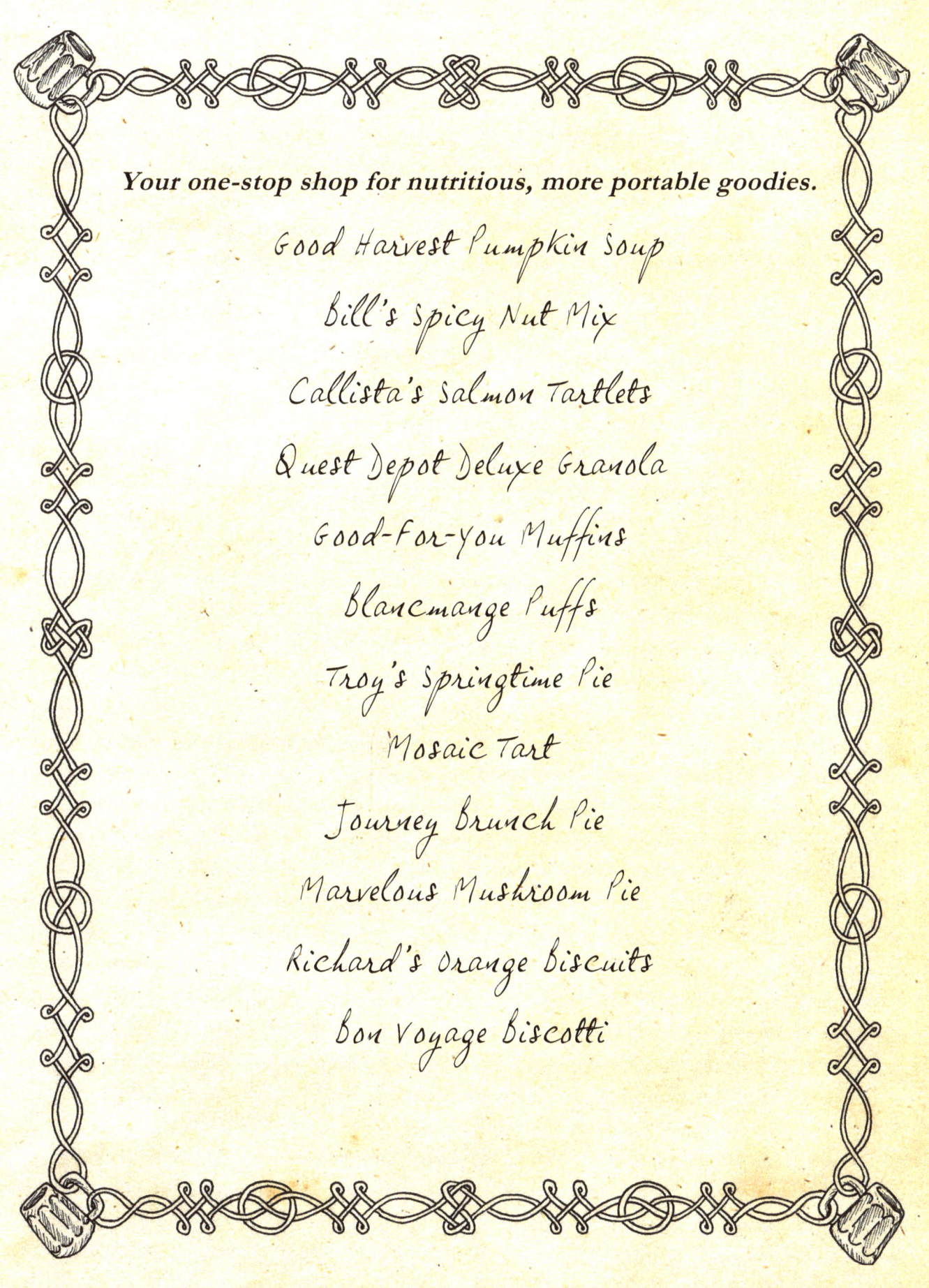

Your one-stop shop for nutritious, more portable goodies.

Good Harvest Pumpkin Soup

Bill's Spicy Nut Mix

Callista's Salmon Tartlets

Quest Depot Deluxe Granola

Good-For-You Muffins

Blancmange Puffs

Troy's Springtime Pie

Mosaic Tart

Journey Brunch Pie

Marvelous Mushroom Pie

Richard's Orange Biscuits

Bon Voyage Biscotti

Quest Depot

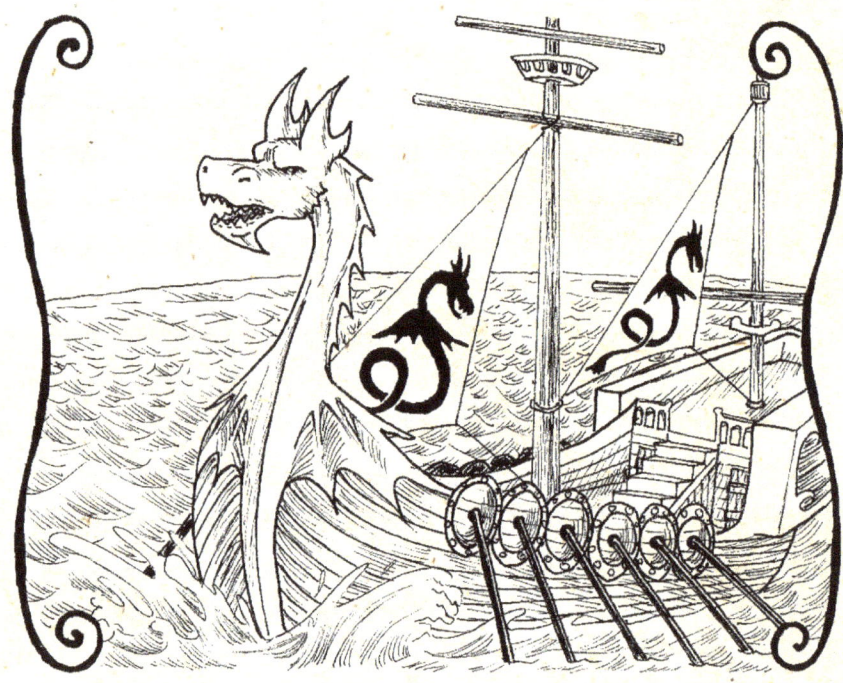

Road trips are better with good food. Everything in this chapter is rather conducive to traveling, whether you are off to slay a dragon or merely driving to the mountains to have a picnic. A little bit of menu planning can prevent you from scrounging relatively unhealthy items when you are traveling (you know, such as vermin and other such critters in a Middle-earth-type setting, or Doritos and Snickers bars when you're driving by yourself to visit far-away family members…).

Good Harvest Pumpkin Soup

We'll start with a light, but intensely flavored, vegetarian soup which is perfect for a thermos—sometimes it's hard to get good vegetable nutrition on the road, but now you can. Sometimes, I had problems getting cans of plain pumpkin (sorry, but I have never been one to mess with fresh pumpkin, even around Halloween), because of a nationwide shortage. This turned out fine, however; an excellent variation is to use 2 pounds of cauliflower (which is about an average head). Remove the core and cut into 1" florets; keep everything else the same.

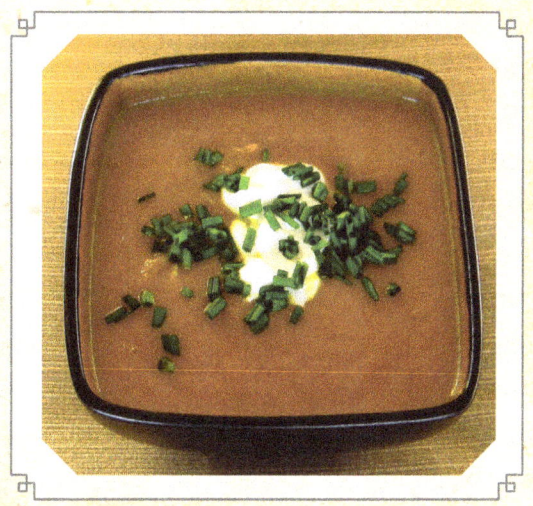

2 tablespoons salted butter
¾ cup shallots, chopped coarsely
1 cup each (peeled and chopped coarsely):
    onion
    carrots
    celery
1 quart vegetable broth
14½-ounce can pumpkin puree (or about
    1¾ cups fresh pumpkin)
2 teaspoons hot Madras curry powder
2 teaspoons sugar
½ teaspoon Savory Seasoning
Light sour cream, about ½ cup
Minced fresh chives, about ½ cup

Melt the butter over fairly high heat in a 3-quart saucepan. Add the shallots, onion, carrots, and celery; sauté 5 minutes. Add the broth, pumpkin, and seasonings. Bring to a boil, lower heat to medium and cook, uncovered, for 20-25 minutes, until the vegetables are very tender; stir occasionally. Blend in 2 batches to complete smoothness. Adjust seasonings, if desired. Garnish with dollops of sour cream and a sprinkling of chives. Cover and refrigerate leftovers. Serves 8 as an appetizer; 4 as a main course.

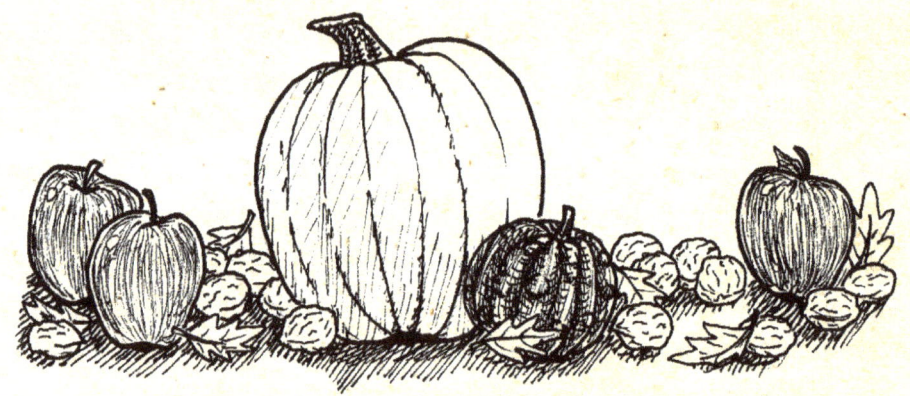

 Now, I happen to be a curry powder fanatic—not that I use it everywhere, but I do love it. I think it reminds me of my childhood, when my Norwegian mom would make curry cream sauce or mix butter and curry with plain white rice. My recipe tester for this thought it was a bit too strong, but everyone has different tastes. If you have doubts, use less and taste it to judge whether it's too spicy.

Bill's Spicy Nut Mix

This addictive snack mix lasts for a few weeks and is a good option to put out around the holiday season; it can also be frozen. Double the three seasonings for extra spice.

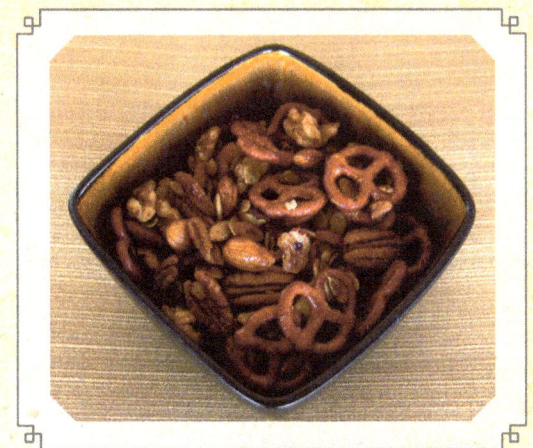

¼ cup salted butter
2 tablespoons soy sauce
1 tablespoon packed golden brown sugar
1 tablespoon honey
½ teaspoon each:
    garlic powder
    cayenne pepper
    pepper
4 ounces each:
    pecan halves
    walnut halves
    whole almonds
    small pretzels
    pumpkin seeds, roasted and salted

Preheat oven to 250°. Coat a 13" by 9" glass baking dish with cooking spray or grease lightly. In a large glass bowl, melt the butter in the microwave on HIGH in 20-second increments until melted. Add the soy sauce, brown sugar, honey, and seasonings and mix well with a whisk. Add the remaining ingredients and mix well. Pour into prepared pan and bake 1 hour. Stir every 15 minutes, and after you remove it from the oven. Cool to room temperature. Store in an airtight container at room temperature. Makes about 6 cups.

 *If you'd like to reduce your carb/gluten intake, omit the pretzels and substitute 4 ounces of some sort of different whole nuts, such as macadamias or cashews.*

Callista's Salmon Tartlets

My younger daughter Callista loves to visit one of our local restaurants where you can have a "high tea." These particular savory, diminutive treats would be a welcome addition to an afternoon tea and they are one of her top five recipes. Bob even likes them!

¼ cup dry white wine, such as Chardonnay
1 tablespoon lemon juice
¼ teaspoon plus ¼ teaspoon Savory Seasoning
6-7 ounces boneless, skinless salmon fillet (thaw as directed, if using frozen fish)
1 cup all-purpose flour
½ teaspoon salt
½ teaspoon dry dill weed (or 1 tablespoon fresh dill, minced)
½ cup soft salted butter
¼ cup 1% milk
3 ounces light cream cheese (Neufchâtel), softened
1 extra large egg
2 tablespoons heavy cream
Dill Mayonnaise, recipe below

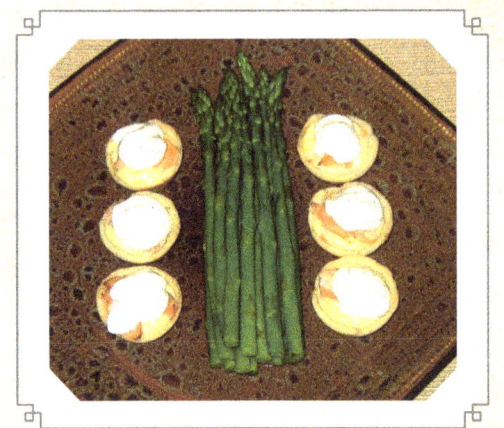

In a small skillet, combine the wine, lemon juice, and ¼ teaspoon Savory Seasoning. Place salmon in pan. Bring to a boil, then simmer on medium heat 5 minutes. Turn salmon over, and simmer another 5 minutes, or until the fish is fully cooked yet still moist in the center. Turn off heat and leave the salmon in the pan.

Preheat oven to 350°. Liberally coat 24 miniature muffin cups with cooking spray. In a large bowl, combine the flour, salt, dill, butter, and milk with a hand mixer on low speed until fully combined. Knead a few times on a lightly floured surface. Divide dough into 24 portions and place one in each cup. Use floured fingers to press dough all the way up the sides. Bake 10 minutes. Remove and maintain oven temperature. Use a shot glass or a rounded spoon to press the pastry cups down, if they are too puffy.

Meanwhile in the same bowl (you don't have to wash the bowl or the beaters), beat the cream cheese until smooth then beat in the egg, cream, and ¼ teaspoon Savory Seasoning until fully mixed. Fill each cup equally with the cream cheese mixture (approximately 1½ teaspoons in each). Using a fork, flake the salmon into 24 mostly equal portions and place one in each cup on top of the cheese. Bake 20 minutes. Cool 10 minutes. Use a sharp knife around the edges to ease removal from pans. Top each with a scant teaspoon of Dill Mayonnaise. Cover and refrigerate leftovers. Makes 24.

Dill Mayonnaise

½ cup mayonnaise
2 teaspoons lemon juice
½ teaspoon dry dill weed (or 1 tablespoon fresh dill, minced)
¼ teaspoon Savory Seasoning

Whisk together all ingredients in a small bowl. Cover and refrigerate leftovers. Makes ½ cup.

Vegetarian Option—Replace the salmon with 1½ cups of thin, fresh asparagus, sliced into ¼" bits. Simmer asparagus for only 3 minutes. Set aside in a fine-mesh strainer to drain well as you prepare everything else and follow all other directions, placing about a teaspoon of asparagus in each cup.

A tablespoon of well-drained, roasted and chopped green chile in the egg mixture would be good—either with the salmon or with the **Vegetarian Option**.

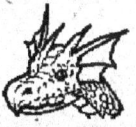

Chapter Four: Quest Depot

Quest Depot Deluxe Granola

Great as a snack, a breakfast cereal, and a topping for ice cream—this yummy granola also pairs well with yogurt. You can also freeze this—let it stand at room temperature 2-3 hours before serving, so the fruit can soften up.

8 ounces old-fashioned oats
2 ounces each:
    pecan halves
    walnut halves
    sliced almonds
¼ cup sunflower seeds, dry roasted and salted
¼ cup dry milk powder
1 tablespoon cinnamon
½ teaspoon salt
¼ cup walnut oil
½ cup honey
6 ounces dried cherries
3 ounces each:
    chopped sugar dates (or chopped dried figs—
        be sure to snip off their stems first)
    dried blueberries
    raisins

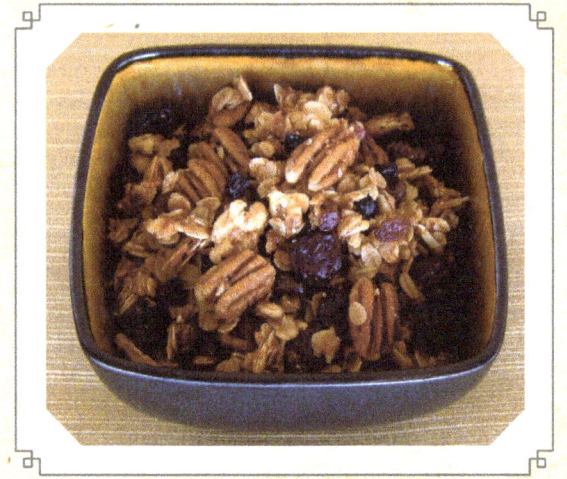

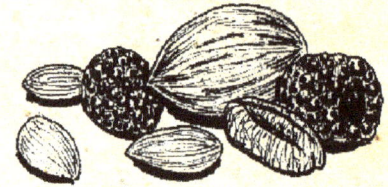

Preheat oven to 350°. Liberally coat a 13" by 9" glass baking dish with cooking spray. In a very large bowl, combine the first eight ingredients. In a 2-cup glass measuring cup, whisk together the oil and honey. Pour over the oat mixture and mix well with a wooden spoon. Pour into the pan (don't bother washing bowl) and bake for a total of 30 minutes. Stir with the wooden spoon at 10 minutes, at 20 minutes, and finally after you remove it from the oven. Let cool in pan for one hour.

Meanwhile, combine the dried fruits in the bowl. Break up the oat mixture with the wooden spoon; pour this into the bowl and mix well. Store in an airtight container at room temperature. Makes about 9 cups.

Good-For-You Muffins

Here are some relatively healthy muffins for the road. They are low in sugar, so they are suitable for savory or sweet purposes.

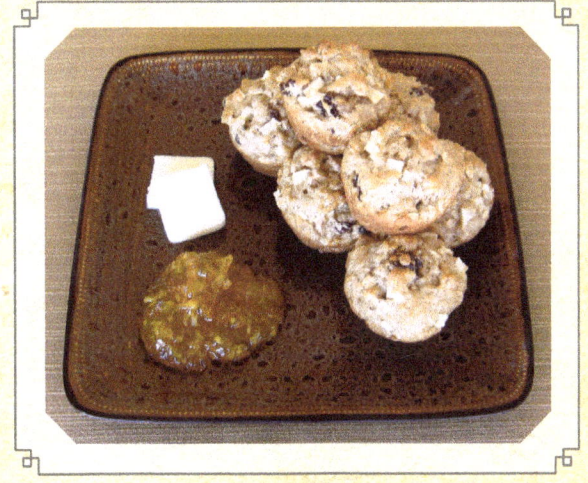

1¼ cups all-purpose flour
⅓ cup wheat flour
⅔ cup old-fashioned oats
¼ cup sugar
¼ cup packed golden brown sugar
1 teaspoon salt
1 teaspoon baking powder
½ teaspoon each:
    baking soda
    cinnamon
    nutmeg
½ cup buttermilk
1 extra large egg
½ cup applesauce
3 tablespoons walnut oil (or vegetable oil)
1¼ cups apple; peeled, cored, and cut into ¼" bits
½ cup raisins (or currants)
2 ounces walnuts and/or pecans, coarsely chopped

Preheat oven to 400°. Coat 12 regular size muffin cups with cooking spray or grease lightly (you could instead use papers, if desired). In a large bowl, combine the flours, oats, sugars, salt, baking powder and soda, and spices. In a 2-cup glass measuring cup, whisk together the buttermilk and the egg well, then mix in the applesauce and oil. Add to the dry ingredients and combine. Add the remaining ingredients and mix just until fully combined. Divide batter into the prepared cups and bake 16-18 minutes, or until they test done in the center. Cool in pan on a rack for about 15 minutes before serving. Cover and store at room temperature. Makes 12.

Chapter Four: Quest Depot

Blancmange Puffs

While waiting around, worrying about what horrible events might unfold in their future, hungry questers would probably like to nibble on something substantial, such as these exotically flavored puffs. For dinner, you could serve 3 or 4 puffs per person, accompanied by a salad or vegetable on the side.

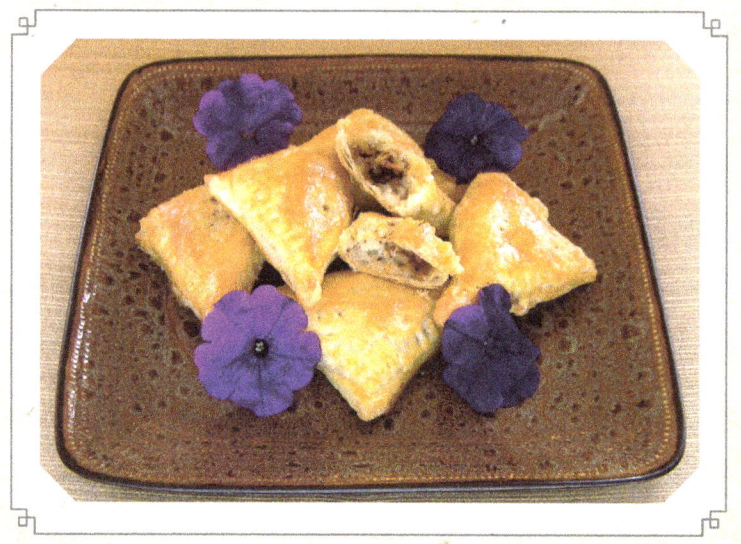

17.3-ounce package puff pastry, thawed according to package directions (such as Pepperidge Farm)
1 tablespoon plus 1 tablespoon salted butter
⅓ cup minced onion
½ teaspoon plus ½ teaspoon salt
½ teaspoon pepper
½ pound boneless, skinless chicken thighs, cut into ¼" bits (partially frozen for easy cutting)[1]
1 cup low-sodium chicken broth
¼ cup long grain rice
1 teaspoon almond extract
3 tablespoons heavy cream
2 teaspoons sugar
1 teaspoon anise seeds
1 extra large egg
1 teaspoon water
Candied Almonds, recipe below

[1] You can use ground chicken, but you will end up with a better texture when you actually dice up your chicken. Plus, I find it easier to obtain chicken thighs rather than ground chicken, at least around my neighborhood grocery stores. If you want your blancmange to be whiter, you can use white meat, but the flavor is richer with dark meat.

In a medium skillet, melt 1 tablespoon butter over rather high heat. Add the onion, ½ teaspoon salt, pepper, and chicken. Sauté until chicken is no longer pink; turn off heat and let stand in pan. In a 1½-quart saucepan, combine the broth, rice, and almond extract. Bring to a boil, stir once, then simmer undisturbed on lowest heat, covered, for 15 minutes. Drain and put rice back in saucepan. Add cream, 1 tablespoon butter, sugar, ½ teaspoon salt, and anise seeds. Combine, then add the chicken mixture to this and let stand 1 hour, uncovered. Season, as desired. Don't bother washing skillet and use it for the Candied Almonds below, which you can make now while the chicken mixture cools.

Preheat oven to 400°. Coat 2 large baking sheets with cooking spray or grease lightly. Take 1 sheet of puff pastry and cut it into 9 fairly equal squares. Put about 1 tablespoon chicken mixture on each square. Put about ½ tablespoon Candied Almonds on top of chicken. Don't overstuff (see below for leftover suggestions). Fold pastry over and make a triangle; pinch edges together and set on 1 sheet. Repeat assembly process with the other sheet. Use fork tines to press edges down on all triangles. Poke the tops of each with fork tines once. In a small bowl, whisk together the egg and water. Brush each triangle with egg wash. Bake 8 minutes; brush with egg wash again. Bake another 8-10 minutes or until golden brown. Let stand 5 minutes before serving. Cover and refrigerate leftovers. Makes 18.

Candied Almonds

2 tablespoons salted butter
1 tablespoon sugar
1 teaspoon anise seeds
¼ teaspoon salt
2 ounces sliced almonds

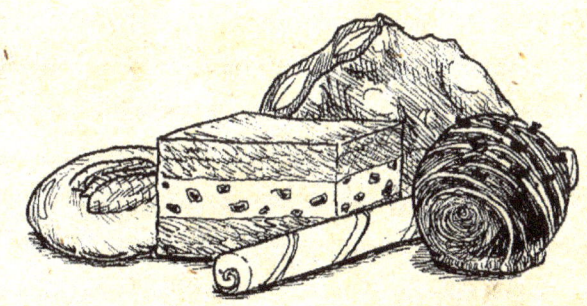

In a medium skillet, melt the butter and mix in the seasonings. Add the almonds and sauté over medium heat 1-2 minutes. Almonds should brown slightly, but be careful not to burn them. Turn off heat and let stand in the pan. When cool, break up nuts gently with a spoon. Any leftover nuts can be used on ice cream or thrown on a salad. Cover and keep leftovers at room temperature. Makes about ⅔ cup.

Being the casual linguist I am, I see the word blancmange and I assume it means "white food." Being the Monty Python fanatic I am, I also picture one of their television sketches in which a giant blancmange suddenly appears on a tennis court and aggressively shoves the players around. I seem to recall this creature is some sort of alien apparently mimicking a relatively modern version of a blancmange, which is a sweet, molded, pudding-type of dessert flavored with almond and can be held together by gelatin (there are variations on this theme; a glance at Wikipedia is helpful here to get the idea).

However, in my food history reading, I discovered that blancmange is a whole different concept, though almonds are the preferred flavor and the food is meant to be as white as possible (I think they mean beige here…). In Life in a Medieval Castle, *Joseph and Frances Gies describe various dishes popular around the twelfth century, whereby usually poultry would be mashed to a paste consistency and mixed with other ingredients and cooked as a custard. Then it would be mixed with items such as rice, almond milk, and sugar, then cooked till it thickened even more. It would be garnished with anise and fried almonds and it was called* **blankmanger** *(112).*

Now, I didn't think a paste of chicken sounded that good, but I was intrigued by the combination of flavors mentioned above and I was determined to create something that really had a medieval influence about it, and thus, I came up with these puffs. At first, you might think the flavors are odd, but I assure you, you will find them a bit addictive. You will probably have some leftover fillings: mix up the nuts and chicken and simply eat it as a snack or lunch.

Troy's Springtime Pie

Though you can obviously make this pie at any time of the year, it is a great dish to serve for an Easter dinner, especially if you have lots of Easter eggs around. If you end up with extra sauce, cook some pasta and combine the two for an impromptu macaroni and cheese.

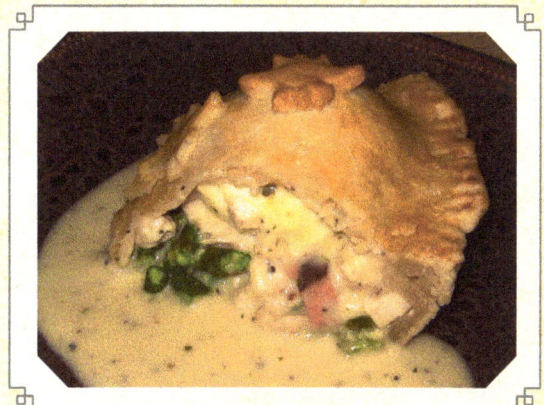

- 8 extra large eggs, hard boiled and peeled in advance
- 2½ cups plus ⅓ cup plus 1 tablespoon all-purpose flour
- 1¾ teaspoons salt, divided
- 5 ounces chilled lard, cut into ¼" bits (or vegetable shortening)
- ¾ cup ice water
- ¼ cup salted butter
- 1 teaspoon Herbes de Provence
- ½ teaspoon pepper
- 2½ cups 1% milk
- ½ pound Gouda cheese, shredded
- 2 cups fresh asparagus (preferably on the thinner side), cut the heads at 1" and the stems at ½" pieces
- 3 ounces cooked ham, cut into ½" dice
- ½ pound cooked chicken, cut into ½" dice
- 1 extra large egg
- 1 teaspoon water

Combine the 2½ cups flour and 1 teaspoon salt in a large bowl. Cut in the lard with a pastry blender until mixture resembles coarse crumbs. Mix in the water, then combine until the dough comes together well and is still moist. Divide dough into a ⅔ and a ⅓ portion. Flatten into discs and wrap each with plastic wrap or put each into covered containers. Refrigerate dough 30-60 minutes.

Meanwhile, melt the butter in a 2-quart saucepan over medium/high heat. Add the ⅓ cup flour, Herbes de Provence, pepper, and ½ teaspoon salt and combine with a whisk until smooth. Add the milk and cook over medium/high heat until sauce is smooth and thicker. Stir in the cheese until melted. Season, as desired. Place the asparagus in a medium bowl. Mix in the remaining ¼ teaspoon salt, 1 tablespoon flour, and ¼ cup cheese sauce. Place the ham and chicken in another medium bowl and combine with ½ cup sauce. Cover remaining sauce and let stand.

Preheat oven to 375°. On a floured surface, roll out the ⅔ portion of dough to approximately 13" and lay in a 9½" glass pie dish. Spread the asparagus mixture all over the bottom. Top with the ham mixture. Arrange the 8 hard boiled eggs evenly over the meat, pressing down slightly. Spread a tablespoon of cheese sauce over each egg. Roll out the ⅓ portion of the crust to about 12" and cover the eggs loosely. Trim and fold the edges over and crimp decoratively. Cut small decorations from the scraps, if desired. Cut ½" slits between the eggs. Whisk together the egg and water and brush all over the pie. Place the decorations over the top and brush them with more egg wash. Bake 25 minutes. Remove from oven and brush with the egg wash again. Bake another 25 minutes until golden brown. Meanwhile, reheat the cheese sauce over a low heat, whisking frequently. Let pie stand 10 minutes before cutting and serve with extra cheese sauce. Cover and refrigerate leftover pie and sauce separately; reheat sauce slowly. Serves 8.

Mosaic Tart

Be sure to cut your vegetables and meat into very small bits. Tired of ham? You could use a 5-ounce can of baby shrimp for variety (give them a rinse, drain them well, and just leave them whole), or 4 ounces of tiny frozen shrimp (thaw as directed).

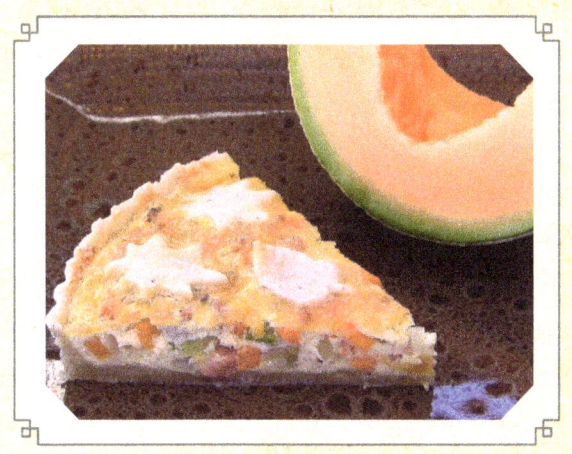

1¼ cups all-purpose flour
¼ teaspoon each:
    Savory Seasoning
    dry thyme
    salt
    pepper
¼ cup soft salted butter
¼ cup water
2 tablespoons salted butter
½ cup each, all cut into ¼" bits:
    onion
    celery
    carrot, peeled
3 ounces cooked ham, cut into ¼" bits
3 extra large eggs
½ teaspoon Savory Seasoning
½ cup half-and-half
2 ounces Gruyere cheese, finely shredded (Jarlsberg or Swiss are fine)

In a large bowl, combine the flour and the following 4 seasonings. Add the ¼ cup butter and water and combine well. Turn out onto a floured surface and knead a few times; flatten into a disk. Turn the bowl over and cover the dough; let rest 30 minutes or so (don't bother washing the bowl afterwards).

Meanwhile in a medium skillet, melt the 2 tablespoons butter rather over high heat. Add the onion, celery, and carrot and sauté 5 minutes. Turn off the heat, mix in the ham, and set aside.

Preheat oven to 375°. Liberally coat a 9½" tart pan with 1" deep removable sides with cooking spray. On a floured surface, roll the dough out to about an 11" circle and lay in the prepared pan. Press lightly up the edges and trim the top flush with

Chapter Four: Quest Depot

the edge of the pan. Save the scraps for decorations. Bake 10 minutes. While the crust is baking, combine the eggs, ½ teaspoon Savory Seasoning, and half-and-half in the large bowl with a whisk until thoroughly blended. Remove crust from oven and sprinkle crust with ⅓ of the cheese. Pour the vegetable mixture evenly over the cheese. Pour the egg mixture over all. Sprinkle with the remaining cheese. Place small pastry decorations as desired. Bake 32-36 minutes, until set in the center. Remove and let stand 10 minutes. Remove pan sides and cut. Cover and refrigerate leftovers. Serves 4-6.

Mix 4 ounces of well-drained, roasted and chopped green chile into the egg mixture.

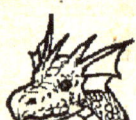

Journey Brunch Pie

This pie combines many breakfast favorites, though it's great for supper, lunch, or brunch. And it would make a delicious picnic dish. Substitute a single ready-made pie crust if you're short on time.

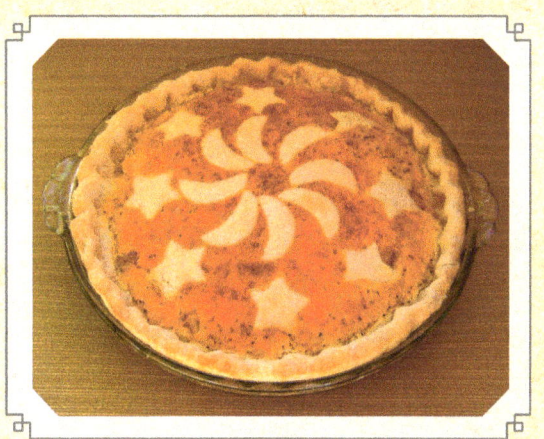

1½ cups all-purpose flour
½ teaspoon plus ¼ teaspoon salt
3 ounces chilled lard, cut into ¼" bits (or vegetable shortening)
6-8 tablespoons ice water
1 tablespoon salted butter
½ pound potato, peeled (or not, depending on the variety you use) and cut into ½" dice
1 cup onion, coarsely chopped
3 ounces cooked ham, coarsely chopped[1]
5 extra large eggs
½ cup half-and-half
1 teaspoon Dijon mustard
1 teaspoon Worcestershire sauce
¼ teaspoon pepper
4 ounces sharp Cheddar cheese, shredded

In a large bowl, combine the flour and ½ teaspoon salt. Cut in the lard with a pastry blender until the mixture resembles coarse crumbs. Add the water in tablespoons, mixing until the dough is incorporated thoroughly; form a smooth ball. Cover bowl with a towel and refrigerate 30-60 minutes.

Meanwhile, melt the butter over rather high heat in a medium skillet. Add the potatoes, onions, and ham. Fry about 8-10 minutes, until the potatoes are golden brown; stir or shake the pan frequently. Let stand in pan.

Preheat oven to 375°. On a floured surface, roll the dough out to about 13" and lay in a 9½" glass pie dish (don't bother washing the bowl; use it to mix the eggs later).

[1] Any other breakfast meat will work here, such as bacon, sausage, or Canadian bacon.

Trim the edge to 1", fold edges under, and crimp decoratively; set aside. Reserve extra dough for decorations, if desired.

In the bowl, combine the eggs, half-and-half, mustard, Worcestershire sauce, pepper, and the ¼ teaspoon salt with a whisk. Pour the ham mixture over the crust; sprinkle with half of the cheese. Pour the egg mixture over all. Sprinkle the remaining cheese over all. Cut pie crust decorations and place on top of cheese, if desired. Bake 46-50 minutes, or until the center is set. Remove from oven and let stand 10 minutes before cutting. Serve hot, warm, or even at room temperature. Cover and refrigerate leftovers; don't freeze. Serves 6-8.

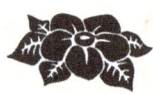 **Vegetarian Option**—Omit the ham and increase the potatoes and onions accordingly, or use your favorite meat substitute. Other vegetables will also work well.

Mix 4 ounces of well-drained, roasted and chopped green chile into the egg mixture.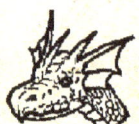

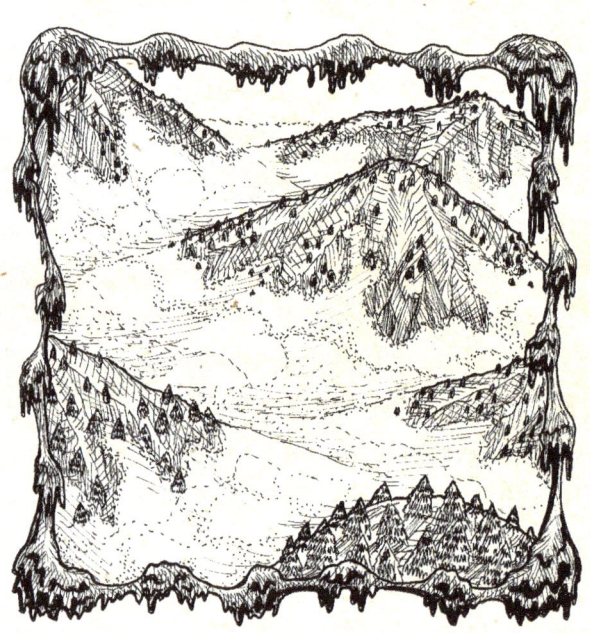

Marvelous Mushroom Pie

Sometimes you just want to skip the meat completely. I can think of a couple of famous halflings who would really have appreciated this pie on their trek to Mordor…

1½ cups all-purpose flour
½ teaspoon salt
3 ounces chilled lard, cut into ¼" bits (or vegetable shortening)
6-8 tablespoons ice water
1 tablespoon salted butter
½ pound fresh mushrooms, thinly sliced
¼ teaspoon plus ¼ teaspoon Savory Seasoning
8 ounces Gouda cheese, shredded
4 extra large eggs
½ cup 1% milk
½ cup heavy cream
¼ teaspoon nutmeg
¼ cup fresh parsley, minced (or 1 tablespoon dry parsley)

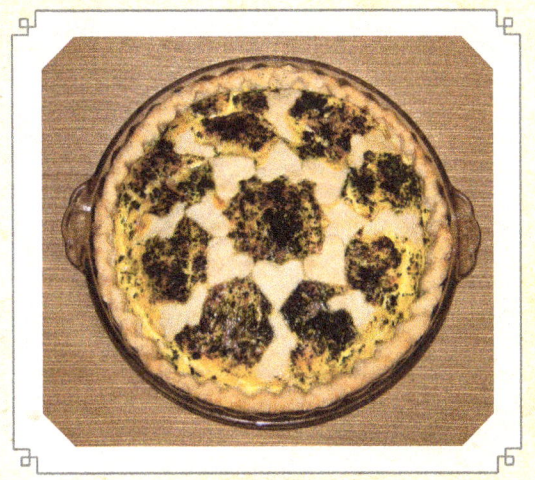

In a large bowl, combine the flour and salt. Cut in the lard with a pastry blender until the mixture resembles coarse crumbs. Add the water in tablespoons, mixing until the dough is incorporated thoroughly; form a smooth ball. Cover bowl with a towel and refrigerate 30-60 minutes.

Meanwhile, melt the butter over rather high heat in a medium skillet. Sauté the mushrooms and ¼ teaspoon Savory Seasoning over rather high heat, stirring frequently. Cook about 6-8 minutes, until all the liquid evaporates; set aside.

Preheat oven to 375°. On a floured surface, roll out dough into a 13" circle. Place in a 9½" glass pie dish. Trim and fold over the edge; crimp as desired. Save scraps for decorations, if you like. In the pie crust bowl (don't bother washing), whisk together the eggs, milk, cream, ¼ teaspoon Savory Seasoning, and nutmeg; set aside. Layer ⅓ of the cheese, ½ the mushrooms, ⅓ of the cheese, the remaining mushrooms, and the remaining cheese over the dough. Pour the egg mixture over. Sprinkle with parsley and place small decorations over all, if desired. Bake 46-50 minutes or until set in the center. Let stand 10-15 minutes before cutting. Serve hot, warm, or even at room temperature. Cover and refrigerate leftovers. Serves 6-8.

Mix 4 ounces of well-drained, roasted and chopped green chile into the egg mixture.

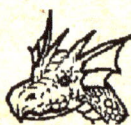

Richard's Orange Biscuits

A minimal amount of ingredients nevertheless results in a wonderful cookie. Sometimes, you just crave simplicity in your baking.

3 large oranges
1 cup plus 1 tablespoon soft salted butter
½ cup sugar
2½ cups all-purpose flour
1½ cups powdered sugar

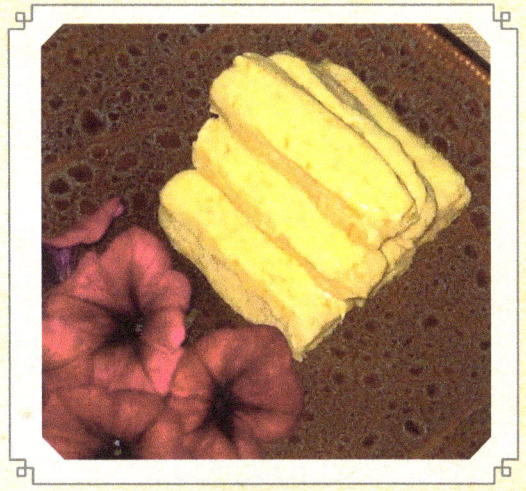

Using a microplaner or fine grater, remove as much of the zest from the oranges as you can. You should have at least 3 tablespoons; set aside. Cut oranges in half and juice them. If necessary, strain the juice; reserve ¼ cup and save the rest in a small bowl.

Preheat oven to 350°. Coat a large baking sheet with cooking spray or grease lightly. In a large bowl, cream the 1 cup butter, sugar, and 2 tablespoons zest on low speed for 1 minute. Add the flour and the reserved ¼ cup juice; mix on medium speed until well combined. On a lightly floured surface, pat out the dough to a 6" by 12" rectangle, about ½" thick. Cut into 36 pieces. Carefully place on the baking sheet. Bake 16-20 minutes, until the cookies are just slightly brown on the bottom. Cool on pan 2 minutes. Carefully place them on a rack and cool 1 hour.

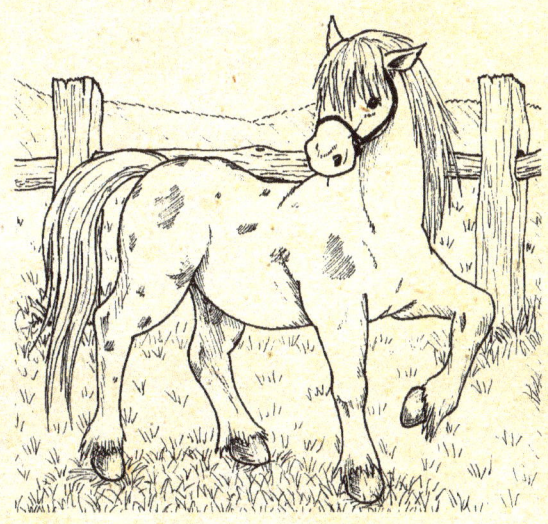

In a medium bowl, whisk together the powdered sugar, 1 tablespoon butter, remaining zest, and 2 tablespoons juice. This should have the consistency more of an icing, not a glaze. You might add a smidge more juice if you think it is too thick. With a recessed or bent spatula, spread about a teaspoon of icing on each cookie and leave on rack over the baking sheet for about half an hour to set. Keep covered at room temperature. Makes 36.

Even though my husband Bob says he dislikes shortbread cookies because he thinks they are boring, he likes these. It must be the icing and the intensely orange flavoring that make these not-so-boring.

Bon Voyage Biscotti

And sometimes you crave a bit more complexity.

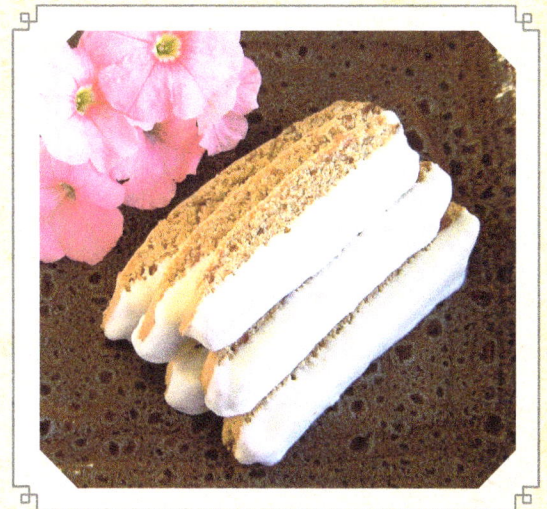

¾ cup soft salted butter
¾ cup packed golden brown sugar
⅓ cup honey
2 extra large eggs, room temperature
2 teaspoons vanilla extract
3½ cups all-purpose flour
1 tablespoon baking powder
1½ teaspoons mace
¾ teaspoon salt
4 ounces pecans, finely chopped
6 ounces dried apricots, chopped into ¼" bits (dried cherries are also good, or use a combination of the two)
1 pound white chocolate, broken into smaller sections (chips are okay)

Preheat oven to 375°. Coat 2 large baking sheets with cooking spray or grease lightly. In a very large bowl, cream the butter, brown sugar, honey, eggs, and vanilla until fully mixed. Add the flour, baking powder, mace, and salt and combine well on a low speed. Add the pecans and apricots and mix another minute or so. Divide dough in half and form each portion into a cylinder about 12-14" long. Place one on each pan. Press gently to flatten the tops until the dough is about 1" thick and 3-4" wide. Bake 25 minutes. Remove and let stand on the sheets 30 minutes.

Preheat oven to 325°. Transfer one portion of baked dough to a large cutting board. With a serrated knife, cut ½" diagonal slices. You'll get about 12 full-sized cookies, then you can cut the remaining ends for shorter, irregularly shaped cookies. Carefully place cut side down on one sheet. Repeat with the other portion on the other sheet. Bake 10 minutes. Carefully turn all the cookies over and bake another 15 minutes (if you break any, don't worry; broken ones can be dipped, too). Cool on sheets 3 minutes. Place all on racks and cool 1 hour. Don't bother washing the pans; when they have cooled off, place a sheet of wax paper on each and set aside.

Meanwhile, place the white chocolate in an 8½" by 4½" glass loaf pan. Microwave chocolate on HIGH in 30-second intervals until fully melted. Dip the bottom half (the browner portion) of each cookie in the chocolate to coat generously. Lay each on wax paper, on one side. Place in the refrigerator until the chocolate hardens, about 1 hour. Store covered at room temperature or keep chilled if the weather is warm. Makes about 24, plus some smaller cookies.

 If you are someone who dislikes white chocolate, you are free to use milk, semi-sweet, or even bittersweet chocolate for dipping. In a comparison test, however, my white-chocolate-hating-taste-testers concluded that the white chocolate was indeed best, and they even thought they could acquire a taste for white chocolate. Maybe.

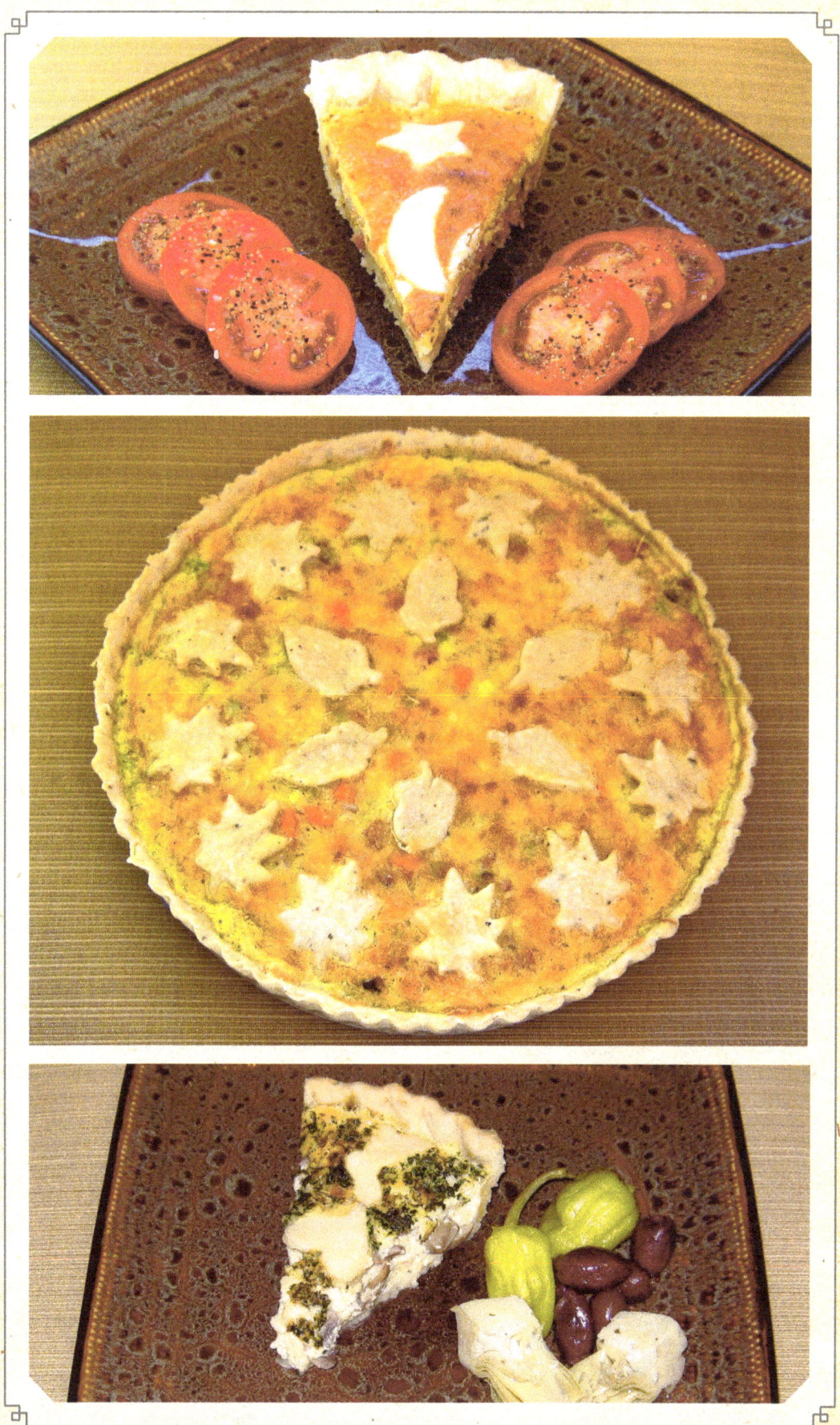

Chapter Five

The Epic-Urean

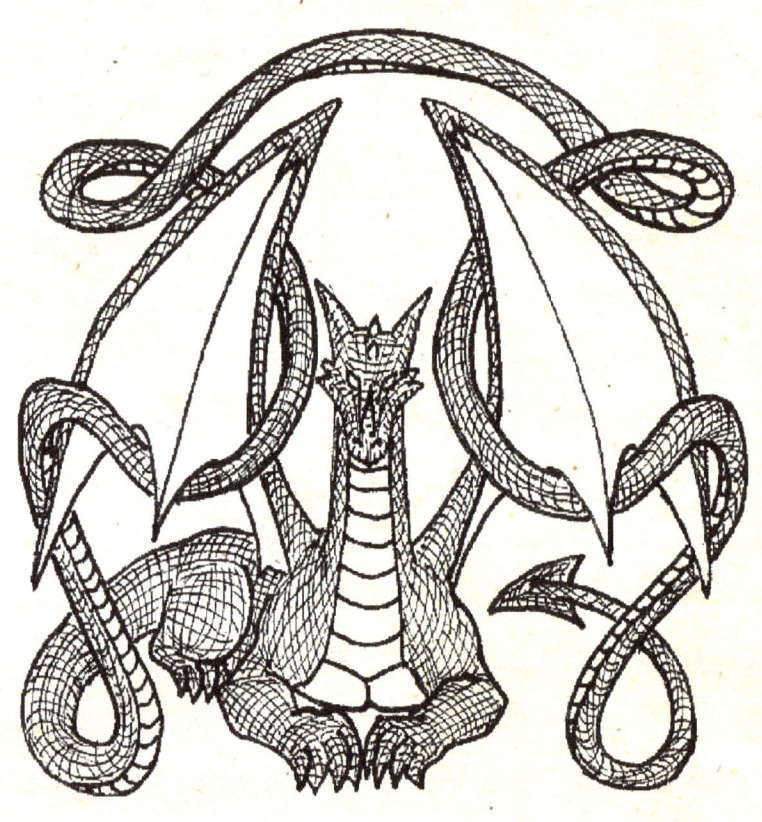

We cater to wizards, mages, witches, and alchemists. That is all we are prepared to say at this time. You will need a password or a spell to get in.

The Exquisite Soup of Master Mage Stormgutz

Aradosa's Rustic Bread & Cheese

Walter's Special Cinnamon Rolls

Beets for Hypomur

Bob's Obsession

Asbjorn's Fish, Chips, and Sauce

Epic-Urean Stew

Sine Qua Non Chicken

Treasured Tidbits

Etta-Evelyn's Angelic Treats

Spidery Spice Cake

Cardamom Berries with Honey Vanilla Ice Cream

Hasty-One-Pot-Cobbler-Pie

One Wizard's Precious Delight

Turquoise Tipple

THE EPIC-UREAN

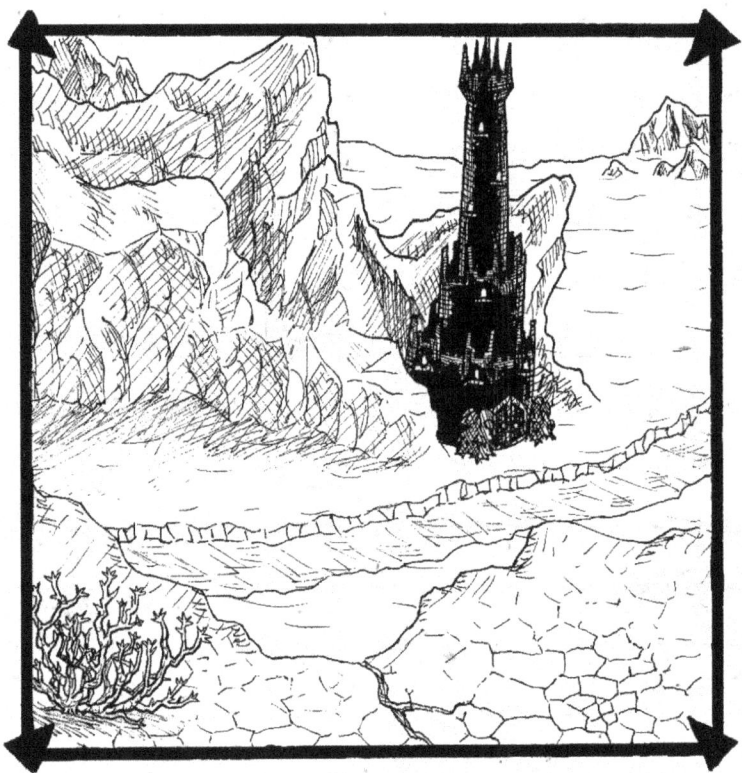

While some of the recipes in this chapter are quite easy, others require some skill; so it seemed appropriate to put them in the restaurant chapter that would cater to people/characters who appreciate a bit of danger in their cooking and like to produce items of a more esoteric nature. Here is where you'll find more exotic colors, flavors, techniques, and a bit of whimsy.

The Exquisite Soup of Master Mage Stormgutz

An extremely comforting soup, perfect for when a wizard has had a busy day doing research and pondering spells. You may substitute other cooked meats for the salmon, such as chicken or sausage; trade extra chicken broth for the clam juice, if desired. Make the croutons first (recipe below) if you prefer them to be rather crispy.

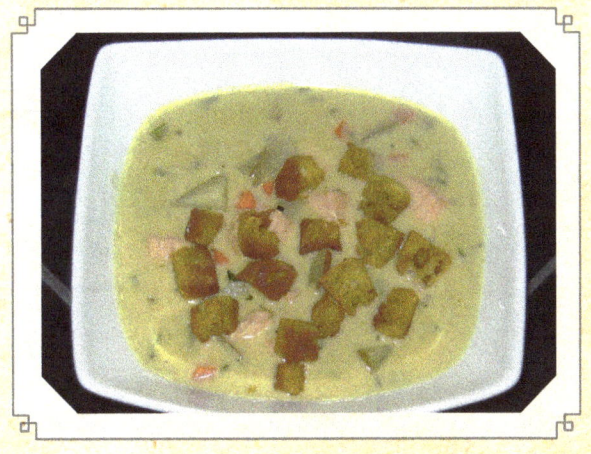

¼ cup salted butter
½ cup each (all cut into small bits):
   celery
   red onion
   carrot, peeled
¼ cup all-purpose flour
16 ounces clam juice
2 [14½-ounce] cans low-sodium
   chicken broth
1 pound red potatoes, unpeeled
   and cut into ½" bits
2 teaspoons hot Madras curry powder
1 teaspoon pepper
½ teaspoon salt
12-16 ounces boneless, skinless salmon fillets, cut into 1" pieces
   (if frozen, thaw as directed)
½ cup heavy cream
½ cup fresh parsley, minced (or 2 tablespoons dry parsley)
Crunchable Croutons, recipe below

In a 4-quart saucepan, melt the butter over moderately high heat. Add the carrot, onion, and celery and sauté 5 minutes. Add the flour and mix in. Add the clam juice, broth, potatoes, and seasonings. Bring to a boil, reduce heat to medium (a gentle boil) and cook, uncovered, for 15 minutes. Stir a few times. Add the salmon and cream; cook another 5-10 minutes, until the potatoes are tender and the fish is cooked through, but still moist. Stir gently. Add the parsley. Adjust seasonings, if desired. Divide into bowls and sprinkle with the croutons below. Cover and refrigerate leftovers; don't freeze. Serves 4-6.

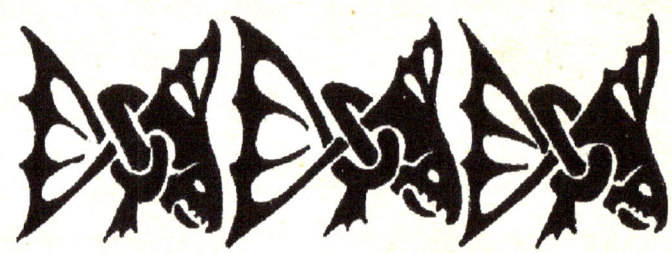

Crunchable Croutons

¼ cup salted butter
1 teaspoon hot Madras curry powder (2 teaspoons, if you love curry)
2 English muffins, split in half and cut into ½" pieces

Preheat oven to 425°. Coat a medium baking sheet with cooking spray or grease lightly. In a large glass bowl, microwave the butter until it melts, using 30-second intervals. Add the curry and combine. Mix in the muffin pieces and combine well. Pour onto prepared sheet and bake 5 minutes. Stir, then bake another 5 minutes. Leave on pan and set aside. Cover and store at room temperature. Makes about 2 cups. These will become crispier if you make them somewhat in advance.

 *This turned into one of my own favorite recipes—it could be because of the curry powder, perhaps. Even Bob tolerates it in a tiny amount.*

Aradosa's Rustic Bread & Cheese

This is another one of my favorites. The bread is rustic and crisp on the outside; leftovers are excellent toasted. There is plenty of cheese for the bread itself, plus extra for other bread products or crackers—pita chips or bagel crisps are good choices. You may also use the cheese in Snotri's Special Ham & Eggs, or Potentially Pungent Potatoes. For your convenience, I have placed the cheese recipe on its own on page xxiv, because sometimes you just need garlic/herb cheese…

1 rather large head of fresh garlic
½ teaspoon walnut oil
3 cups bread flour
1 teaspoon baking soda
1½ teaspoons plus ½ teaspoon salt
½ cup plus ¼ cup fresh chives, minced
¼ cup plus 2 tablespoons fresh sage, minced
1½ cups buttermilk, room temperature
8 ounces light cream cheese (Neufchâtel), softened
1 cup Ricotta cheese
1 ounce Parmesan or Romano cheese, finely shredded
½ teaspoon pepper

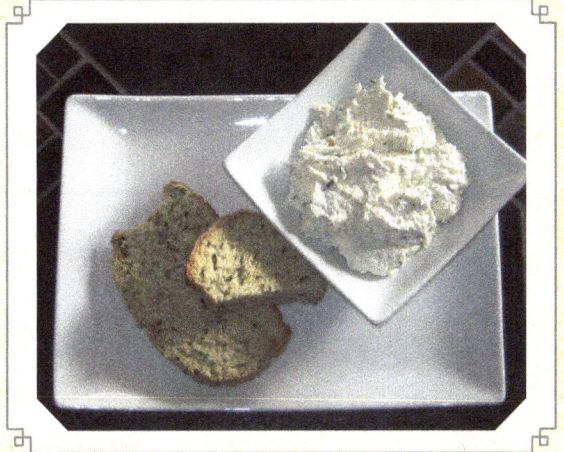

Preheat oven to 450°. Cut off the top ¾" of the garlic and place root-side down on a 12" square of aluminum foil. Drizzle with the oil and enclose loosely. Set on a medium baking sheet (you'll use this again later) and bake 35 minutes. Let cool in the foil 30 minutes. Squeeze out the cloves onto the foil and mash coarsely with a fork or chop into small pieces. Set aside.

Preheat oven to 425°. Coat the medium baking sheet with cooking spray or grease lightly. In a large bowl, combine the flour, soda, 1½ teaspoons salt, ½ cup chives, and ¼ cup sage. Add the buttermilk and combine well with a wooden spoon. Knead on a lightly floured surface a few times, form into a ball, then place on the pan. Using a very sharp knife, slash a 1" deep, large X on the top. Bake 33-37 minutes until golden brown. Let it stand 15 minutes on the sheet. Transfer to a rack and cool 30 minutes before cutting into wedges or slices. Store at room temperature or refrigerate. Serves 8-10.

While the bread is cooling: in a large bowl (I just use the rinsed and dried bowl from the bread dough), beat the cream cheese with a hand mixer until smooth. Add the remaining cheeses, herbs, ½ teaspoon salt, and pepper. Mix well, then add the garlic and mix. Season, as desired. Cover and refrigerate leftovers. Makes about 2 cups.

I mention using a very sharp knife in the recipe. When I was working on taking photographs for my website, I had baked the bread and had used some other knife, maybe a serrated one. Then the bread baked and instead of opening up nicely, the loaf looked rather strange. I thought it looked like cells dividing. My neighbor definitely thought it looked like bread, but it also looked like a weird, large mushroom. Callista, the scientist, thought it looked like the two hemispheres of the brain, and then she also alluded to other items I won't mention, since I consider this cookbook PG-rated. The main thing to remember is that even if your bread comes out of the oven looking lop-sided, mutant bread is still perfectly edible. One just can't always predict exactly how things will bake—altitude, attitude, and weather can and will affect your end product.

If you don't want to use all of the fresh herbs in the bread (for whatever reasons), either omit them or use 3-4 tablespoons of Herbes de Provence (see page xxii for a recipe) or any other herby seasoning mix.

Walter's Special Cinnamon Rolls

These rolls are a truly decadent combination of flavors. I figure they must be healthy since there are oats and raisins in them, right?

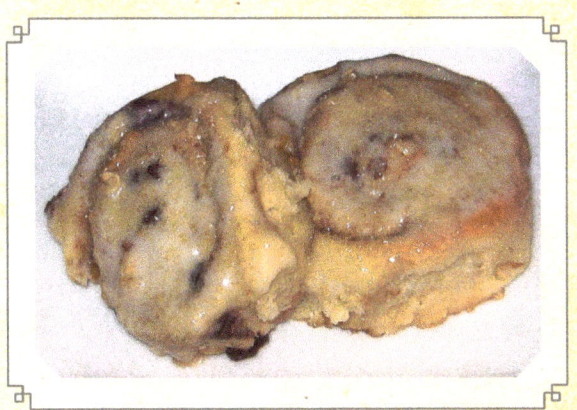

1 cup plus ¼ cup 1% milk
6 tablespoons plus ¼ cup salted butter
¼ cup sugar
1 teaspoon salt
4 cups bread flour
1 package active dry yeast
2 extra large eggs, room temperature
¾ cup old-fashioned oats
1 cup raisins (or currants)
1 cup packed golden brown sugar
1 tablespoon cinnamon
3 ounces sliced almonds, chopped coarsely
2 ounces semi-sweet chocolate, cut into ¼" bits
2 ounces white chocolate, cut into ¼" bits[1]
¼ cup soft salted butter
2 ounces light cream cheese (Neufchâtel), softened
2 cups powdered sugar
1 teaspoon vanilla extract
2 tablespoons turbinado (raw) sugar
You'll need a strand of waxed dental floss (about 18")

In a 1½-quart saucepan, combine the 1 cup milk, 6 tablespoons butter, sugar, and salt. Cook over medium heat, whisking until the butter melts. Turn off heat and cool to 120°. Place 2 cups flour and yeast in a large bowl and combine. Add the 120° milk mixture and the eggs. Beat on a medium speed for about a minute. Add the remaining flour and beat well for 2 minutes. Change to a dough hook and mix 5 minutes on the lowest speed, until you have a smooth dough. Cover bowl with a towel and let rise in a relatively warm, draft-free place for 1 hour.

---

[1] For both chocolates, you could instead use chips for convenience. You could even switch your chip flavors around—try toffee pieces and bittersweet chips.

Meanwhile, melt the ¼ cup butter and set aside. In a medium bowl, combine the oats, raisins, brown sugar, cinnamon, almonds, and chocolates; set aside. After the hour is up, press the dough down. Place it on a floured surface, cover with the same towel, and let it rest for 10 minutes. Liberally coat a 2" deep 15" by 11" glass baking dish with cooking spray or grease and set aside.

Roll the dough out on a floured surface to a rectangle, about 17-18" wide and 15-16" deep. Pull gently at the corners to achieve a mostly rectangular shape. Brush the melted butter all over the dough. Sprinkle with the oat mixture and press into the dough. Starting at the bottom, roll up the dough and pinch seam to close. Cut the roll into 15 portions by placing the dental floss around the bottom of the roll, then crossing it on top to slice through the dough easily. Carefully place in the pan in 3 rows of 5; collect any stray filling and sprinkle over all. Cover with the towel again and let rise another 30 minutes.[1]

Preheat oven to 375°. Bake 26-30 minutes until the rolls are lightly golden. Remove and let cool 15 minutes. Meanwhile, combine the soft butter and cream cheese in a large bowl. Using a hand mixer, beat until well combined. Add the powdered sugar, ¼ cup milk, and vanilla and beat on high speed for a couple of minutes. Spread all over the rolls. Sprinkle the turbinado sugar equally over all, then serve while warm. Store leftovers covered at room temperature or chill; microwave for a just-baked effect. Makes 15.

 *This is another treat that my white-chocolate-haters (who are really now merely dislikers) agreed tastes really good with white chocolate.*

[1] **STOP HERE** if you want to make these in advance. Cover the pan with plastic wrap and refrigerate overnight. Then let stand at room temperature 30 minutes before proceeding to bake. This is a good way to impress guests with freshly baked cinnamon rolls without making them wait for all the rising time.

Beets for Hypomur

You can certainly cook your own beets for this. You will need about 2 pounds of fresh beets, boiled or roasted until knife tender, peeled, and then cut into whatever shape you prefer. Then you can also do a quick sauté of the greens for a no-waste side dish. Wash them well, shake off the excess water, and cut them into 1" slices. Heat a tablespoon each of butter and water in a large skillet; sauté over high heat just until your greens have wilted. Mix with some flavored vinegar and salt and pepper to taste. Or, just use two 15-ounce cans of sliced beets (drained) if you're lazy or busy. I understand.

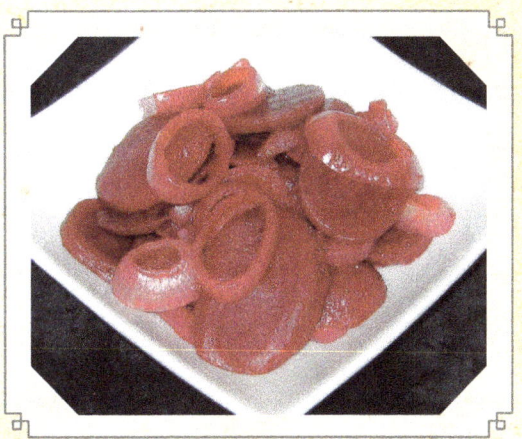

⅓ cup water
⅓ cup white vinegar
2 tablespoons sugar
½ teaspoon each:
    salt
    cinnamon
    ground cloves
About 4 cups cooked beets (peeled; small whole, sliced, or cubed beets are fine)
½ pound boiler onions; peeled, cut into ¼" slices, and separated into rings

In a 3-quart saucepan, combine the water, vinegar, sugar, and seasonings with a whisk. Bring to a boil. Add the beets and onions and cook over medium heat, covered, for 5 minutes; stir once halfway through. Turn off heat; mix, then cover and let stand 30 minutes. Transfer to a 6-cup glass container; cover and refrigerate at least 1 hour before serving; stir a couple of times. Serve with a slotted spoon. Cover and refrigerate leftovers. Serves 6-8.

Bob's Obsession

The following is the perfect accompaniment for fish and chips, but is also great for lots of other occasions.

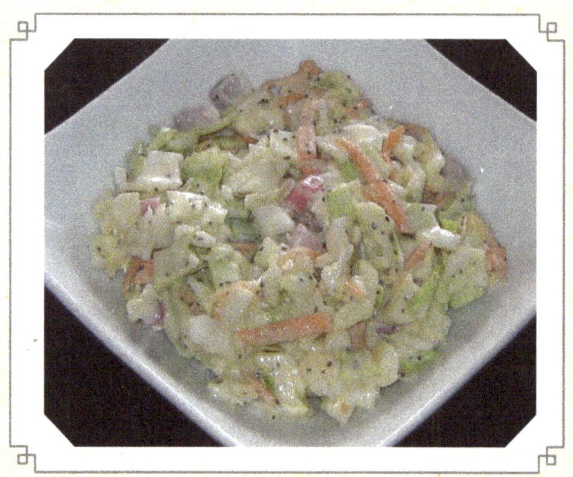

¾ cup mayonnaise
2 tablespoons sugar
2 tablespoons white vinegar
1 teaspoon celery seed
½ teaspoon salt
½ teaspoon pepper
4-5 cups green cabbage, cored and diced (about half of a smallish head)[1]
½ cup onion, coarsely chopped
½ cup carrot, peeled and shredded

Place mayonnaise, sugar, vinegar, and the 3 seasonings in a large bowl. Whisk until thoroughly combined. Season, as desired. Add the remaining ingredients and combine well. Cover and refrigerate leftovers. Can last 2-3 days, depending on your cabbage. Serves 6-8.

---

[1] Be sure to use fresh, whole cabbage here—pre-shredded cabbage will make your coleslaw watery. Red cabbage will also work. Use whatever color onion you like; scallions are also fine.

 *This coleslaw could only be named after Bob, since he obsesses over it. He said that didn't seem like a very good name for a fantasy book, but I asked him, "Well, what about Peter? Or Edmund? Or Sam? Those don't seem like fantastical names, yet those are characters in fantasy stories."*

As I said previously (Herby Cabbage Sauté on page 63), this is Bob's favorite food in my entire repertoire. I don't know why—after all, it's just coleslaw; not too sweet, not too creamy. I make it once a month, using right around five cups of cabbage, then I usually have around five cups leftover for other things. Bob would probably engrave this on my tombstone: She was a good wife and she made excellent coleslaw.

Frankly, I think it's rather strange. The girls and I get bored with having it so often (Bob would actually like it to be served weekly—sheesh...). I like to experiment with different types of slaw, but he always requests this one. I'm smart enough to schedule this recipe on a regular basis, however, since it always makes him happy. You might agree with his assessment or not, but you won't be able to change his mind about it.

Asbjorn's Fish, Chips, and Sauce

This is my one and only deep-fried recipe in the cookbook, mainly because I think deep-frying is best left to people who have large deep-fryers, like restaurant owners. Besides, you know it's unhealthy for you. One thing I hate about deep-frying recipes is that they always say something vague, such as, "oil for deep-frying," and you never really know how much oil is enough, so I'm being specific in my quantity here; it's just the right amount.

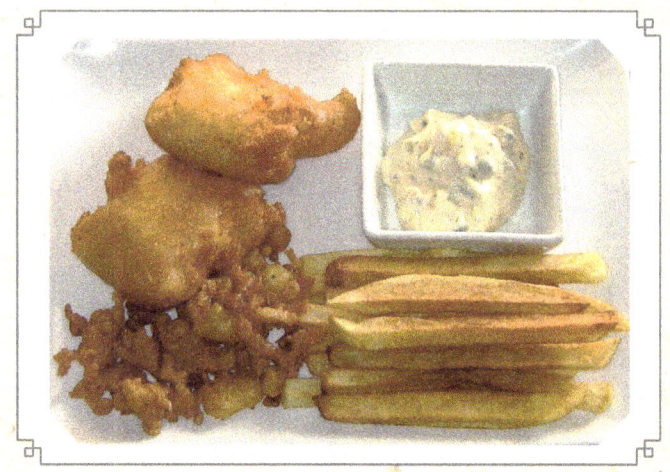

1 cup all-purpose flour

½ teaspoon salt

½ teaspoon pepper

¼ teaspoon cayenne pepper

¼ teaspoon baking powder

1 cup lager or white ale beer, room temperature

1½ pounds potatoes, preferably russets

4 rather similarly sized boneless, skinless white fish fillets, such as cod, halibut, or tilapia (1-1¼ pounds total)[1]

48 ounces vegetable oil

Extra salt

Malt vinegar

Farsi's Tartar Sauce, recipe below

In a medium bowl, combine the flour, seasonings, and baking powder. Whisk in the beer slowly; let stand. Peel the potatoes and cut into ½" strips. Preheat oven to 350°. Line 2 large baking sheets each with a double layer of paper towels. Pour oil into

[1] Pat dry fresh or frozen fish with a couple paper towels. If using frozen, as I usually do, thaw according to the package directions.

[2] Of course, you can use a home deep-fryer, if you happen to have one. I refuse to get one, because it would only tempt us (by us, I really only mean Bob, who is devoted to Tater-Tots—baking tots is fine!) to use it more than we should, then there is the matter of oil disposal—once you've fried fish, you would definitely not want to use that oil again.

a 6-quart saucepan and heat to 375-380°.[2] When your thermometer reaches the desired temperature, carefully add half of the potatoes. Fry until golden brown; stir occasionally with a slotted spoon. With the slotted spoon, remove to one prepared sheet. This will probably take 6-8 minutes. Let oil come back to 375°. Repeat with the remaining potatoes. Sprinkle with salt. Place potatoes in oven.

Meanwhile, raise oil temperature again to 375°. Using tongs, dip each fillet into the beer batter, coating well, then lower carefully into the hot oil. Fry about 3-4 minutes, then flip over and fry another 3-5 minutes, until golden brown and (you hope) fully cooked, yet still moist inside. Depending on the size of your fillets, you might have to fry the fish in 2 batches; maintain oil heat. Remove fish with tongs and place on the other prepared sheet; put in oven. After the fillets are done, use the slotted spoon to drizzle dollops of leftover beer batter into the oil to make crispies. When these are golden brown (3-4 minutes), remove with slotted spoon to another couple of paper towels (you may sprinkle salt on these, if desired). Remove potatoes and fish from oven. Season again, if necessary. You may pass malt vinegar for sprinkling on the fish. Serve with Farsi's Tartar Sauce and/or ketchup. Cover and refrigerate leftovers; crisp them for a while in your regular oven for best re-heating results, not your microwave. Serves 4.

Farsi's Tartar Sauce

- 1 cup mayonnaise
- 2 tablespoons sweet pickle relish
- 2 tablespoons small capers, drained well
- 1 teaspoon sugar
- 1 teaspoon malt vinegar
- ½ teaspoon each:
    - salt
    - pepper
    - cayenne pepper
    - garlic powder

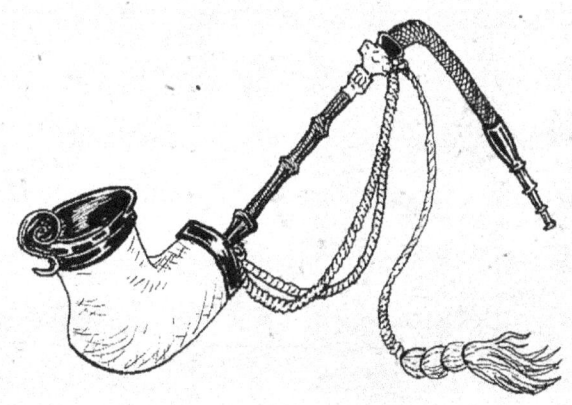

Chapter Five: The Epic-Urean

Combine all ingredients in a small bowl and chill. Season, as desired. Cover and refrigerate leftovers. Makes about 1¼ cups.

Perhaps you are wondering why there is an unusual-looking pipe next to my tartar sauce recipe. Is it just because halflings and other fantasy characters apparently like to smoke whenever they get the chance? That might be true, but this particular pipe belonged to my Norwegian grandfather, Asbjorn, for whom this recipe is named. It currently hangs on the wall in my study. The Norwegian word for grandfather is **bestefar**. *When I was a toddler, I had trouble pronouncing the word. Somehow, I shortened it to "Farsi," though I pronounced it more like fa-see. The name stuck, even for my younger sister, and we always called him Farsi. He certainly liked his fish!*

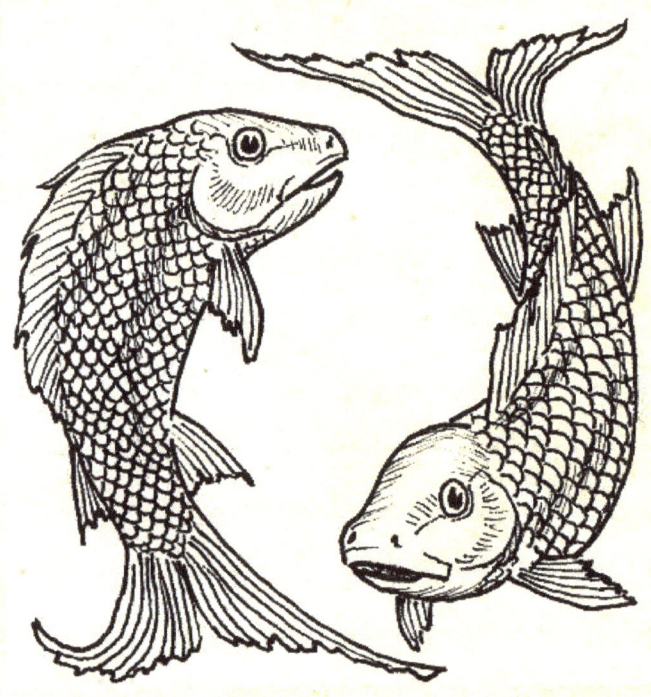

Epic-Urean Stew

This is one of those stews that tastes even better the next day, so be glad if you have leftovers. If you use a 3-quart saucepan for the onions, then you could use this pot to cook some potatoes for mashing. See Mini-Mashers (page 11) if you would like a recipe for basic mashed potatoes. **Start your marinade the night before.**

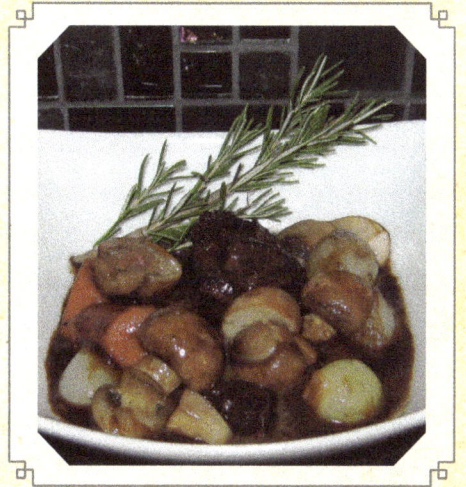

- 750 ml. bottle dry red wine, such as Cabernet Sauvignon or Merlot
- 3 large bay leaves
- 1 teaspoon dry thyme (or 3 fresh sprigs, each about 4" long)
- 1 teaspoon crushed rosemary (or 2 fresh sprigs, each about 4" long)
- 3-3¼ pounds boneless beef chuck, cut into 1½" pieces (trim off any large bits of fat)
- 1 tablespoon Kitchen Bouquet
- ½ cup apple butter[1]
- ¼ cup all-purpose flour
- ¼ cup walnut oil
- 8 fairly large cloves of fresh garlic, sliced paper thin
- 3 cups water
- ½ pound pearl onions, any color
- 1 pound carrots, peeled and cut diagonally into 1" chunks
- 1½ teaspoons plus ½ teaspoon Savory Seasoning
- ½ teaspoon pepper
- ¼ cup salted butter
- 1 pound fresh mushrooms (whole buttons or larger sizes; cut these into halves or quarters)
- Mashed potatoes and/or crusty bread

In a 6-quart saucepan, combine the wine, bay leaves, thyme, and rosemary. Add the meat. Cover with the lid and refrigerate overnight. Stir a couple of times.

---

[1] If you have trouble obtaining apple butter, try combining ½ cup applesauce with 1 tablespoon sugar and 1 teaspoon cinnamon.

Four hours before serving: with a slotted spoon, remove meat to a large bowl. Pour marinade into a 4-cup glass measuring cup. Add Kitchen Bouquet and apple butter to the marinade; mix and set aside. Add flour to the meat and stir it up, so that most of the meat is coated. Rinse out the saucepan; coat it liberally with cooking spray. Add oil to the saucepan and turn heat to rather high. Brown half of the meat for about 5 minutes, stirring frequently. With a slotted spoon, remove meat to a 3-quart medium deep skillet (later, rinse this and save for the mushrooms). Repeat with the remaining meat. Any marinade left in the bowl can be added to the 4-cup glass measuring cup. Remove remaining meat to skillet.

Sauté the garlic in the remaining oil for 30 seconds, then add back all the meat with any accumulated juices. Add the marinade mixture and bring to a boil. Turn burner to its lowest simmer; cover and cook 2 hours. Stir about every 30 minutes, scraping up brown bits.

Meanwhile in a 3-quart saucepan, blanch the onions for a couple of minutes in the 3 cups water. Remove with a slotted spoon and let cool for a while; discard water. Cut off the ends and peel; set aside.

Add the carrots to the meat; cover and simmer on lowest heat another 30 minutes. Add the onions, 1½ teaspoons Savory Seasoning, and pepper; turn heat up one notch and simmer another 30-45 minutes, uncovered, until the carrots are tender. Stir occasionally. Remove bay leaves and any fresh herb sprigs and discard. Adjust seasonings, if desired.

About 10 minutes before serving time, melt the butter in the 3-quart medium deep skillet over rather high heat. Add the ½ teaspoon Savory Seasoning and mushrooms and sauté about 5 minutes, stirring frequently. You may add these to the finished stew, or serve on top of each serving as a garnish. Serve with mashed potatoes and/or crusty bread. Cover and refrigerate leftovers. Serves 6-8.

Sine Qua Non Chicken

The next item is a perfect casual Sunday dinner, and pairs nicely with salads or other green vegetable options. You might have some chicken leftover, but I find that four or five people can easily finish off the whole meal. This is one recipe you should definitely make a point of reading through completely, and it is helpful to set out all of your ingredients in advance—though that's good advice for any recipe, I suppose. I hate it when I forget to do this, only to realize I should have been marinating meat overnight or refrigerating something for three hours before proceeding… but here it is, dinnertime. Oops. **Start this two and a half hours before serving.**

6 tablespoons salted butter, divided
3 generous (5") sprigs each:
    fresh thyme
    fresh rosemary
    fresh sage
A whole chicken with giblets, right
    around 5 pounds
1 tablespoon salt, divided
1 teaspoon pepper, divided
½ teaspoon garlic powder
3 cups plus 12 cups water
3 tablespoons all-purpose flour
2 tablespoons heavy cream
½ teaspoon poultry seasoning
2 rather large heads fresh garlic (optional)
1 teaspoon walnut oil (optional)
1 pound carrots, peeled and cut into 2" chunks
1 pound fingerling potatoes
Kitchen twine

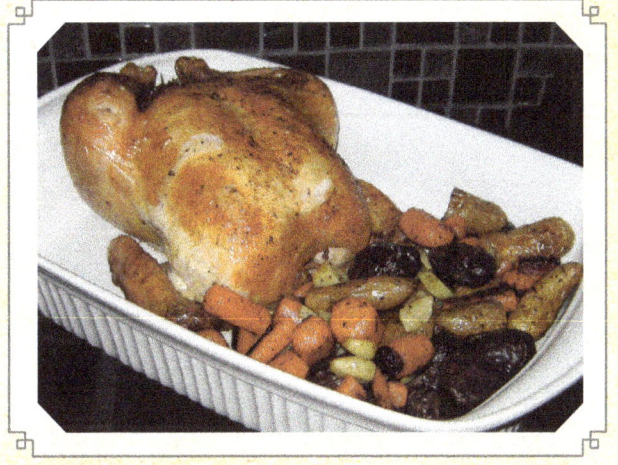

Preheat oven to 450°. Use a 4-cup glass measuring cup for everything. Lay 2 feet of heavy-duty foil crosswise in a 13" by 9" glass baking dish; coat foil with cooking spray. Place 1 tablespoon butter and one sprig of each herb in the middle of the prepared pan. Rinse chicken and pat dry with paper towels. Place the giblets in a 2-quart saucepan and set aside. Place the chicken breast side up in pan. Place 1 tablespoon butter and one sprig of each herb within the bird's chest cavity. Fold skin over cavity and tie the legs together with 12" kitchen twine. Combine ½ teaspoon salt, ½ teaspoon pepper, and the garlic powder in a small bowl and sprinkle all over chicken. Enclose loosely with foil. Roast 1 hour.

Meanwhile, add ¼ teaspoon salt and 3 cups water to the giblets. Bring to a boil, then cook over medium/high heat, uncovered, for 40 minutes. Place a fine-mesh strainer over the 4-cup glass measuring cup and pour the broth into this. You should end up with 1½ cups broth. Either discard the giblets, mince them and add to the broth, or give some to a lucky pet. Set broth aside. Rinse out saucepan and reserve.

Optional: cut off the top ¾" of each garlic head. Place the garlic root-side down on a 12" piece of regular foil and drizzle with the oil. Enclose loosely and place in a 9" square pan. Roast at 450° for 35 minutes. Remove and set aside for about 30 minutes (don't bother washing the pan). Open up the foil and squeeze out the cloves (you may need to snip off a bit more of the peel to get all of the garlic out). Leave the cloves on the foil and set aside.

Meanwhile, microwave 2 tablespoons butter in a small bowl until melted. Add ¾ teaspoon salt and ¼ teaspoon pepper. Coat the 9" square pan with cooking spray and place the carrots and potatoes in this. Drizzle with the butter mixture and combine. Place the remaining fresh herb sprigs on top and roast 30 minutes. Remove the sprigs, mix the vegetables, replace the herbs and roast another 20-30 minutes, until the vegetables are sharp knife tender.

After 1 hour of roasting, remove the bird and loosen the foil. Spoon baste. Leave the foil open and roast another 30 minutes. Baste again and roast another 30 minutes. Thigh temperature should reach 180°. When done, remove from the oven, enclose with the foil and let rest 10-15 minutes, while you finish the gravy.

Melt the remaining 2 tablespoons butter in the 2-quart saucepan. Add the flour, whisking until smooth. Add the cream, ½ teaspoon salt, remaining pepper, and the poultry seasoning. Whisk in the reserved giblet broth and cook over medium heat, whisking frequently, until the gravy is thicker and smooth, about 5 minutes. Adjust seasonings, if desired.

Cut and discard the twine. Carve up the chicken and serve the gravy on the side. Mix the vegetables with the garlic (if you are using it). Place all of the herb sprigs in a

6-quart saucepan. After dinner, place the skin, bones, carcass, and any pan drippings into this saucepan. Add the remaining 1 teaspoon salt and the 12 cups water. Bring to a boil, then cook over medium heat 1 hour, uncovered. Cool in the saucepan 1 hour, then strain this into a very large bowl and discard all the solids. You should end up with 6-8 cups of rich chicken stock which you can cool and freeze to use later (see below). Cover and refrigerate leftovers. Serves 4-6.

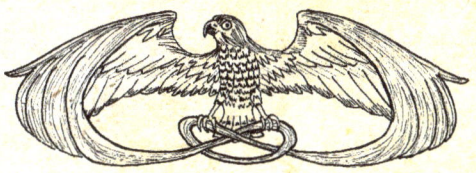

Chicken Dinner Plan

The stock above is perfect to use in recipes such as Six of One Half a Dozen Soup, Wisdom Chicken Soup, and Rabbit Braised with Herbs.

If you have some leftover boneless meat, you can throw it in soups, or make things like Courageous Low-Carb Chicken or Grape & Chicken Cups.

Here is a good plan of attack:

- Make all of Sine Qua Non Chicken for a Sunday dinner and freeze the stock.
- Use up any leftover meat on Tuesday.
- A month later, thaw the stock and enjoy it then (be sure to skim and discard any large areas of fat that may have accumulated on the stock).

Quicker Chicken Dinner Plan For Really Busy People

- Keep the vegetables and garlic the same (if using).
- Substitute a 14½-ounce can low-sodium chicken broth in the giblet gravy.
- Purchase a high quality 3-pound roasted chicken—place some fresh herbs in the cavity, cover with foil, and roast at 450° for about an hour or so.
- Cook the vegetables as specified in the recipe.
- You can still make a pot of stock out of the skin, bones, and herbs.

You might question the inclusion of so much roasted garlic here, but it is a completely optional addition. One of our favorite restaurants serves an entire head of roasted garlic with almost every entrée (this is an expensive surf and turf-type of special occasion place). I happen to love it, though I will admit that sometimes garlic can be unpredictable and it might launch an assault on your digestive system. So, if you hate garlic or you don't want to risk the consequences, omit it or only use one head of garlic.

A member of the **allium** *family*, garlic is an ancient plant recorded as early as 2300 BC in the Near East civilizations (Tannahill 47). Since it has wonderfully smelly qualities, it was popular in food preparation to mask other, rather questionable foods, such as meats that were probably well past their prime. Garlic sauces were often prepared to eat with various types of poultry: Wilson writes that medieval cooks believed items such as a roasted goose past its prime couldn't be digested well without a good garlic sauce, followed by exercise and liquor (122). Seems odd advice for digestion and dieting; maybe one should eat a garlic goose, follow it with some gin, then go for a walk—that could work, I suppose, though I think I'd be more prepared for a nap after something as heavy as all that.

Treasured Tidbits

Sometimes wizards have to take certain people as prisoners to gain information. Sometimes torture is involved, but occasionally a different approach can be more effective. Instead of constant, horrible pain, a wise wizard might try a gourmet approach, especially if his prisoner happens to be fond of fish.

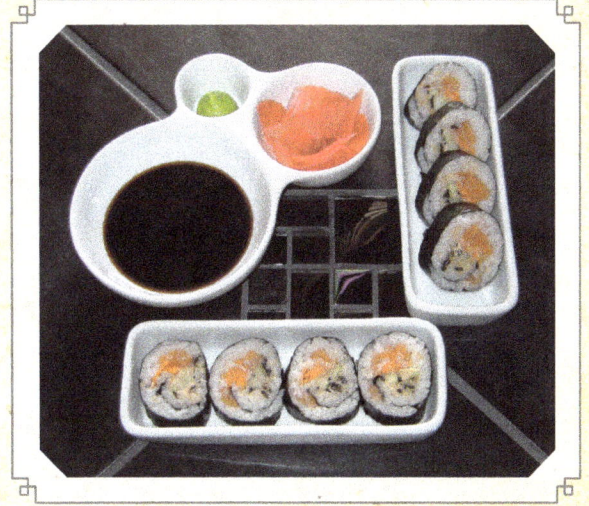

So, just like a mage on a quest for knowledge, I obsessed over sushi creation for a while. Some of my reading about the subject sounded strangely, and perhaps unnecessarily, ritualistic—especially regarding rice preparation—that's part of why my instructions sound a bit strange (stranger than usual, I mean…). Yet, I wanted to make this a simpler process that did not require me to go to sushi school for 10 or 20 years.

If you have never attempted making sushi, here is a good recipe to start with if you are curious. You can expect that your first attempt will certainly not be as perfect as a restaurant's sushi is. My second attempt was a big improvement, so you will need to resign yourself to a few practice sessions. This is perhaps the longest recipe in the cookbook and is full of options and anecdotal information, so you'll have to find some courage to face it—it's definitely a good idea to read through the entire recipe before you tackle it. You can consider it a culinary quest.

A bamboo rolling mat and wooden paddle set are very helpful here and I highly recommend purchasing them. You could probably use parchment paper to assist the rolling and a wooden spoon, if you don't have a sushi-making kit.

If you have never eaten sushi before, give it a try. Perhaps you will find that these little tidbits will ultimately become something you might crave; they might even become (dare I say it?) **PRECIOUS** to you.

Make the pickled ginger, or *gari*, the night before, so the flavors can intensify!

Pickled Ginger (Gari)

¼ pound fresh ginger[1]
½ teaspoon salt
2 tablespoons rice vinegar
2 tablespoons seasoned rice vinegar
1 tablespoon sugar
1 tablespoon plus 1 cup water
5 drops of red food coloring[2]

Using a vegetable peeler, peel the ginger and slice as thinly as possible. You will need a total of ½ cup sliced ginger. Lay on a small plate and sprinkle with the salt. Let stand 30 minutes.

Meanwhile, combine the vinegars, sugar, 1 tablespoon water, and food coloring in a 1-quart saucepan with a whisk. Bring to a boil and cook 30 seconds. Pour into a 1-cup glass container and let stand (don't bother washing the saucepan).

In the saucepan, bring the 1 cup water to a boil. Add the ginger and cook over a medium heat for 15 minutes. Drain, then add to the prepared brine. Cover and store overnight in the refrigerator. Lasts for a few days; store leftovers covered in the refrigerator. Makes ½ cup.

---

[1] Try to get a hunk of ginger that has as few small branches as possible. This can be tough; you might have to buy a larger piece just to get a relatively straight piece that is easy to peel and slice. You can also find pickled ginger already made in various grocery stores, if you want to skip this particular step. If you happen to grow your own, or if you have a source that sells young ginger, you can simply use the whole root—peel and all, if it is very tender. Young ginger has a rosy tint to it; food coloring is used merely to mimic this color.

[2] This ingredient is completely optional—if you have an objection to the rather small amount of red food coloring listed here, feel free to omit it; the taste of the *gari* will not be affected. You could also substitute a teaspoon or so of beet juice, if you have some around. Or look for some young ginger!

Sushi Rice

1 cup sushi rice (no substitute)
1¼ cups water
½ teaspoon salt
2 tablespoons seasoned rice vinegar

Rinse the rice with cold water in a fine-mesh strainer. Place in a 1½-quart saucepan with the water. Bring to a boil and stir once. Reduce heat to the lowest setting, cover and cook undisturbed for 17 minutes. Turn off the heat and let stand undisturbed, covered, for 15 minutes. Using a wooden spoon or paddle, place rice in a 9½" glass pie dish; add the salt and vinegar. Mix in gently. Do not use any metal utensils from now on (except for your cutting knife). Cool until rice is at room temperature (about 1 hour). Do not chill. Do not use burned rice, if there is any (I've never had any). Do use rice on the same day. Cover with a cloth napkin if you are not using immediately.

Why not use metal (except for your cutting knife)? Apparently, metallic utensils and bowls will perhaps impart a subtle, and undesirable, taste to the rice and the sushi. I've never risked using metal stuff because I definitely don't want my sushi to taste like metal.

Vinegar Water

¼ cup water
2 tablespoons rice vinegar

Combine both in a non-metallic bowl. You will use this for glue, dipping your fingers, and moistening a towel or cloth napkin to wipe off your knife between cuts. Set aside right next to your workstation. Makes ⅓ cup.

Sushi

About ⅔ of a large cucumber, peeled, seeded, and cut into long, thin strips

1 medium carrot, peeled and cut into long ribbons using a vegetable peeler

¼ pound sashimi-grade raw salmon; boneless, skinless, and cut into ¼" strips[3]

1 tablespoon black sesame seeds, lightly toasted

2 tablespoons mayonnaise

1 teaspoon Sriracha chili sauce

3 [8" by 8"] toasted *nori* (seaweed) sheets

Prepared *wasabi* paste

Soy sauce

Gari, recipe above

[3] Sashimi-grade, raw, and previously frozen salmon was most easily available to me, but remember I'm land-locked. However, raw fish can be problematic, and the *wasabi* accompaniment is served with sushi to help you ward off bacteria. Be sure to use sashimi-grade fish (tuna is a good option). **NEVER** use raw, soft, white fish for sushi (these types of fish are prone to excessive bacteria—for more extensive fish facts and suggestions, please consult a sushi cookbook—or just play it safe with salmon).

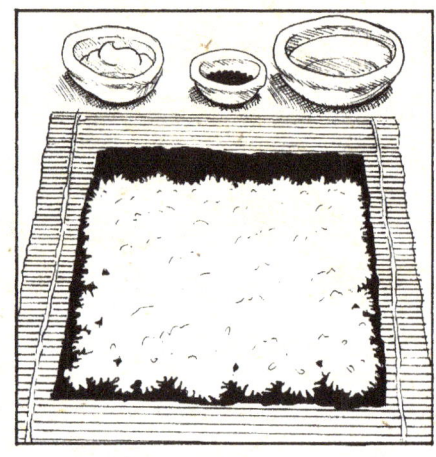

Be sure you have your room temperature rice and your vinegar water ready to go. Place the prepared vegetables and fish on a plate. Place the sesame seeds in a tiny bowl. Combine the mayonnaise and Sriracha in a small bowl. Have a clean, non-metallic plate ready for your rolls. Place a bamboo mat on a large cutting board. Place one sheet of *nori*, shinier side down, on your mat. Frequently moisten your fingers with the vinegar water while you work. Spread ⅓ of the rice all over the *nori*, leaving 1" empty at the top.

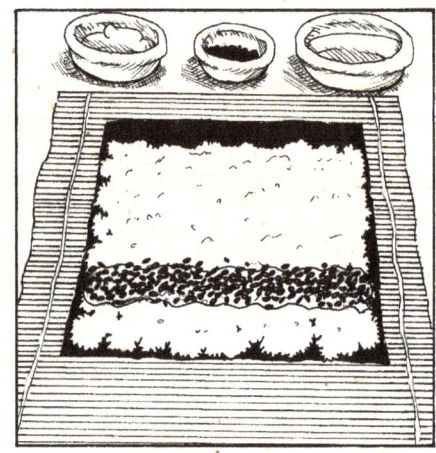

Spread ⅓ of the mayonnaise mixture horizontally along the bottom third. Then sprinkle ⅓ of the sesame seeds on top.

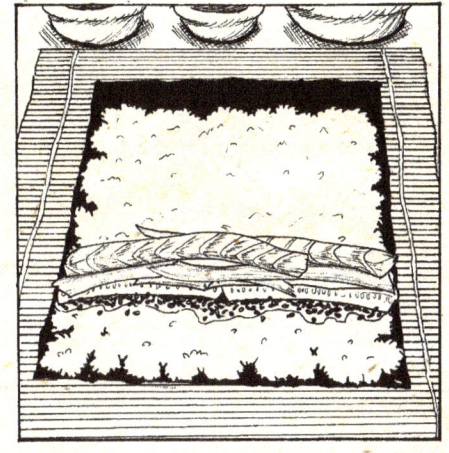

Place ⅓ of the strips of cucumber, carrot, then salmon along the top of the sesame seeds. Use your fingertips to spread vinegar water along the top 1" of the *nori* (which will have a tendency to curl).

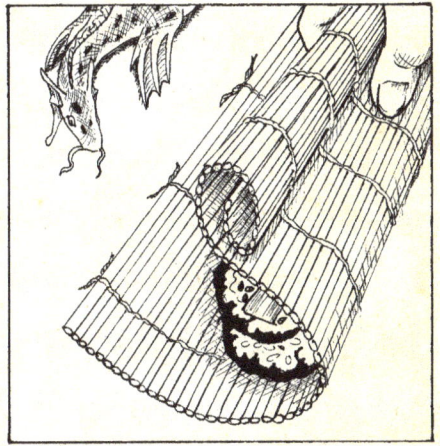

Using your fingers to hold the filling down, start rolling your bamboo mat as tightly as you can (remember not to be too discouraged if your first attempt seems a bit loose). Roll completely out of the mat and spread more vinegar water along the outer seam of the *nori* to glue it closed. Place seam-side down on a non-metallic plate.

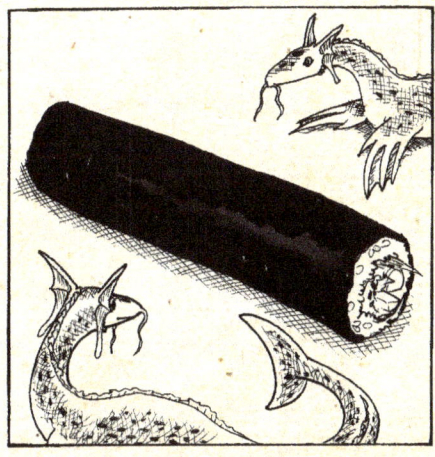

Repeat with the remaining ingredients. Remove bamboo mat from cutting board. By this time, you will be ready to cut the first roll you assembled. Place this roll on the cutting board, seam-side down.

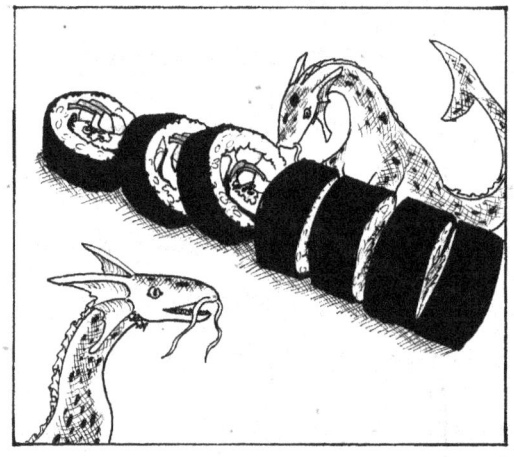

Use a very sharp, non-serrated knife to make your cuts. Moisten a towel or cloth napkin with vinegar water and use this between cuts to wipe your knife. Cut roll into 8-10 slices and lay these on a serving plate (non-metallic, of course). I usually cut more like 9 or 10 slices since I prefer sushi to be thinner and easier to eat in a single bite. Continue with the other rolls. Place the end pieces on the plate with the cut edge down; it's okay for some raggedy bits to show on the top.

Serve immediately. Or, you may cover all lightly with a cloth napkin or plastic wrap and refrigerate. Serve with soy sauce, *wasabi* paste, and *gari*. You can eat sushi with chopsticks or your fingers. Sushi is best eaten the day it is prepared, though the next day is still okay—sushi should never smell "fishy." Keep leftovers covered and refrigerated. Makes 24-30 pieces, enough to serve anywhere from 2-4 people as an entrée. They are excellent to put out at a party, especially since you can have them ready in advance.

If you are not ready to try raw fish, here are some different avenues to pursue. The only thing to remember is you only need about ¼ pound or 1 cup to make all three rolls. A few strips of cooked crab, lobster, shrimp, or crab substitute work well. A few heated shrimp tempura also work (remove tails).

A few strips of cooked chicken also work—you can use those packaged varieties in any flavor. You could use teriyaki chicken or beef. Try some pork chop strips, or wrap up some leftover Thanksgiving turkey. Just make sure that all of your cooked meats are relatively dry; you don't want to utilize copious amounts of gravies or sauces in your rolls. You can even use breaded chicken tenderloins—heat a couple according to package instructions, cut into strips, and roll them up while the meat is still warm. Serve immediately to enjoy a warm/cold contrast or go ahead and chill before serving.

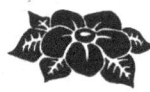 **Vegetarian Option**—Omit the fish. You can then exercise some creativity, perhaps depending on what sort of fresh or canned produce you have around. You won't need much, however, just a few leaves or

strips to replace the fish. Here are some good choices: a few spinach leaves, a couple of thinly sliced fresh mushrooms, a few strips of avocado, some strips of bell pepper, a few sliced, canned water chestnuts or bamboo shoots (drained first). Just be sure not to overload your rolls and keep your fillings sort of in strips. Do not use foods that are bulky or liquidy such as tomatoes, and do not use foods such as peas or corn (though a few fresh snow pea pods would be okay).

Since I live in New Mexico, we are fortunate to have sushi-joints that serve green chile tempura sushi—perhaps that's a radical concept, but we always order a roll. This would involve tempura-frying strips of roasted green chile. You would still be vegetarian if you did this. Knowing my dislike of deep-frying, you can imagine that I would much rather go out and simply order this type of roll with the other sushi items…

A really desperate and feral prisoner who loves fish would probably just devour all of these sushi bits in about three minutes, but generally this serves three in a more leisurely fashion. Chloë, Callista, and I share this for dinner; afterwards, we feel content and light about what we ate, plus we end up with clear sinuses. Bob usually opens up a can of chili because raw fish and seaweed are definitely not his favorite things in the world.

Etta-Evelyn's Angelic Treats

These do take some time to make, but remember this is the wizard section of the cookbook. On the plus side, these are one of the only sweets I can actually say is quite decadent, yet low-fat! I don't get to say that very often in this cookbook...

2 ounces sliced almonds
¾ cup cake flour
1 cup powdered sugar
1 cup egg whites, room temperature
1 teaspoon each:
    cream of tartar
    vanilla extract
    almond extract
¼ cup honey
Glaze of Enchantment, recipe below

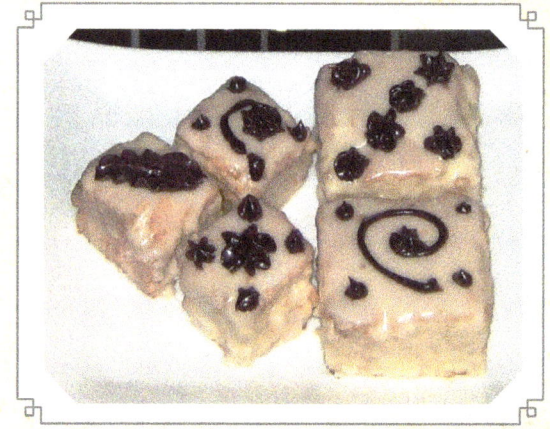

Lightly toast the almonds. Let them cool, then grind them in a small food processor. Combine with the cake flour and powdered sugar in a medium bowl. Set aside. Spray a small amount of cooking spray in a 9" square pan. Line the bottom of the pan with parchment paper and spray paper lightly. Place a 12" square of aluminum foil on a large cooling rack, then set rack on a large baking sheet.

Preheat oven to 350°. In a very large bowl, combine the egg whites, cream of tartar, and the extracts. Beat with a whisk attachment on rather high speed until peaks form. While whisking, slowly add the honey and continue to whisk until smooth and stiffer. By hand with a spatula, fold in the flour mixture gently but thoroughly. Spread in the prepared pan evenly; bang pan twice on the counter to remove air bubbles. Bake 26-30 minutes or until center springs back when touched lightly. Run knife around edge and turn pan over onto the foil. Leave alone for 1 hour. Make the glaze near the end of this hour. Remove pan and discard paper. Turn cake over onto a cutting board (you can just eat this as a cake now; sprinkle some powdered sugar on the top, cut, and serve next to a scoop of ice cream or have as a plain snack). Discard foil. Cut the cake into however many portions you would like—9 to 36. Place pieces back on the rack over the baking sheet.

Using a fork underneath, hold each piece of cake over the icing bowl. Use a spoon to cover the top and sides of each cake with the glaze well. Carefully place on the rack, using a recessed (bent) spatula or another fork to help you. Use recessed spatula to spread glaze more evenly, if necessary. Repeat with all. Let stand on the rack for 1 hour. Choose one of the Decorating Options below and decorate all of the cakes. These can be served immediately or they can stand for a while. Store covered at room temperature or chill. Makes 36 small treats, or 9 substantial cakes (or you can cut 12 or 18).

Glaze of Enchantment

2 pounds powdered sugar
⅔ cup 1% milk
1 tablespoon vanilla extract
1 tablespoon almond extract

Place the sugar in a very large bowl. Combine the remaining ingredients in a 1-cup glass measuring cup and add to the bowl. Beat on low speed with a whisk attachment to combine. Then beat on high speed for a few minutes to mix thoroughly. There is plenty of glaze to cover all of the cakes generously, regardless of the size you end up cutting. Cover and refrigerate leftover glaze, which can be used on other baked goods.

Decorating Options:

Easy option: Place 1-2 tablespoons cocoa powder in a fine-mesh strainer. Sprinkle over all the cakes. Use a doily or stencil if you would like a design on bigger cakes.

Moderate option: Purchase 2 small icing tubes in the colors of your choice. Draw abstract designs on the tops of the cakes or attempt to draw various designs if you are feeling artistic.

A bit harder option: Microwave 3 ounces bittersweet chocolate in a zipped, snack-size plastic bag until fully melted. Let it cool for a few minutes. Cut a tiny hole in one corner and squeeze the chocolate into designs.

Spidery Spice Cake

I imagine wizards like to joke around about past battles and monsters, especially when the danger is over. You can think about what spiders generally like to eat when you make this cake.

¼ cup plus 1 tablespoon soft salted butter

¾ cup sugar

1 extra large egg, room temperature

1½ cups all-purpose flour

1 teaspoon baking powder

1 teaspoon cinnamon

½ teaspoon baking soda

¼ teaspoon each:
  ground ginger
  ground cloves
  nutmeg
  salt

¾ cup buttermilk, room temperature

½ cup applesauce, room temperature

1 tablespoon of red food coloring[1]

1 teaspoon vanilla extract

½ cup raisins (or currants)

2 ounces pecans, chopped coarsely

½ cup apple butter[2]

1 ounce light cream cheese (Neufchâtel), softened

1 cup powdered sugar

2 tablespoons 1% milk

1 ounce semi-sweet chocolate

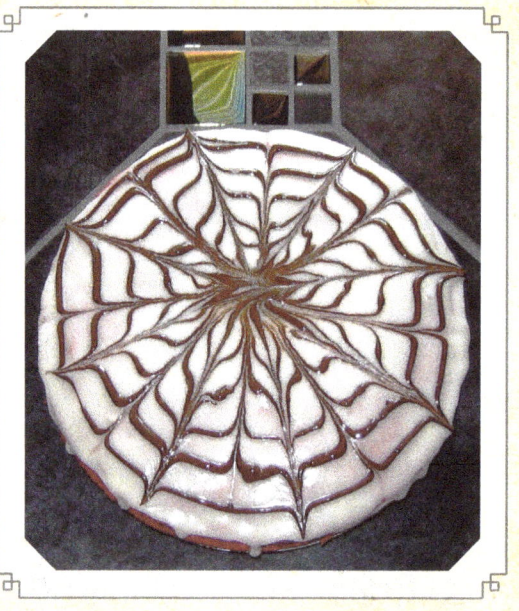

[1] This ingredient is completely optional—if you have an objection to the rather small amount of red food coloring listed here, feel free to omit it; the taste of the cake will not be affected.

[2] If you have trouble obtaining apple butter, try combining ½ cup applesauce with 1 tablespoon sugar and 1 teaspoon cinnamon. Or you may find many recipes online if you want to pursue a homemade option. However, ½ cup of just about any flavor of spreadable jam or curd will also work well with this cake.

Preheat oven to 350°. Coat a 9" heavy aluminum round pan with cooking spray or grease lightly. In a large bowl, cream together the ¼ cup butter, sugar, and egg until fluffy. In a medium bowl, combine the flour, baking powder and soda, and the 4 seasonings (don't wash bowl; use later). In a 2-cup glass measuring cup, whisk together the buttermilk, applesauce, food coloring, and vanilla. Starting with the dry ingredients, add ⅓ of the flour mixture, then half of the buttermilk mixture, alternating dry and wet, and ending with dry. Beat well; scrape down sides if necessary (if this appears curdled, don't worry). Add the raisins and pecans and beat well. Pour into prepared pan and bake 36-40 minutes, until the center tests done. Cool 15 minutes on a rack. Run knife around edge, turn out of pan, and place cake bottom on rack. Cool 1 hour.

Place cake on a serving dish. Carefully split cake in half horizontally and set the top aside. Spread apple butter on bottom half, then carefully replace the top half. In a medium bowl, combine the cream cheese and 1 tablespoon butter well using a hand mixer. Add the powdered sugar and milk and beat well. Spread over the cake top with a recessed or bent spatula. It is okay to let some icing drizzle over the sides. Let it stand while you melt the chocolate.

Place the chocolate in a snack-size plastic bag and zip closed. Microwave at 15-second intervals until fully melted (this will probably take about a minute). Snip a small hole in one corner and use this as a pastry bag to decorate the cake.

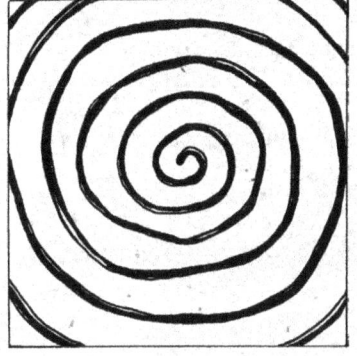 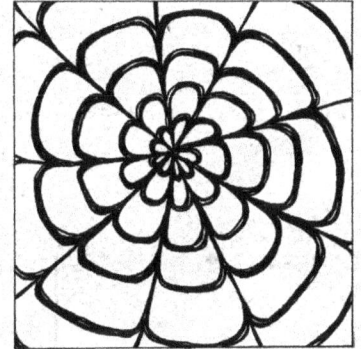 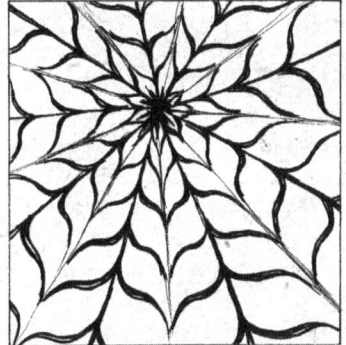

Starting in the center, draw concentric circles all around the top of the cake about ½" apart.

Then use a butter knife or a toothpick to pull the chocolate from the outside edge toward the center at about 2" intervals (at the edge).

Next, starting at the center, pull the knife to the edge between the previous lines. Wipe off the knife or toothpick occasionally, since it will collect icing.

Refrigerate about 30 minutes to set the icing before cutting. Cover and store at room temperature or refrigerate. Serves 8.

Chapter Five: The Epic-Urean

Cardamom Berries with Honey Vanilla Ice Cream

I also imagine wizards are rather stressed out most of the time. They have to deal with political maneuvering, bad weather conditions, forces of evil that are too awful to comprehend, and occasional blunders by the people (yes, I'm thinking of Pippin Took) they have chosen to accompany them on serious missions. Wizards would probably appreciate relaxing with this flavorful dessert. Though good anytime, this is a quintessential summertime dessert, especially if you pair it with the ice cream.

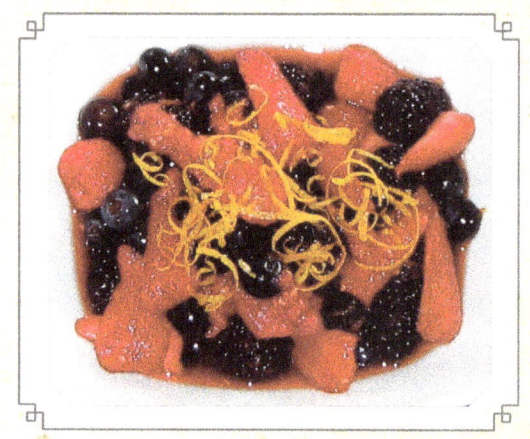

2 pounds assorted fresh berries; such as raspberries, blueberries, blackberries, or strawberries (stem and quarter strawberries; leave the other ones whole)[1]
½ cup honey
2-3 tablespoons fresh orange zest, finely grated[2]
2-3 tablespoons fresh orange juice
½ teaspoon ground ginger
½ teaspoon ground cardamom
Optional: ¼ cup raspberry-flavored liqueur, such as Chambord (or more, if desired)
Honey Vanilla Ice Cream, recipe below

Place berries in a large bowl. In a 1-quart saucepan, combine the honey, orange zest and juice, and the spices. Over medium heat, whisk just until the spices dissolve and the honey melts. You may add the liqueur with the honey and heat it to soften the alcohol flavor, if desired, or add the liqueur after heating. Pour over the fruit and combine. Let stand 1 hour; stir a few times. Serve alone in bowls; pour over ice cream or cake slices (such as pound cake). Cover and refrigerate leftovers. Serves 6-8.

[1] Use only fresh berries. You may use any combination of berries, or even just one.
[2] You'll need one giant orange, or two medium ones to get the zest.

Honey Vanilla Ice Cream

1¼ cups heavy cream
1 cup 1% milk
½ cup egg substitute
¼ cup honey
½ cup sugar
1 tablespoon vanilla extract
1½ cups Cardamom Berries
Optional: ½ cup raspberry-flavored liqueur, such as Chambord (or more to taste)

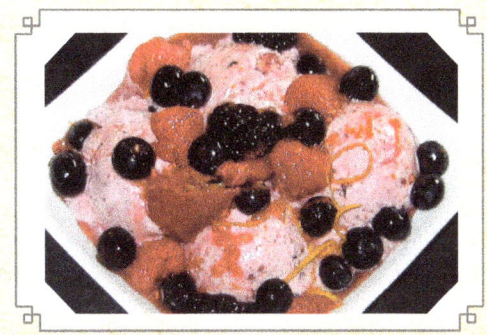

Make sure the cream, milk, and egg substitute are chilled well. Follow manufacturer's instructions regarding the preparation of your particular ice cream maker. In a 4-cup glass measuring cup, combine the cream, milk, egg substitute, honey, sugar, and vanilla and whisk until the sugar dissolves. Pour into a 6-cup electric ice cream maker; turn on and let mix for 30 minutes. Puree the berry mixture (strain this if you hate seeds). Pour berries and optional liqueur into the ice cream and mix another 5 minutes. You may now choose one of these options:

1) Pour into glasses and serve immediately as a smoothie.
2) Pour into a 7-cup container, cover, and freeze for 2-3 hours for a soft serve.
3) Freeze for 5-6 hours for a firmer consistency (stir a few times).

Serve with additional Cardamom Berries as a sauce over the top, if desired. Cover and freeze leftovers; keeps for a few days. Serves 6-8.

Sorry to give you even more options, but you could also leave the ice cream as a plain vanilla flavor and forget about the berry recipe completely. Now, this is a delicious vanilla ice cream on its own. But you could also go crazy flavoring it with other liqueurs, such as ½ cup of Frangelico, Amaretto, Grand Marnier, Kahlúa, or Bailey's—the possibilities here are up to you. Come to think of it, about 4 ounces of lightly toasted and finely chopped nuts would really complement this vanilla/liqueur ice cream, such as pecans, walnuts, almonds, or hazelnuts. After the ice cream has mixed 30 minutes, add any of these variations and mix an additional 5 minutes. Keep in mind, your ice cream might not become extremely firm if you add alcohol, but that is okay.

Crème de Cacao and miniature chocolate chips? Coconut rum and lightly toasted sweetened coconut? Stop me now!

Hasty-One-Pot-Cobbler-Pie

As I said previously, wizards like to dabble with danger and the caramel sauce following this dessert fits the bill. Wizards are also busy and don't like to spend too much time doing mundane things like dishes.

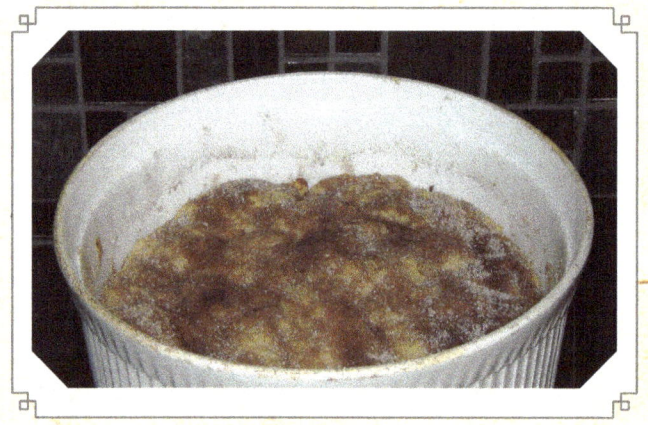

2 tablespoons salted butter
2 tablespoons lemon juice
6 cups apples, peeled, cored, and sliced thinly
⅓ cup plus ⅓ cup sugar
¼ cup plus ¾ cup all-purpose flour
1 teaspoon cinnamon
¼ teaspoon plus ½ teaspoon salt
3 ounces sliced almonds, lightly toasted
¼ teaspoon baking powder
2 tablespoons half-and-half
2 teaspoons almond extract
½ cup soft salted butter
1 tablespoon cinnamon sugar
Crackling Caramel Sauce, recipe below

Preheat oven to 375°. Coat a 2-quart round casserole dish with cooking spray or grease lightly. In a 4-quart saucepan, combine the 2 tablespoons butter and the lemon juice over high heat. Add the apples; cover and cook over medium heat 5 minutes. Stir a couple of times. Add ⅓ cup sugar, ¼ cup flour, 1 teaspoon cinnamon, and ¼ teaspoon salt into the apples and combine. Add in the almonds, then pour this into the prepared dish. Rinse and dry the saucepan.

In the same saucepan, mix the ⅓ cup sugar, ¾ cup flour, ½ teaspoon salt, baking powder, half-and-half, almond extract, and ½ cup butter until well combined. Place tablespoon-sized portions of dough all over the apples. Bake 25 minutes. Spray top lightly with water, then sprinkle the cinnamon sugar all over the top. Bake another 9-11 minutes, until golden brown. Let stand on a rack about 1 hour before serving. Meanwhile, rinse and dry the saucepan and prepare the caramel sauce. You may serve ice cream or whipped cream with the cobbler-pie, if desired. Store covered at room temperature or refrigerate. Serves 6-8.

Crackling Caramel Sauce

1½ cups sugar
¾ cup water
1½ cups heavy cream, room temperature

In a 4-quart saucepan, combine the sugar and water with a large whisk. Bring to a boil over high heat until sugar dissolves. Lower heat to medium and cook without stirring. Swirl saucepan occasionally and use a wet pastry brush around the inside of the saucepan to prevent the sugar from crystallizing too much on the sides. Cook until the sugar is a lovely amber color—this can take anywhere from 15-25 minutes (the darker the color, the more bitter and burnt the taste).

Be sure to **WATCH** this carefully—do not leave this sauce unattended (you don't have to hover over it exactly, but don't stray too far from the kitchen, especially near the end of cooking). Lower heat slightly and slowly pour in the cream, whisking all the time. Use a potholder to cover your whisk handle—this will spatter! Sauce will look like a sticky mess, at first.

Keep whisking over a medium heat until all the hard bits dissolve, about 5 minutes. Turn off the heat; cover and let stand about 30 minutes; it will thicken. Cover and refrigerate leftovers; reheat slowly. Makes about 2 cups; plenty for the cobbler-pie and some ice cream or other desserts later on as well.

One Wizard's Precious Delight

If a certain witch could get her hands on this recipe, she would imbue the sweet concoction with esoteric spells to induce obsession. She would then feed it to a callow boy, compelling him to betray his beloved siblings. Will eating this candy drive you to commit horrific acts? Or will it merely make you gain a few pounds over a weekend binge? There is only one way to find out.

Do be sure to read the entire recipe before you begin, especially the part about starting **THREE DAYS BEFORE SERVING**. Remember, this is the wizard's chapter, and this might seem to be a complicated dish, but it's easy once you get past the initial preparation.

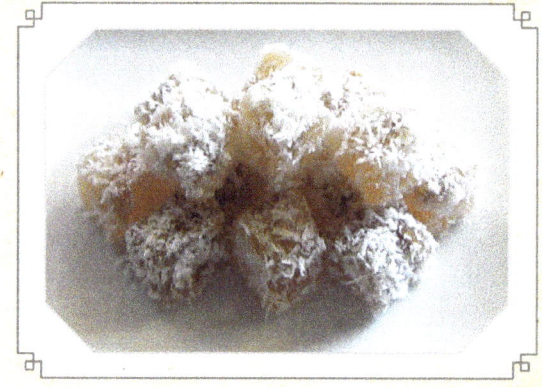

- 1 ounce shelled, roasted, and salted pistachios
- 1 ounce walnut halves
- 1 ounce whole hazelnuts
- 2 cups sugar
- ½ cup plus 1 cup water
- ½ cup cornstarch
- ½ teaspoon citric acid
- 1½ teaspoons orange extract (or other flavor)[1]
- 1½ teaspoons cinnamon extract (or other flavor)[2]
- A few drops of food coloring, if desired (only 2 or 3 drops are needed)
- Powdered sugar for dusting
- **Various Coatings,** listed below

*** THREE DAYS BEFORE SERVING ***

Chop the nuts rather finely. Combine in a small bowl and set aside. Coat a 9" by 5" loaf pan with cooking spray and set aside. Combine the sugar and ½ cup water in a 1-quart saucepan. Bring to a boil, whisking until the sugar dissolves. Then keep the liquid at a **STEADY, MODERATE BOIL** on medium/low heat. Use a pastry brush

---

[1 & 2] You may experiment with other flavors; rose water, vanilla, almond, and mint are traditional. You may also try using a no-sugar-added fruit juice for the 1 cup water; apple is a nice alternative.

dipped in water to brush the inside of the pot occasionally to prevent the sugar from crystallizing on the sides.

Insert a candy thermometer and cook without stirring until the temperature reaches 260-265° (hard ball stage). This will take a while, perhaps 20-40 minutes, depending on various circumstances, but:

DO NOT IGNORE IT.

DO NOT MULTI-TASK, EXCEPT TO DO THIS:

Set up a hand mixer with a whisk attachment; set aside. Place the 1 cup water, cornstarch, citric acid, extracts, and food coloring (if using) into a 3-quart saucepan. Combine all with a medium-sized whisk, then place on the stove without turning on the heat. When the sugar mixture reaches the 260° mark, turn heat to the lowest setting and remove the thermometer.

IMMEDIATELY: Turn heat on the cornstarch mixture to rather high. Cook on high, whisking constantly until fully mixed and starting to boil and thicken. It will become **VERY** thick.

IMMEDIATELY: Lower the heat a couple notches. Switch to the hand mixer and mix on low speed until the mixture becomes creamy. This might become a bit messy, so try to keep the mixing under control.

IMMEDIATELY: Slowly pour the hot syrup into the cornstarch mixture while mixing on low speed until fully integrated over medium heat. Turn off heat and mix in the nuts with the hand mixer on low speed. Pour into the prepared pan. Place on a rack until completely cool. Cover lightly with a lightweight towel or cloth napkin and let stand overnight.

 *The hard part is over! It is smooth sailing from here.*

*** TWO DAYS BEFORE SERVING ***

Sprinkle some powdered sugar on a cutting board. Flip the candy out onto the board. Cut into 45 (5 by 9) pieces using a pizza slicer or other sharp knife. Line a medium baking sheet with wax paper or parchment paper. Sprinkle some powdered sugar on the pan. Place the candy pieces on the pan, ¼" apart, uncovered, so they can dry out a bit. Cover with the same cloth only overnight.

*** ONE DAY BEFORE SERVING ***

Turn all the pieces over and let stand, covered lightly.

*** DAY OF SERVING ***

Choose your coating from the Various Coatings listed below and dip each candy.

Various Coatings (choose one or use half of two variations, as desired; place your chosen coating in an appropriate shallow bowl for dipping):

½ cup powdered sugar sifted with ½ tablespoon cornstarch
¼ cup unsweetened cocoa powder sifted with 2 tablespoons powdered sugar
½ cup lightly toasted sesame seeds
½ cup unsweetened coconut flakes (as seen in the photo above)
8 ounces melted semisweet chocolate (Cool a bit, then dip each candy and place on the same parchment sheet. Refrigerate, uncovered, just until the chocolate sets.)

Dip each candy into your desired coating, covering on all sides. You can press the candy into your coating to help make it stick. Set on a plate. Turkish Delight needs to breathe and stay dry. Keep finished candies covered loosely with a lightweight cloth napkin or towel at room temperature. Or wrap loosely in lightweight wax or parchment paper and place in a small box that is tied with a silk ribbon (the color is up to you). Do not keep the candy in completely airtight containers, because the sugar content will start to melt and you'll end up with wet candy. The weather and overall humidity will affect your candies. Makes 45 pieces.

Turkish Delight. Many people first encounter this mysterious sweet upon reading The Lion, The Witch and the Wardrobe *by C. S. Lewis. In the novel, Lewis's White Witch conjures up "several pounds" of the stuff and Edmund Pevensie proceeds to make a pig of himself. What makes it so special? Is it simply a matter of magic? Does the candy have an ability to transform itself into whatever perfect candy the eater might desire? Could it even be a type of sweet* meat? *Or is the character of Edmund Pevensie merely a victim of war-time deprivation; so desperate to gorge on sugar that he would sell out his family?*

My first foray into fantasy literature was the Narnia series; all seven chronicles, though my favorites were (and still are) The Horse and His Boy *and* The Magician's Nephew. *Long ago, I asked my mother if we could buy some Turkish Delight and she found the American-made "Aplets and Cotlets" by Liberty Orchards. A box of these fruity confections often became THE never-fail Christmas gift for my parents when my sister and I were at a loss as to "what can we get mom and dad? They already have everything…"*

I like Turkish Delight, but to me it is no substitute for a luxurious collection of milk chocolate-nut-caramel-type candies. I might sell my soul for chocolate, but not Turkish Delight. Would I ever sell out my sister? No; it would NEVER happen, no matter what. Obviously, this recipe was not included in my original cookbook, since it is Narnian, not Middle-earthian. It has such exotic and seductive connotations, yet it is definitely an acquired taste for some. As a jaded adult trying to develop a recipe, I bought a few varieties of Turkish Delight straight from Turkey. Many were rather disappointing not only in their appearance, but also their taste. Others were lovely and delicious. My local Middle Eastern grocery stocks about 30 varieties. Sampling a few of these candies led me to create the following recipe, and I will continue my Turkish Delight story there. And if you happen to find this candy recipe too stressful, go ahead and skip to the next one—you'll get some Turkish Delight flavor without all the fuss.

Turquoise Tipple

Here's an exotic-looking cocktail that's a comforting sweet treat after a long day poring over illegible manuscripts. Come to think of it, wizards are a lot like grad students…

Before you pour your drink, you might want to garnish your glass: place a tablespoon or so of orange juice on a small plate. Place a tablespoon of sugar on another small plate. Carefully roll the outside of your glass in the juice, then carefully roll in the sugar. Let glass dry while you mix the cocktail. Or, keep it simple with just a slice of orange on the side.

1 ounce coconut rum (such as Malibu)
1 ounce hazelnut liqueur (Frangelico)
½ ounce each:
    simple syrup (available in liquor stores)
    vanilla vodka (Smirnoff or Absolut)
    blue Curaçao (Hiram Walker)
    half-and-half
6 drops orange bitters (Angostura)
3-4 ice cubes

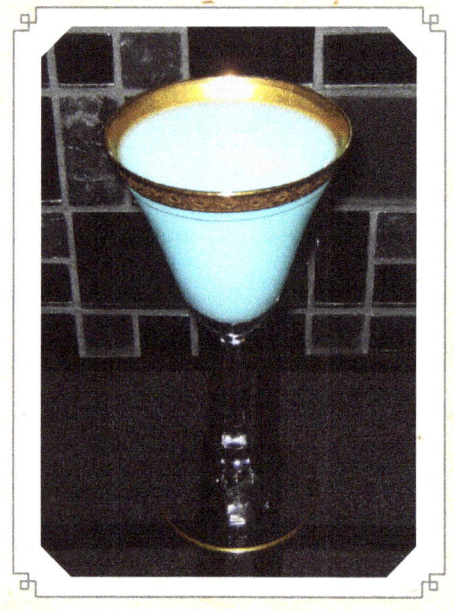

Place all ingredients in a cocktail shaker. Shake well for 20-30 seconds, then strain into a coupe glass. Or you may serve over a few new ice cubes in a rocks or old-fashioned glass. Serves 1.

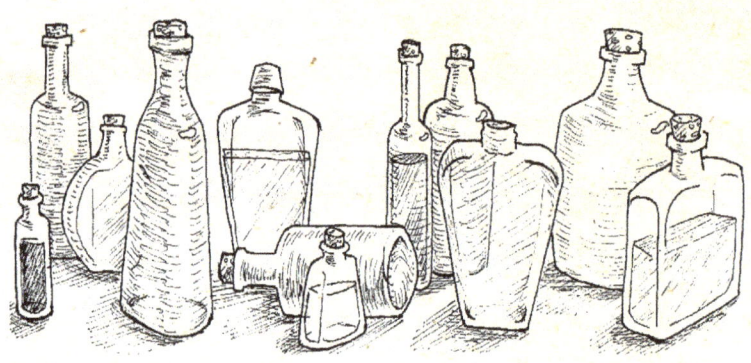

As a girl reading The Lion, The Witch and the Wardrobe, *I always associated Turkish Delight with the color turquoise. Maybe this was because I live in New Mexico, where turquoise is a dominant color in large things such as the sky and small things such as jewelry, but it was also simply because of the beginning sounds of the words Turkish and turquoise—I was a child making connections.*

When I was contemplating including Turkish Delight in my re-tooled cookbook, I remember buying a rather non-descript box of the candy. I was surprised by how boring the sweets looked—beige and white. They even tasted kind of boring. Can a candy taste like "beige and white"? Yes, it certainly can. They were nothing like the Liberty Orchards confections I mentioned in the previous recipe, but also nothing like future varieties I tried. However, the ingredients listed on this "boring box of Turkish Delight" sounded like they would make a fabulous drink, in theory. And they do. Of course, you can use clear Curaçao and the cocktail will visually resemble that "boring box," but my childhood vision is more festive-looking. I thought of naming it Turkish Delight, but well, I really wasn't in the mood to visit the Land of Copyright Law again, just in case…

Chapter Six

Glitnír's Hall

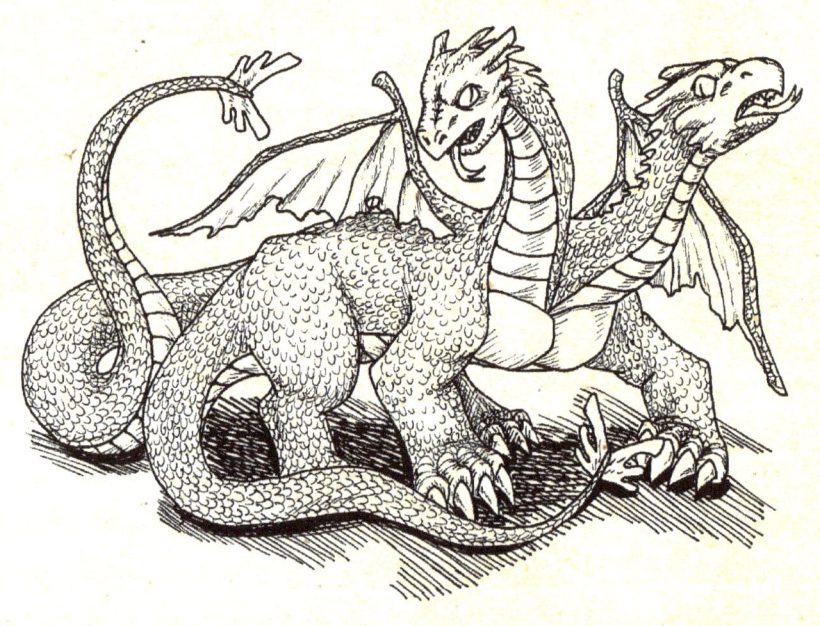

Wholly hearty food for dwarves.

Thrúd's Hearty Split Pea Soup
Rádgrid's Stuffed Mushrooms
Göll's Gorgeous Seed Cake
Skeggjöld's Boozy Beans
Mushrooms of Mist
Hlökk's Trenchers
Hild's Mushroom Bacon Dish of Might
Snorri's Special Ham & Eggs
Geirahöd's Pork Pie of Battle
Reginleif's Favorite Chicken
Pumpkin Streusel Pie for Randgrid
Hrist's Nutmeggers
Skögul's Spice Cookies
Herfjötur's Fancy Bread Pudding

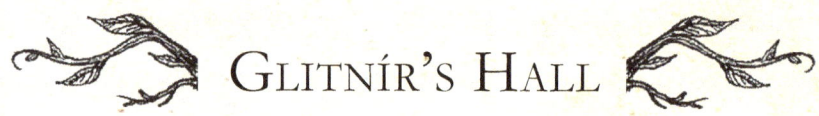

GLITNÍR'S HALL

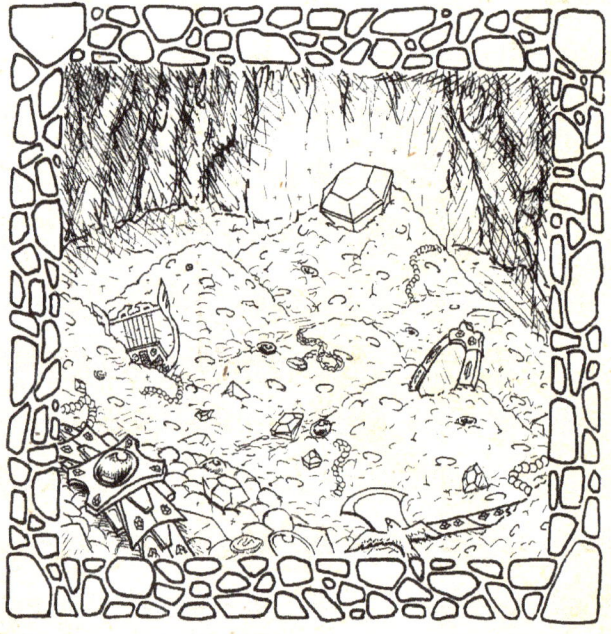

Originally, I did not have a specific chapter just for dwarves until now, but I really like the way this restaurant came together. If you are looking for some sort of bready product you can take with you on long voyages (something like Tolkien's *cram*), this cookbook will not specifically supply one. I will suggest you do this: follow the proportions listed on a box of biscuit mix. Turn your oven about 10° hotter than the directions recommend. Bake your biscuits for about two minutes more than suggested. Do not consume until at least one day after baking, and preferably only when you are desperately hungry after a long hike. I know I'm not stoic enough to do this; I would prefer to make Head-in-the-Clouds Biscuits (page 59). This is a much more pleasant experience.

I have borrowed my names here from *The Prose Edda*, a unique and mythological Icelandic work written by Snorri Sturluson (1179-1241). I heard of some other author who did the same thing when naming his characters… but, since the copyright was not renewed, the *Edda* is part of the public domain and free for other writers to use.

Thrúd's Hearty Split Pea Soup

Dwarves probably appreciate large slabs of meat; I bet hams would be popular. If you cook up a large spiral-sliced ham, you'll end up with a substantial ham bone leftover. Pair this with some leftover cabbage and you'll be able to make a really hearty soup.

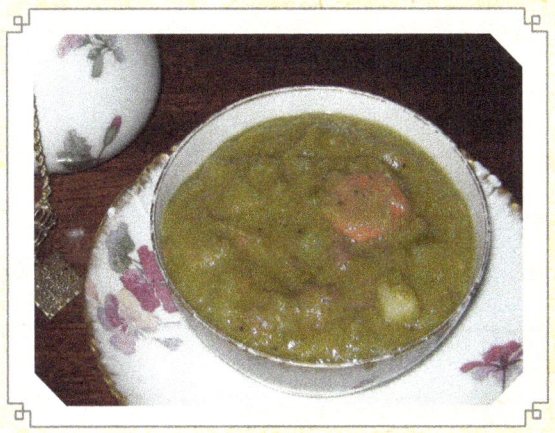

2 quarts low-sodium chicken broth
3-4 cups onions, diced
1 pound split peas, rinsed and sorted
1 very meaty ham bone[1]
1½ cups celery, cut into ¼" slices
1½ cups carrots, peeled and cut into ¼" slices
1 pound potatoes, peeled (or not) and cut into ¾" cubes
4-5 cups cabbage, coarsely chopped
1 teaspoon pepper
1 teaspoon dry marjoram (or 2 tablespoons fresh marjoram, minced)
½ teaspoon salt

In a 6-quart saucepan, combine the broth, onions, peas, and ham bone. Bring to a boil, then lower heat to a simmer, cover, and cook 45 minutes. Turn the bone over halfway through cooking. Remove the bone (brush off any stray onions and peas and return them to the pot) and place it in a large bowl to cool off. Add the remaining ingredients to the saucepan; bring to a boil again. Reduce heat to low, cover, and simmer 20 minutes.

Meanwhile, remove as much meat as you can from the bone and chop coarsely. You should end up with anywhere from 2 to 4 cups of meat. Add this to the soup and raise heat to medium. Cook, uncovered, for 10-15 minutes, until your vegetables are tender. Stir occasionally. Blend 3 cups until smooth and add this back to the saucepan. Adjust seasonings, if desired, but be careful doing so since you can't really tell how salty your ham might be. Cover and refrigerate leftovers; don't freeze, because

[1] Use about a 2-pound bone from a 10-12 pound ham. I usually make this soup after I have baked a spiral-cut ham for some holiday; then I strip it, while leaving quite a bit of meat on the bone.

your potatoes might end up mushy. It will keep well in the fridge for a week or so. Serves 8-10.

 *Here's one of the places where I sneak in leftover cabbage (maybe I shouldn't let Bob read this…). You can always add a little water or broth to this, if it becomes too thick as a leftover. A perfect soup for cold weather, and goes well with almost any sort of bread product you can imagine.*

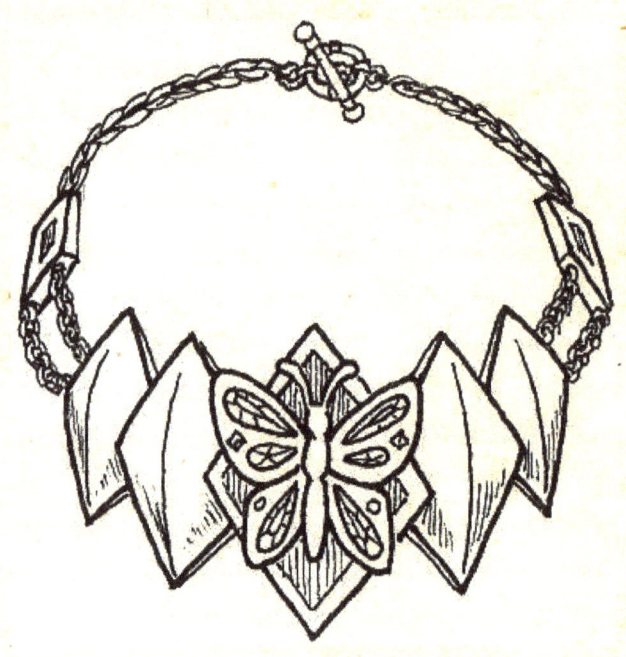

Rádgrid's Stuffed Mushrooms

Serve these with a salad for dinner or as a savory knife-and-fork appetizer at a party.

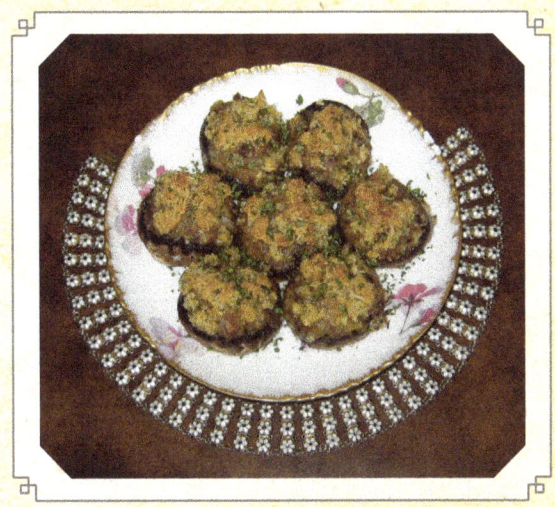

16 fresh mushrooms, each about 2½" in diameter
1 tablespoon salted butter
½ cup minced shallots
½ pound hot bulk pork sausage
1 extra large egg
1 ounce plus 1 ounce Parmesan or Romano cheese, finely shredded
2 tablespoons plus 2 tablespoons seasoned dry bread crumbs
1 teaspoon Worcestershire sauce
½ tablespoon heavy cream
½ teaspoon Savory Seasoning
2 tablespoons salted butter, melted and cooled a bit
Some minced fresh parsley or chives for garnish, if desired (about ¼ cup)

Clean mushrooms and remove stems; set caps aside. Chop all the stems finely. In a medium skillet, melt 1 tablespoon butter over high heat. Add the stems and shallots; sauté over high heat until they are dry, stirring frequently. Let stand in pan 30 minutes.

Preheat oven to 375°. Coat a 9" square pan with cooking spray or grease lightly. In a medium bowl, combine the sausage, egg, 1 ounce cheese, 2 tablespoons bread crumbs, Worcestershire sauce, cream, and Savory Seasoning well with your hands. Add the shallot mixture and combine well. Distribute meat mixture evenly onto each mushroom cap; use a spoon to smooth the tops and place caps rounded side down in pan. In a small bowl, combine the remaining bread crumbs and cheese with the melted butter. Sprinkle a teaspoon of this mixture on top of each mushroom. Bake 45 minutes. Use tongs to remove from pan; discard cooking liquid. Garnish, if desired. Cover and refrigerate leftovers. Makes 16; serves 4 as an entrée.

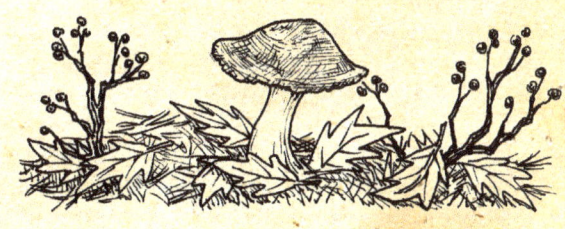

Göll's Gorgeous Seed Cake

This cake is not too sweet and would be a lovely snack or breakfast item with coffee, tea, milk, or hot chocolate. You could also enjoy it with a beer, if you are so inclined.

- 1 cup all-purpose flour
- ½ cup cake flour
- ½ cup sugar
- 2 teaspoons baking powder
- ½ teaspoon salt
- ½ tablespoon plus 1 tablespoon poppy seeds
- ½ tablespoon plus 1 tablespoon sesame seeds, lightly toasted
- 1 tablespoon plus 2 tablespoons salted, dry roasted sunflower seeds
- ¼ cup plus ¼ cup soft salted butter
- ½ cup light sour cream, room temperature
- ½ cup buttermilk, room temperature
- 1 extra large egg, room temperature
- ¼ cup packed golden brown sugar
- ¼ cup old-fashioned oats

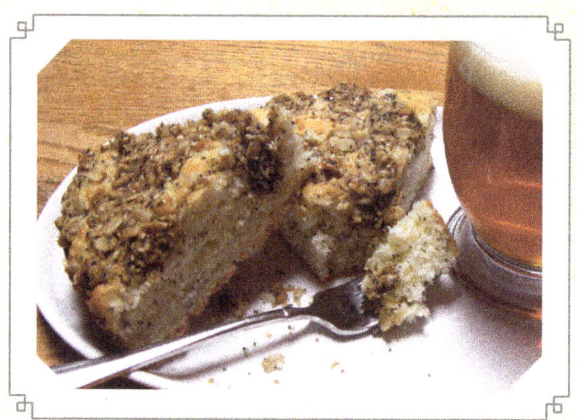

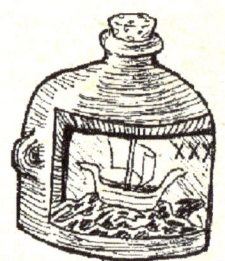

Preheat oven to 350°. Coat a 9" springform pan with 2" deep sides with cooking spray or grease lightly. In a large bowl, combine both of the flours, sugar, baking powder, salt, ½ tablespoon each of the poppy seeds and sesame seeds, and 1 tablespoon of the sunflower seeds. Add and mix in ¼ cup of the butter and the sour cream. In a 2-cup glass measuring cup, whisk together the buttermilk and the egg, then mix this into the dry ingredients well. Spread in prepared pan. In a medium bowl, combine the brown sugar, oats, and the remaining seeds. Add the remaining ¼ cup butter and combine with your hands. Sprinkle this evenly in clumps on top of the batter. Bake 37-41 minutes or until the center tests done. Place on a rack and cool at least 30 minutes before removing pan sides and cutting. Keep leftovers covered at room temperature. Serves 6-8.

Skeggjöld's Boozy Beans

When it comes to dry beans, your cooking time might vary. Remember, I live at a high altitude and might need to cook beans longer than people at sea level. If your beans get done sooner than you expect, you can always just leave them covered on the stove.

1 pound small dried beans (such as navy, lima, or Great Northern)
Water to cover beans plus 3 quarts water
¾ pound premium bacon, cut into ½" pieces
4 cups onion, diced
½ cup packed golden brown sugar
½ cup spicy brown mustard
¼ cup ketchup
2 tablespoons molasses
2 tablespoons dry mustard
2 teaspoons salt
2 teaspoons pepper
1 teaspoon cayenne pepper
3 cups dark or amber beer[1]
1 cup whiskey

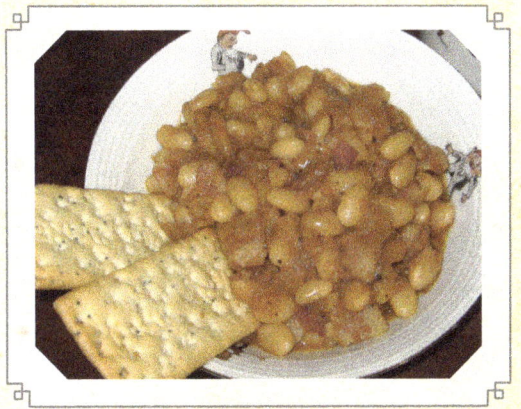

[1] My own current favorite is Negra Modelo dark beer and I have used Jack Daniels for my whiskey. Obviously, you have tons of choices here, so just use your favorites. A stout or chocolate beer might work well, paired with some bourbon or scotch. You probably wouldn't want to use incredibly expensive products—they're best just for drinking.

Place the beans in a 6-quart saucepan with enough water to cover them by 1". Cover and soak overnight. Drain; rinse and sort. Add back to the saucepan with the 3 quarts water. Bring to a boil, then simmer, covered, over lowest heat for 2 hours, stirring occasionally. Drain beans, then rinse out the saucepan; don't bother washing it. Coat the saucepan with cooking spray. Sauté the bacon and onion over high heat, stirring frequently, until the bacon starts to brown, about 20 minutes. In a 2-cup glass measuring cup, combine the brown sugar, mustard, ketchup, molasses, and the 4 seasonings with a whisk. Add to the saucepan. Slowly pour in the beer and then add the whiskey and beans. Bring to a boil, then cover and set on a low simmer for 30 minutes. Uncover and simmer 30-45 minutes, until the beans are tender, thick, and creamy. Stir frequently, scraping up brown bits. Adjust seasonings, if desired. Cover and refrigerate leftovers. Serves 8-10.

Mushrooms of Mist

A perfect side dish for any entrée. If you can get button mushrooms, just leave them whole. I have to get over my obsession with button mushrooms, especially since I can't seem to find them very often.

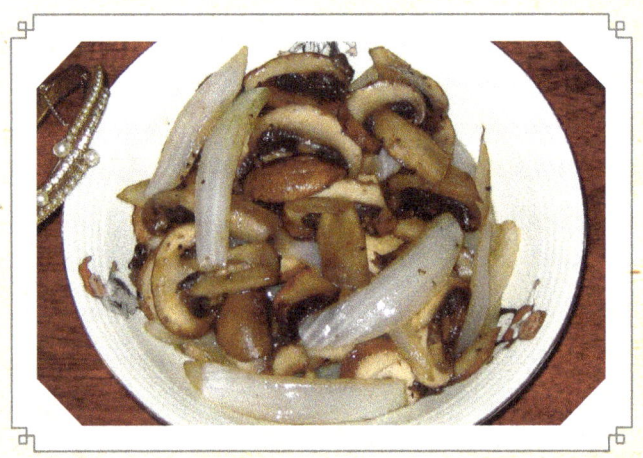

1 tablespoon salted butter
A ½ pound onion, cut into ½" slivers
½ pound fresh mushrooms (whole buttons, or cut other mushrooms into ¼" slices)
⅛ teaspoon each:

    pepper   onion salt
    garlic salt   celery salt

In a 3-quart deep skillet, melt the butter over high heat. Add the onion and mushrooms; cook over medium/high heat, covered, for 3 minutes. Uncover and add seasonings. Raise heat to high and cook for about 3-4 minutes, stirring frequently, until the moisture has mostly evaporated. Adjust seasonings, if desired. Cover and refrigerate leftovers. Serves 2-4, depending on your other dishes. It could just serve one dwarf or even one halfling if he were really in the mood just to eat a big bowl of savory mushrooms…

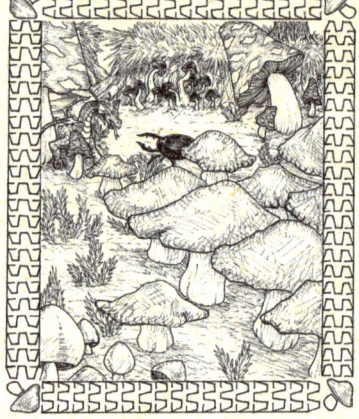

Hlökk's Trenchers

Here's a yummy, casual supper dish or a substantial snack. You can leave the bread out and simply use this as a mushroom gravy over steak or whatever you like.

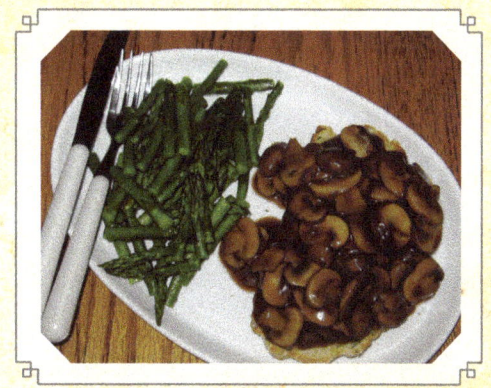

1 tablespoon salted butter
½ pound fresh mushrooms, thinly sliced
14½-ounce can low-sodium beef broth
2 tablespoons all-purpose flour or Wondra
1 teaspoon Worcestershire sauce
¼ teaspoon each:
    Savory Seasoning
    pepper
    Kitchen Bouquet
4 slices of fresh bread, about 1" thick (such
    as sourdough, French, or Italian; about 4" by 5")
Some soft salted butter or spreadable margarine

In a 3-quart deep skillet, melt the butter over high heat. Add the mushrooms and sauté over rather high heat for 3 minutes, stirring frequently. Whisk together the broth, flour, Worcestershire sauce, and seasonings. Add to the skillet and bring to a boil. Reduce heat to medium/low and cook 15-20 minutes, uncovered, until it thickens to a nice sauce; stir occasionally. Adjust seasonings, if desired.

Meanwhile, toast the bread slices, then spread each with butter or margarine. Place on plate and ladle mushrooms and gravy equally all over toasts. Cover and refrigerate leftovers separately. Serves 2 as a main dish; 4 as a side dish.

I take this idea from the medieval period, whereby a thick piece of stale bread would become a sort of plate, or "trencher." A selfish guest would usually finish his meal by eating his trencher after it had absorbed all of the sauce or gravy. Other generous guests would be kind enough to donate his/her trencher to the poor or to any canines hanging around (Tannahill 190). If your trencher became too soggy, you would get another one. I think using an actual plate and using toasty fresh bread are improvements here, and I would never think of you as greedy if you eat your trencher. I think it's odder to eat off of something, then give it to someone else, but that's just me. My dog really appreciated getting to lick the plate clean, however.

Hild's Mushroom Bacon Dish of Might

This is actually the first dish I invented for my undergraduate cookbook project, though it has changed from the original slightly. To me, this is quintessential fantasy food that would appeal to anyone who relates to dwarves or halflings. Yes, it is heavy on the bacon, but you wouldn't eat it every day, would you? Serve a big salad with it, or pair it with any of the vegetable side dish recipes included in the cookbook.

- 1 quart plus 2 tablespoons water
- 1 pound potatoes, cut into ¾" chunks (peeled or not; it depends what kind of potatoes you use)
- ¾ pound premium (regular fat) bacon, cut into 1" pieces
- 1 tablespoon reserved bacon fat
- 1 tablespoon salted butter
- 1½ cups onion, cut into ¼" slivers
- ½ pound fresh mushrooms (whole buttons or cut into ¼" slices or halves)
- ½ teaspoon salt
- ½ teaspoon pepper

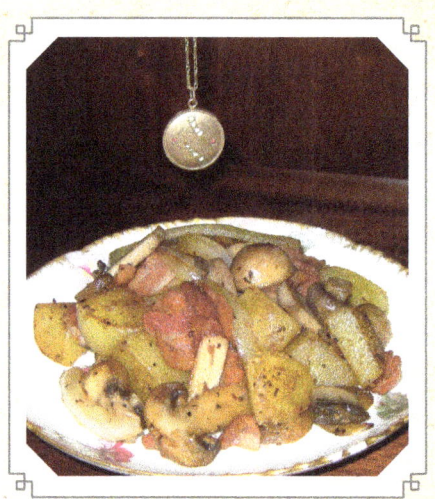

In a 5-quart deep skillet, combine the 1 quart water and the potatoes. Bring to a boil and cook for 5 minutes. Drain; don't bother washing pan. In the same skillet, fry the bacon over rather high heat, stirring frequently and scraping up the brown bits, until it is thoroughly cooked, but still rather chewy, not too crispy. With a slotted spoon, remove bacon to paper towels to drain. Reserve 1 tablespoon of the rendered fat. Discard or reserve the remaining fat for other uses (again, don't bother washing pan).

Add the reserved bacon fat and butter to the pan and melt over rather high heat. Add the onions and potatoes and fry uncovered over rather high heat, stirring frequently, until the potatoes start browning at the edges, about 8-10 minutes, scraping up any brown bits. Add the mushrooms and fry another 2 minutes. Add the 2 tablespoons water, cover and cook over moderately high heat for 2 minutes. Uncover, add salt and pepper, and continue cooking over medium heat until most of the liquid evaporates, another 1-2 minutes, stirring often. Mix in the bacon and serve. Season, as desired. Cover and refrigerate leftovers. Serves 4.

Mix 4 ounces of well-drained, roasted and chopped green chile into the dish near the end of cooking.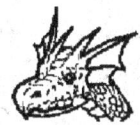

 *As a sort of concession to the good-health-gods, I was going to say this serves 4-6, but who am I kidding? If you don't serve anything with this and you have a bacon-loving companion (like Bob) who actually said, "This is the kind of food that makes me sad when I'm done eating it," you'll be lucky to serve 2 with a bit leftover.*

What to do with those leftovers? Turn them into a breakfast, either first or second: cook one or two eggs, any style. Sprinkle some shredded Cheddar cheese over the potatoes, microwave to heat and serve alongside your eggs. You could also mix some diced green chile, jalapeños, or salsa into the potatoes. Or: scramble one or two eggs and combine with your leftover potatoes. Wrap this up in a flour tortilla (you could even add some pinto beans to this…) and enjoy out of hand. Make it more substantial by setting this burrito on a plate, then smother it with salsa, red or green chile sauce, and cheese; heat in the microwave until the cheese has melted—now you'll need a knife and fork. You might recall I live in New Mexico, right?

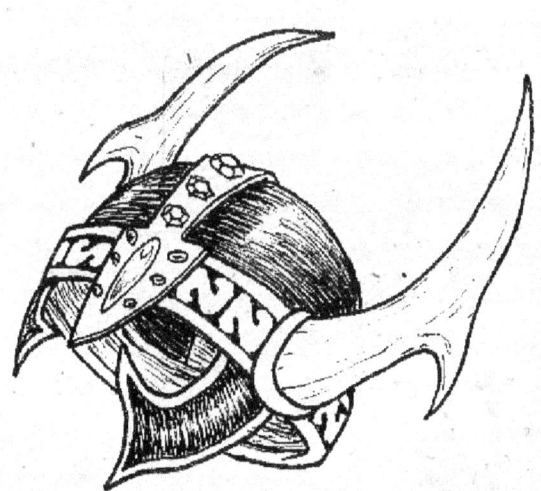

Snorri's Special Ham & Eggs

Creamy, delicious eggs like these will make your breakfast or brunch special. Instead of the ham, you may use a few slices of Canadian bacon or even thin pork chops here. Allow a few minutes extra cooking time for pork chops.

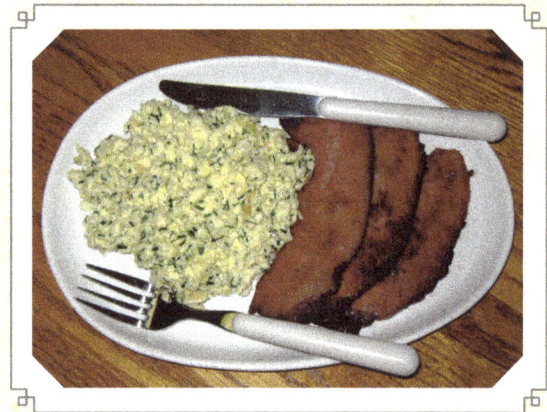

- 1 tablespoon plus 1 tablespoon salted butter
- 1 tablespoon packed golden brown sugar
- ¾ pound cooked ham slices
- 6 extra large eggs
- ¼ cup heavy cream
- ½ teaspoon Savory Seasoning
- ½ cup minced fresh chives
- 5-6 ounces spreadable herb/garlic cheese (⅔ cup)[1]

In a large skillet, melt 1 tablespoon butter and brown sugar over medium/high heat. Add the meat and fry until a golden brown on both sides. Turn heat to very low and cover.

Meanwhile in a large bowl, whisk the eggs, cream, and Savory Seasoning until combined well. In another large skillet coated with cooking spray, melt the remaining tablespoon of butter over medium/high heat. Pour the egg mixture into the skillet and cook over medium/high heat until just beginning to scramble, stirring occasionally and gently with a spatula. Sprinkle with the chives and add the cheese, breaking it into smaller pieces or mashing it as you mix it in. Continue scrambling until the eggs are fully cooked and fluffy. Don't brown them (though if you do, they're still quite edible). Adjust seasonings, if desired. Serve alongside the ham and accompany with items such as toast, biscuits, scones, or English muffins. Keep leftovers covered in refrigerator. Serves 3-4, or perhaps just one terribly hungry dwarf...

[1] Something like Boursin cheese would be great here; just use a 5.2 ounce package, any flavor. For a simple and delicious homemade option, please see Aradosa's Cheese on page xxiv.

 **Vegetarian Option**—You can fry up your favorite breakfast-meat substitute if you like, or just prepare the eggs and slather extra jam/honey/butter on your bread product of choice.

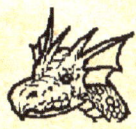

Mix 4 ounces drained, roasted, and chopped green chile into the eggs with the chives and cheese. A ½ cup or so of your favorite salsa would also be nice for variety.

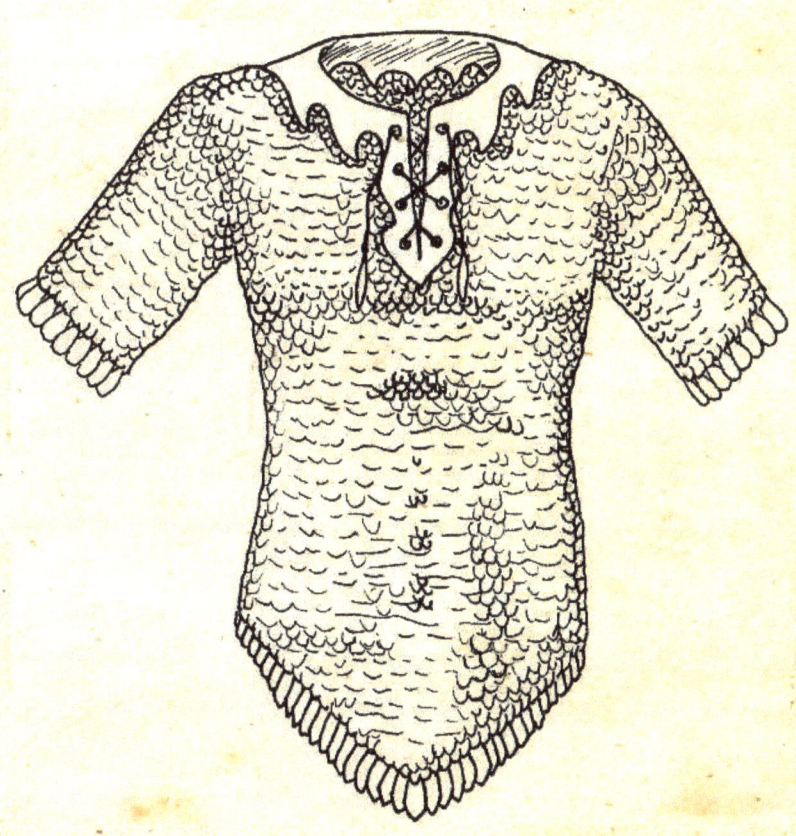

Geirahöd's Pork Pie of Battle

If making a pie ends up being too much trouble on a busy day, you could omit the pastry here (or substitute two ready-made pie crusts, though you probably won't have much leftover to decorate it—that's okay) and simply turn this into a stew by adding a 14½-ounce can of low-sodium chicken broth. Cook it for about 10 more minutes on a low simmer, covered. As a stew, this will probably serve more like 3-4 people. Flour tortillas or corn bread would be delicious with the stew.

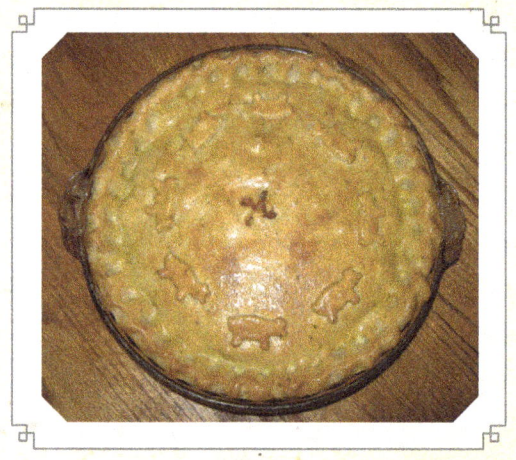

2¼ cups all-purpose flour
¼ cup cornmeal
1 teaspoon salt
1 teaspoon dry thyme (or 2 tablespoons fresh thyme, minced)
¼ cup chilled salted butter, cut into ¼" bits
3 ounces chilled lard, cut into ¼" bits (or vegetable shortening)
¾ cup ice water
1 tablespoon salted butter
1 cup onion, diced
1 pound pork tenderloin, cut into ½" cubes
½ cup dry white wine, such as Chardonnay
½ teaspoon each:
    Savory Seasoning   onion salt
    dry thyme   garlic salt
    onion powder   pepper
    garlic powder
½ cup fresh or frozen corn
½ cup fresh or frozen lima beans (or peas)
14-ounce can petite diced tomatoes, undrained
1 tablespoon all-purpose flour or Wondra
1 extra large egg
1 teaspoon water

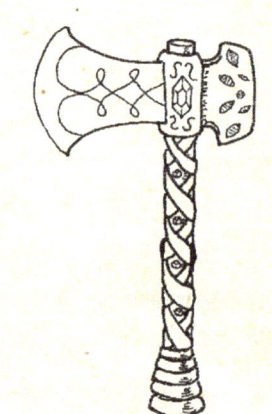

In a large bowl, combine 2¼ cups flour, cornmeal, 1 teaspoon each of salt and dry (or fresh) thyme. Add the ¼ cup butter and lard and mix in with a pastry blender, until the mixture resembles coarse crumbs. Add ice water and combine well with a wooden spoon. Divide into ⅔ and ⅓ portions and flatten into round disks. Put in covered containers or cover each with plastic wrap and refrigerate 30-60 minutes.

Meanwhile, coat a 3-quart medium deep skillet with cooking spray, then sauté the 1 tablespoon butter, onion, and the pork over medium/high heat just until there is no longer any pink color. Add the wine and cook over high heat until it is almost dry. Add the next 7 seasonings, corn, lima beans, tomatoes, and 1 tablespoon flour and mix in. Bring to a boil, then cook uncovered over a medium heat for 5 minutes. Stir a couple of times. Let stand; it should still be moist and saucy. Adjust seasonings, if desired.

Preheat oven to 375°. On a floured surface, roll out the large disk to a 13" circle and place in a 9½" glass pie dish. Pour in the stew. Roll out the smaller disk to about 12" and place on top. Trim edges, fold over and crimp decoratively, reserving scraps. Cut a small X in the center. With pie crust scraps, cut small decorations. In a small bowl, whisk together the egg and 1 teaspoon water. Brush top of pie with egg wash and apply decorations—egg wash these as well. Bake 30 minutes. Brush top of pie with egg wash again and bake another 16-20 minutes, until golden brown. Let stand 10 minutes before cutting. Serve hot, warm, or even at room temperature. Cover and refrigerate leftovers; reheats well. Serves 6-8.

Vegetarian Option—Replace the lard in the pie crust with vegetable shortening. Keep everything the same, except replace the meat with 3 cups of assorted diced vegetables and add an extra tablespoon of flour to thicken the sauce. Good choices would be summer squashes, broccoli, cauliflower, bell peppers, or just additional onion, corn, lima beans, and/or peas.

If you wanted to cave in to my New Mexican suggestions, add about 4 ounces of diced green chile, drained, roasted, and chopped to the meat, either in the pie or in the stew.

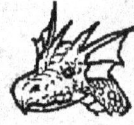

Other protein choices work as well, such as beef, or chicken. Just for variation, I've poured salsa and sprinkled Cheddar cheese over a heated leftover slice—microwave again to melt the cheese.

Reginleif's Favorite Chicken

Use a smoked paprika to enhance the flavor in this wonderfully rich dish.

- 2 tablespoons plus 1 tablespoon salted butter
- 8-10 boneless, skinless chicken thighs (2-2½ pounds)
- Salt & pepper
- ¾ cup shallots, cut into ¼" crosswise slices
- ½ pound fresh mushrooms, cut into ¼" slices
- 1 tablespoon paprika
- 14½-ounce can low-sodium chicken broth
- 1 cup half-and-half
- ½ cup heavy cream
- 1 tablespoon all-purpose flour

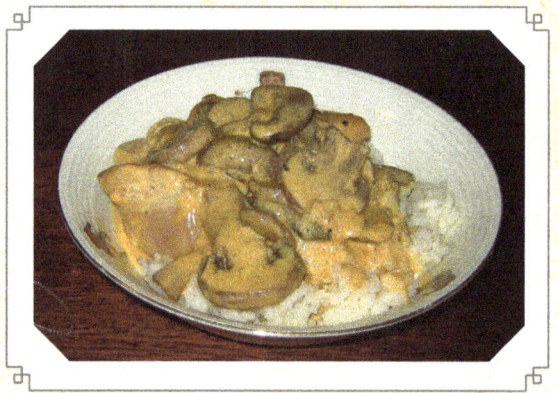

Trim off noticeable fat from the chicken thighs. In a 5-quart deep skillet, melt the 2 tablespoons butter over rather high heat. Place chicken in skillet; sprinkle with salt and pepper. Sauté over high heat 5 minutes. Turn over; season with more salt and pepper and sauté another 5 minutes, until both sides of the thighs are golden brown. Occasionally shake the pan to prevent chicken from sticking. Remove to a plate; re-use skillet without washing it. Add the 1 tablespoon butter, shallots, and mushrooms. Sauté 3 minutes on moderate heat, while scraping up the brown bits. Add the paprika and broth and bring to a boil. Whisk the remaining ingredients in a 2-cup glass measuring cup. Add the cream mixture and chicken with any accumulated juices to the skillet. Cook over medium/high heat for about 20 minutes until sauce has reduced somewhat and is slightly thicker. Turn chicken over and spoon sauce over each. Reduce heat to low and cook 10 more minutes. Adjust seasonings, if desired. Serve with rice, egg noodles, mashed potatoes, or crusty bread. Cover and refrigerate leftovers. Serves 4-6.

Pumpkin Streusel Pie for Randgrid

This is for people (like myself) who think regular pumpkin pie is boring. So I jazzed it up and now it is the perfect fall dessert, especially at a holiday such as Thanksgiving—make it the night before, then you can cross one thing off of your list.

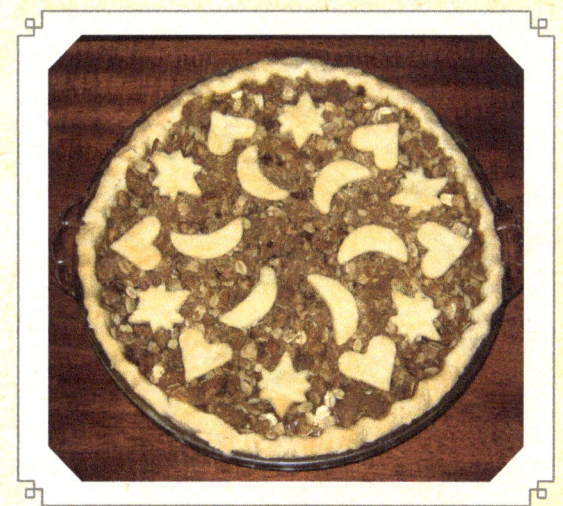

1½ cups plus ¼ cup all-purpose flour
½ teaspoon plus ½ teaspoon salt
3 ounces chilled lard, cut into ¼" bits
   (vegetable shortening is fine)
6-8 tablespoons ice water
1 tablespoon cinnamon
2 teaspoons ground ginger
½ teaspoon each:
   ground cloves
   nutmeg
   allspice
2 tablespoons salted butter
2 tablespoons plus ½ cup sugar
6 ounces pecan halves
14½-ounce can pumpkin puree (about 1¾ cups)
3 extra large eggs
½ cup heavy cream
2 teaspoons vanilla extract
⅔ cup old-fashioned oats
½ cup packed golden brown sugar
¼ cup soft salted butter

In a large bowl, combine the 1½ cups flour and ½ teaspoon salt. Cut in the lard with a pastry blender. Add the water in tablespoons, mixing until the dough is incorporated thoroughly. Knead a few times on a floured surface. Flatten dough into a disk and place in a covered container or wrap in plastic. Save bowl for later use. Refrigerate 30-60 minutes.

For the spice mix: in a small bowl, combine the remaining ½ teaspoon salt, cinnamon, ginger, cloves, allspice, and nutmeg and set aside.

In a medium skillet, melt the 2 tablespoons butter over medium/high heat. Add the 2 tablespoons sugar and 1 teaspoon spice mix and stir to dissolve. Add the pecans and sauté 2-3 minutes, stirring frequently. Set aside to cool for a few minutes, then chop the nuts coarsely and set aside.

Preheat oven to 375°. On a floured surface, roll out the pie crust to about 13" and lay in a 9½" glass pie dish. Trim and fold over the edge; crimp decoratively. Cut decorations from scraps, if desired.

In the large bowl, whisk together the pumpkin, eggs, cream, ½ cup sugar, vanilla, and 1 tablespoon of the spice mix. Then mix in half of the reserved nut mixture. Pour into the prepared pie crust and bake 25 minutes.

Meanwhile in a medium bowl, combine the oats, ¼ cup flour, brown sugar, the remaining spice mix, and the remaining nut mixture. Add the soft butter and combine well with your hands. Sprinkle all over the pie to cover all of the pumpkin. Place decorations on top of streusel, if desired. Bake another 25 minutes. Cool on rack at least 2 hours before cutting. Serve with whipped cream. Cover and store at room temperature or refrigerate. Serves 6-8.

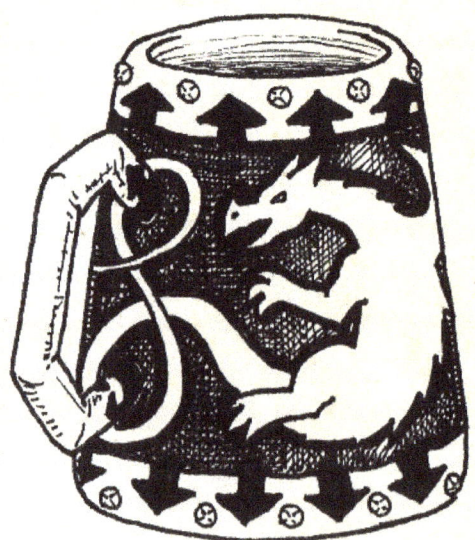

Hrist's Nutmeggers

Excellent holiday cookies, these will really remind you of the winter holiday season while they bake. Any extra nutmeg sugar is great on hot cereals, or you can combine it with cinnamon sugar for a different flavor.

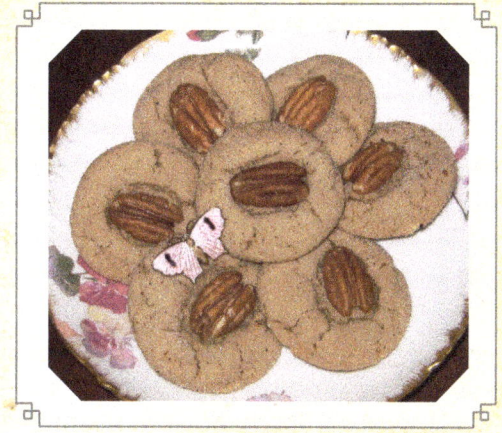

- ½ cup soft salted butter
- 1 cup packed golden brown sugar
- 1 extra large egg, room temperature
- 1¾ cups all-purpose flour
- 1 teaspoon plus ½ teaspoon nutmeg
- 1 teaspoon baking soda
- ½ teaspoon salt
- 2 tablespoons sugar
- 36 nice pecan halves

Preheat oven to 375°. Coat 2 large baking sheets with cooking spray or grease lightly. In a large bowl, combine the butter, brown sugar, and egg on medium speed until creamy. Add the flour, 1 teaspoon nutmeg, soda, and salt and combine well. In a small bowl, combine the sugar and ½ teaspoon nutmeg. Divide dough into 36 pieces, and roll into balls, about 1¼" diameter. Roll each in the sugar/nutmeg mixture. Place on sheets 1½" apart. Set a pecan half on top of each. Bake 7-9 minutes. Cool on pans 1 minute; remove to racks. Store covered at room temperature. Makes 36.

Skögul's Spice Cookies

These are a fragrant variation on one of my favorite treats, Mexican Wedding Cookies.

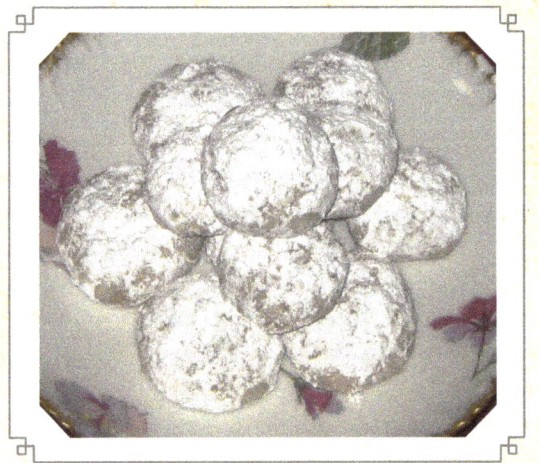

- 4 ounces pecan halves, toasted lightly and cooled
- ½ cup all-purpose flour
- ½ cup cake flour
- ½ cup plus ¾ cup powdered sugar
- ¼ teaspoon each:
    - salt
    - nutmeg
    - cinnamon
    - allspice
    - ground cloves
    - ground ginger
- ½ cup soft salted butter
- ½ teaspoon vanilla extract
- 2 tablespoons heavy cream

Place the pecans in a large food processor and pulse until they are fully ground. Add the flours, ½ cup powdered sugar, and all the spices. Process until combined. Add the butter, vanilla, and cream and pulse thoroughly. Scrape into a 2-quart covered container. Refrigerate 1 hour.

Preheat oven to 400°. Coat 2 large baking sheets with cooking spray or grease lightly. Divide dough into 36 pieces then roll into balls, about 1¼" diameter. Place 1" apart on sheets. Bake 8-10 minutes. Remove; let sit on pans 30 minutes.

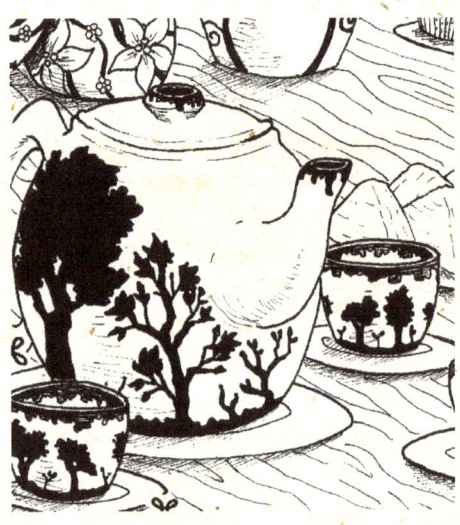

Meanwhile, rinse out and dry the 2-quart container. Place ¾ cup powdered sugar in container. Put a quarter of the cookies in this; cover, and roll them around gently in the sugar. Place cookies carefully on a rack over a cookie sheet. Repeat with the remaining cookies, 9 at a time. You can sprinkle any remaining powdered sugar over the tops of the cookies, using a fine-mesh strainer. Store covered at room temperature. Makes 36.

Herfjötur's Fancy Bread Pudding

For this dessert, I usually buy the giant croissants from Costco (where else?). Other rather light-textured, unsliced, bread products will also work, as long as you can cut them into 1½" chunks (try panettone or challah). Serve with whipped cream, ice cream, or dessert sauces (chocolate and caramel are nice). A tablespoon of various liqueurs might also be good, if you like.

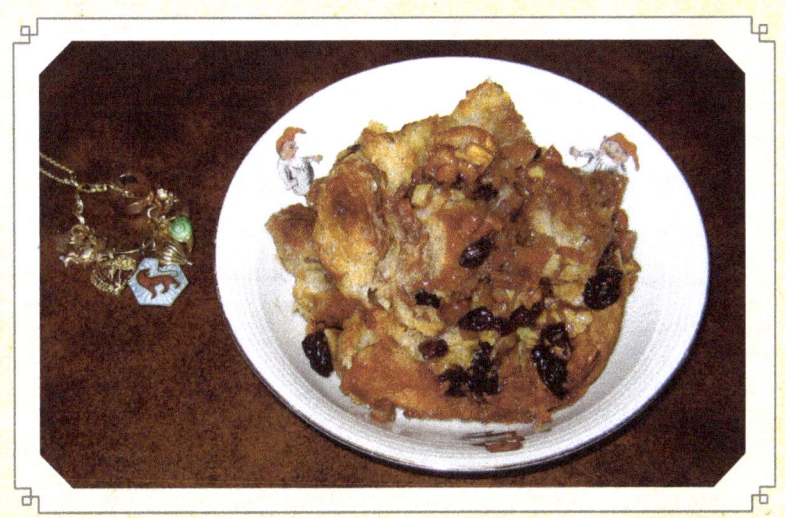

2 cups half-and-half
¾ cup egg substitute
1 extra large egg
¼ cup sugar
½ teaspoon each:
    cinnamon   nutmeg   ground cardamom
¼ teaspoon each:
    salt   allspice   ground cloves
1 pound large croissants
½ cup salted butter
¾ cup packed golden brown sugar
½ cup maple syrup (light is okay)
½ teaspoon vanilla extract
½ teaspoon salt
4 ounces raisins
4 ounces pecans, coarsely chopped

In a large bowl, combine the half-and-half, egg substitute, egg, sugar, and the 6 seasonings. Whisk until fully combined. Cut the croissants into 1½" chunks. Place them in the bowl and mix until all the croissants are coated with some egg mixture. Let stand.

Preheat oven to 350°. Liberally coat a 13" by 9" glass baking dish with cooking spray. In a 2-quart saucepan, combine the butter, brown sugar, and syrup over medium heat. Whisk occasionally until the brown sugar has dissolved and the butter has melted. Add the remaining ingredients and set aside.

Stir the croissant mixture, then pour evenly into the prepared dish. Pour the butter mixture over all and mix slightly. Bake 40-44 minutes, or until set in the center and golden brown. Let stand 30 minutes before serving. Cover and chill or store at room temperature. Serves 8-12.

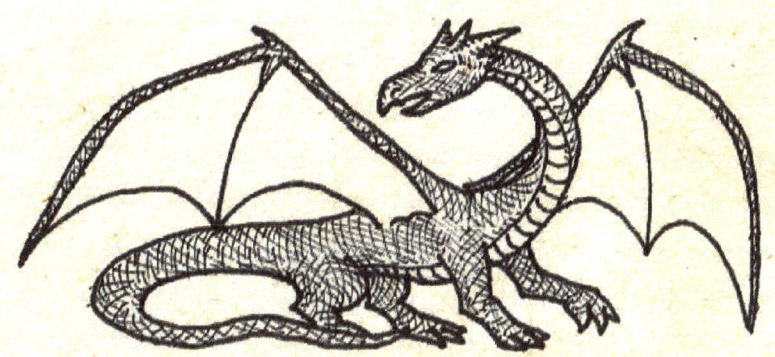

Chapter Seven
Monstrous Morsels: The Hot Spot for Egregious Enemies

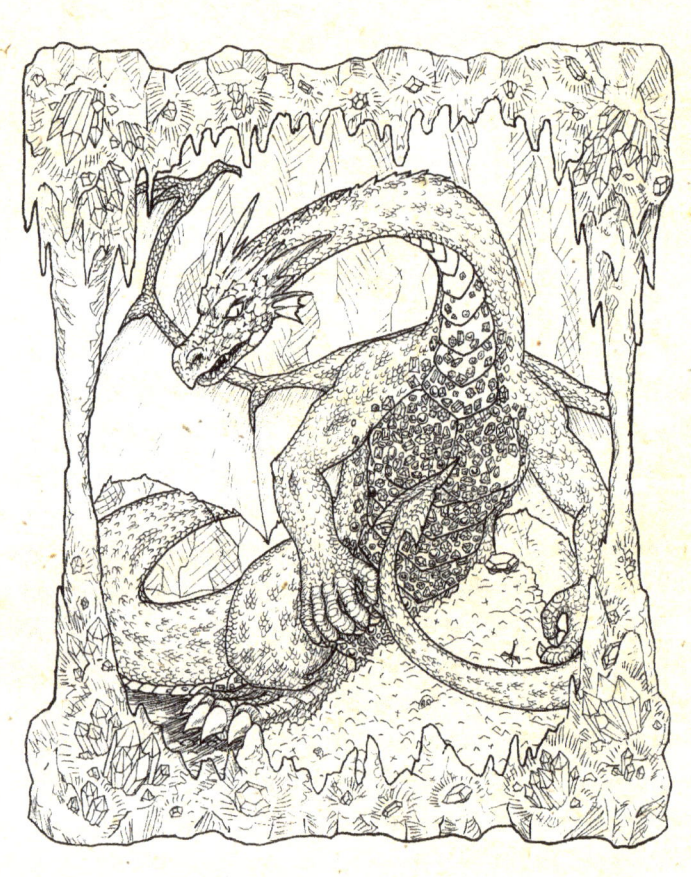

Are you a troll? An orc? A goblin? Zombie, by chance? Do you make others uncomfortable when you just try to eat a peaceful meal at their establishments? You'll feel at home here.

Fungus Liquid

Zeldôshâkh's Gnarly Bones

Must Eat Brain Food...

Pig & Curd on Bread

Glürbin's Gutless Wonders

Meat on Metal Stick

Raskofim's Roadkill

Gündürnüb's Grüb

Chunks & Gobbets

Clôxiga's Crunchable Salmon

Tshigwú's Bit o' the Flank

Cold Dead Livid Bread

Sweets for Sbileng

Queevhô's Bleedin' Treats

Monstrous Morsels

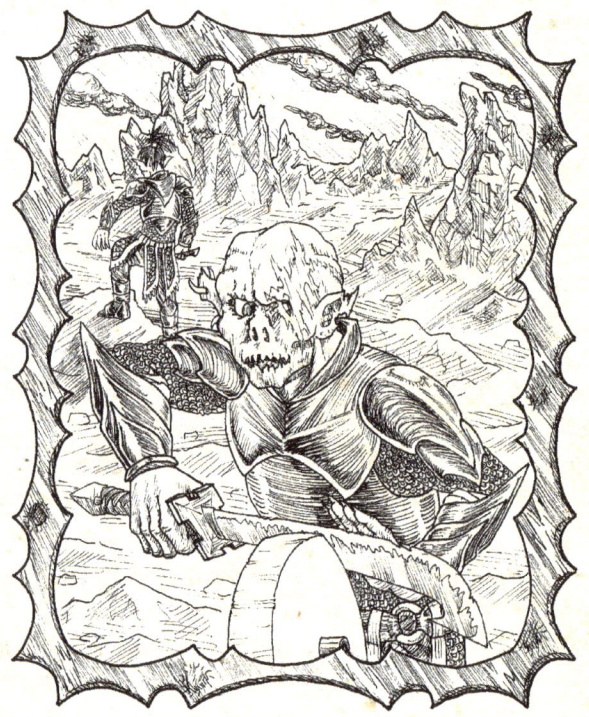

You'll be relieved to know I have given you more polite names for all of the recipes included in this chapter, in case you serve these dishes to people who might not have a warped sense of humor. Originally, I was thinking of adopting a sort of persona to introduce the recipes for this restaurant—I thought it would be fun to act like a female orc or goblin who longs to elevate her brethren and help them appreciate better quality foods; i.e., food that has actually been cooked for a while, not just torn out of someone's torso and devoured on the spot. But even a female orc would have to know that sometimes that's all a poor orc can manage, being off at war so often. I was going to call her Zeldóshâkh. Perhaps Zeldóshâkh heard about the dubious choices that some of her fellow orcs make while trying to dine on the road and she's decided to put her own, more sophisticated, spin on these items. However, as my mind kept conjuring up an orcish "lady" who would speak with a particular type of voice accompanied by various grunting noises, I decided it was better to let you envision your own version of a pedantic female goblin giving cooking instructions to class up her cousins.

Fungus Liquid
(a.k.a. Mushroom Bacon Bisque)

You have to imagine that life as an orc is pretty brutal. But even your average monster needs to find some comfort in his (or her—it's really hard to picture female orcs, isn't it?) crudely made bowl after a long day of slaughter. The only objection an orc could make here would be that there are way too many vegetables in this soup and not enough meat.

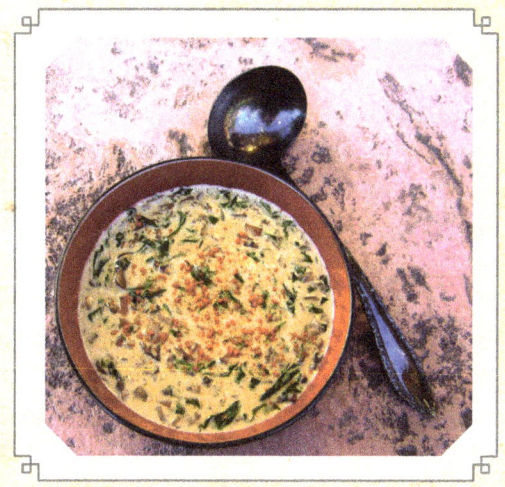

2 tablespoons salted butter
2 ounces good quality precooked bacon, cut into ¼" slices
1 tablespoon minced garlic
1 cup red onion, coarsely chopped
1½ pounds fresh mushrooms, coarsely chopped
⅓ cup all-purpose flour
14½-ounce can low-sodium beef broth
2 tablespoons cream sherry
1 tablespoon Worcestershire sauce
1 teaspoon dry thyme (or dry summer savory)
½ teaspoon each:
    Savory Seasoning   paprika
    pepper   salt
5-6 ounces fresh baby spinach, coarsely chopped
1 cup heavy cream
Additional paprika for garnish

Melt butter over medium/high heat in a 4-quart saucepan. Add the bacon and fry 2-3 minutes. Remove with a slotted spoon and place on a paper towel; set aside. Add the garlic, onion, and mushrooms to the saucepan; cover and cook over medium/high heat 5 minutes. Stir a few times. Uncover and add the flour, mixing well. Add the broth, sherry, Worcestershire sauce, and seasonings. Bring to a boil, then cook over medium/low heat, covered, 5 minutes. Add the spinach and mix in well, then add the cream. Bring to a nice simmer and cook uncovered over medium/low heat for

10 minutes, stirring occasionally. Add the bacon. Adjust seasonings, if desired. Ladle into bowls and sprinkle with additional paprika. Cover and refrigerate leftovers. Serves 3-4.

Add 4 ounces of roasted and chopped green chile, with juice, near the end of cooking.

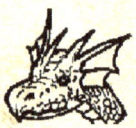

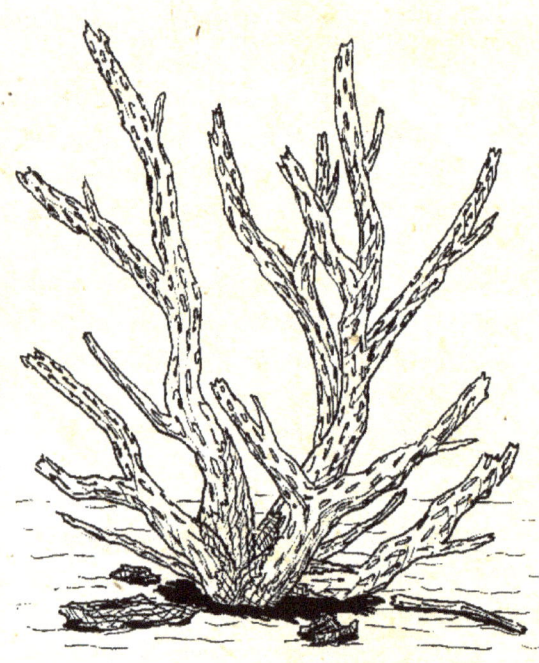

Zeldôshâkh's Gnarly Bones
(a.k.a. Spicy Breadsticks)

Some monsters have a good sense of humor and would appreciate the food puns in this chapter.

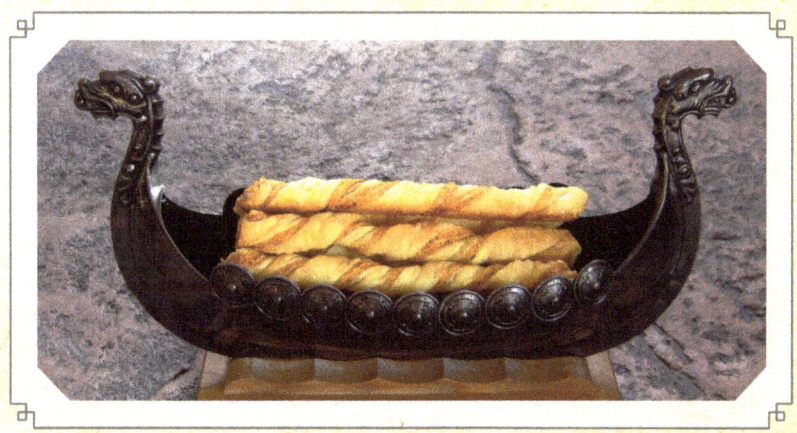

17.3-ounce package frozen puff pastry sheets, thawed according to package directions (such as Pepperidge Farm)
2 ounces Parmesan or Romano cheese, finely shredded
2 ounces Gruyere cheese, finely shredded (Swiss or Jarlsberg are also fine)
½ teaspoon cayenne pepper
½ teaspoon pepper
2 tablespoons salted butter, melted and cooled a bit
All-purpose flour

Preheat oven to 400°. Coat 2 large baking sheets with cooking spray or grease lightly. Combine the 2 cheeses in a medium bowl. Combine the seasonings in a tiny bowl. Unfold 1 pastry sheet and place on counter, with the creases running vertically. Brush ¼ of butter in the middle section, sprinkle with ¼ of the pepper mixture, then sprinkle with ¼ of the cheese mixture. Press into pastry. Fold the right side over the cheese then repeat the layering on top of this section. Fold the left side over this and press together, especially at the edges.

Flip pastry over and rotate, so it now faces you horizontally. Place on a lightly floured surface. Roll the pastry out to a rectangle that is about 16" wide and 7" deep. Using a pizza slicer, cut once in the center vertically, then cut horizontally into 6 strips at approximately 1" intervals. Hold the ends of each and twist a few times, then place 1" apart on prepared sheet. Press the ends onto the sheet. Repeat with the other pastry sheet. Bake 15-17 minutes. Let stand on pans 5 minutes before serving. Cover and store at room temperature. Makes 24.

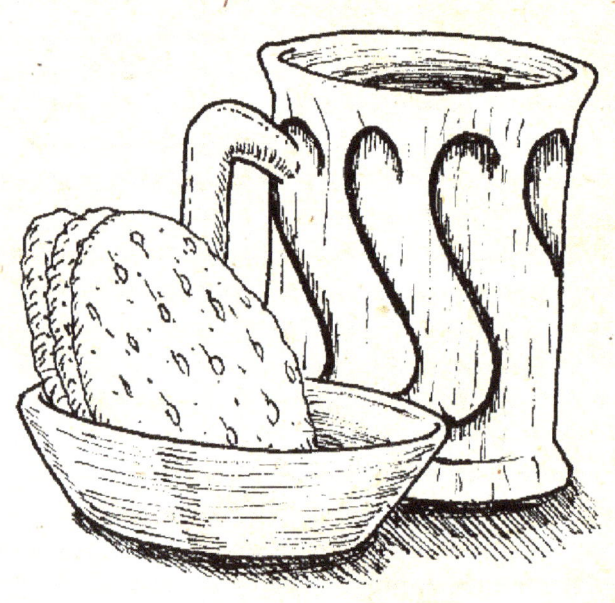

Must Eat Brain Food...
(a.k.a. Cauliflower Cheese)

The next item is a solid side dish and not meant to be like a soufflé. If a zombie had even the tiniest inkling of consciousness left in his/her brain, he/she would undoubtedly appreciate the obvious double entendre in this recipe.

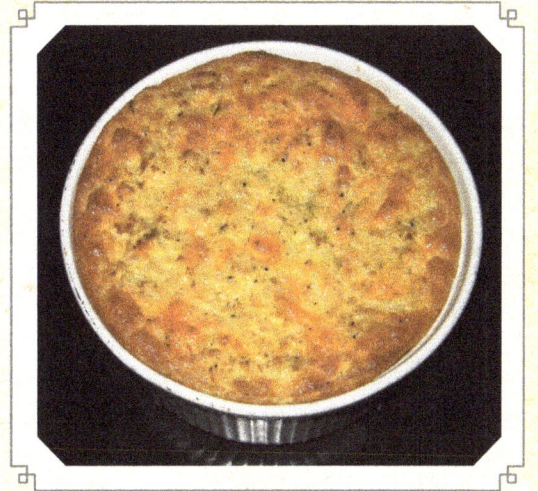

An average head of fresh cauliflower, cut into 1-2" florets (about 2 pounds, cored)
6 cups water
2 tablespoons salted butter, melted
¼ cup heavy cream
2 extra large eggs
2 tablespoons all-purpose flour
1 tablespoon baking powder
½ teaspoon salt
½ teaspoon pepper
¼ teaspoon nutmeg
4 ounces sharp Cheddar cheese, shredded

Preheat oven to 375°. Coat a 1-quart round casserole dish with cooking spray or grease lightly. Place cauliflower in a 4-quart saucepan with 6 cups water; bring to a boil. Lower heat to medium and cook 15 minutes, or until cauliflower is fork tender. Drain; return to the saucepan and mash coarsely, so there are still some small chunks of cauliflower left (some cooking liquid will remain—that's okay). Add the butter to the saucepan. In a 2-cup glass measuring cup, combine the cream, eggs, flour, baking powder, and seasonings with a whisk. Add this to the saucepan, then add the cheese. Pour into the prepared dish and bake 45-55 minutes, or until a knife inserted in the center comes out mostly clean; the center should be set. Let it stand 10 minutes before serving. Serve hot or warm. Cover and refrigerate leftovers. Serves 6.

Add 4 ounces roasted and chopped green chile, well-drained, with the eggs.

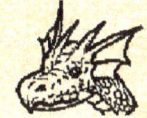

Chapter Seven: Monstrous Morsels

Pig & Curd on Bread
(a.k.a. Brie & Bacon Panini)

This sandwich is designed especially for trolls, though in a scaled-down proportion. While a whole sandwich would probably be fairly substantial for a human being, this would merely be an *amuse-bouche* for your average troll...

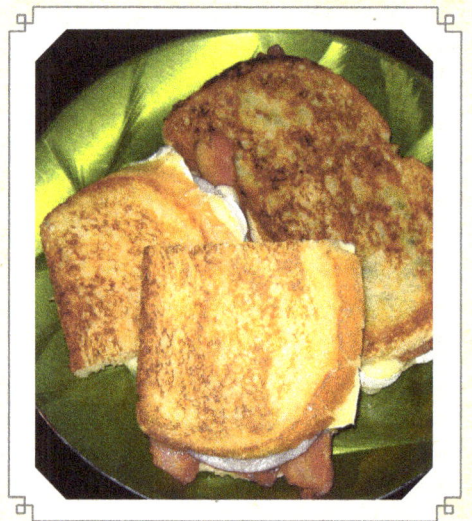

- 2 tablespoons small capers, drained well
- 1 tablespoon mayonnaise
- 2 teaspoons Dijon mustard
- 2 teaspoons prepared horseradish
- 4 slices sourdough or multi-grain bread, about ½" thick, 4" by 5"
- 7-8 ounces Brie, Camembert, or Limburger cheese, cut into ¼" slices (use the rind as well; you might not use all of it)
- A large red onion—cut 4 slices from the center, ¼" thick
- 6 slices good quality bacon, cooked until crispy (precooked variety is okay)
- 3-4 tablespoons soft salted butter, or spreadable margarine

Combine the first 4 ingredients in a small bowl and set aside. Lay 1 slice of bread on a cutting board and layer it with half the cheese, 2 slices of onion, and 3 strips of bacon. Spread half of the mustard mixture on another slice of bread and place this side down on top of the bacon. Press down all over the sandwich. Spread the top with about a tablespoon of butter. Repeat with the remaining ingredients. Heat a griddle to medium/hot.

CAREFULLY[1] place each sandwich on hot griddle, butter side down, and press down all over with your hands or a spatula. Now butter the tops of each. When golden brown (2-3 minutes should do), CAREFULLY flip each over. Press down all over again with spatula and fry the other side until it is golden brown, another 2-3 minutes. Cut in half and serve. Cover and refrigerate leftovers. Serves 2-4.

[1] You can certainly use a sandwich press if you like (hence my term, *Panini*), but a common griddle will cook both at once and a press might only accommodate one at a time. I stress the word carefully in the recipe, since this is loaded with stuff and you don't want it all to fall out.

 **Vegetarian Option**—Omit the bacon or replace it with the vegetarian bacon substitute you like best. A few strips of roasted red pepper would also be good (pat dry with a paper towel).

A few strips of roasted green chile could make a killer sandwich.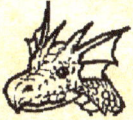

This is quite a pungent sandwich which is great on its own or as an accompaniment to soup. Limburger seems most fitting for trolls because of its smell (meaning no offense to trolls, of course…); however, I find it to have a rather mild flavor. You might disagree; in a casual sampling of Limburger cheese in my mother's kitchen, six people had different opinions on its flavor though everyone did agree it was definitely stinky. Bob likes this particular sandwich with Brie and sourdough. Callista dislikes raw onion, so I usually leave the slice off of her portion.

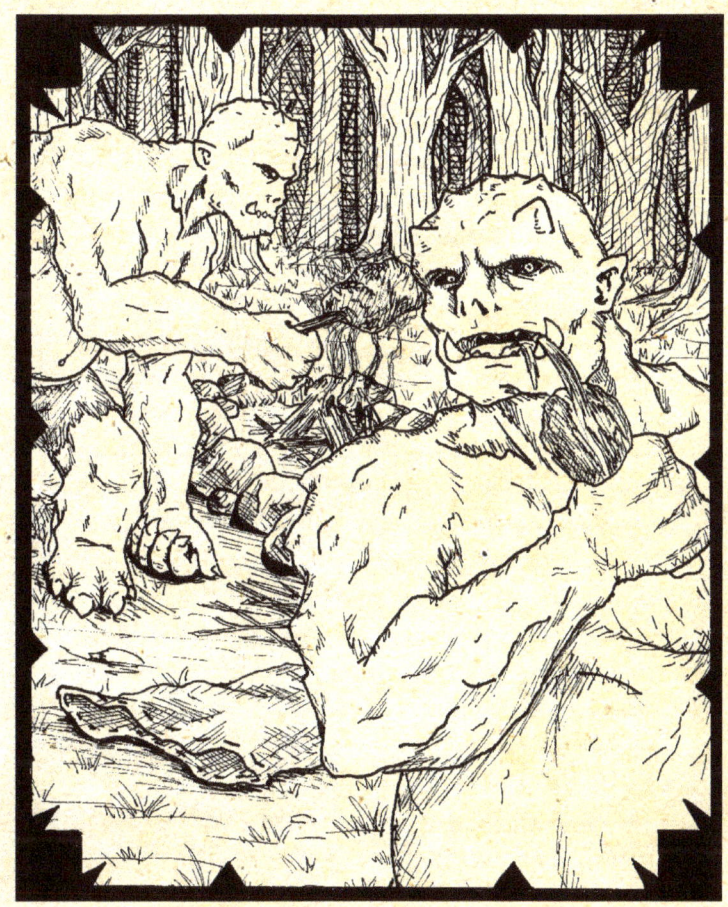

Some trolls prefer an even smellier version:

Want Stinkier Sandwich
(a.k.a. Bleu & Bacon Panini)

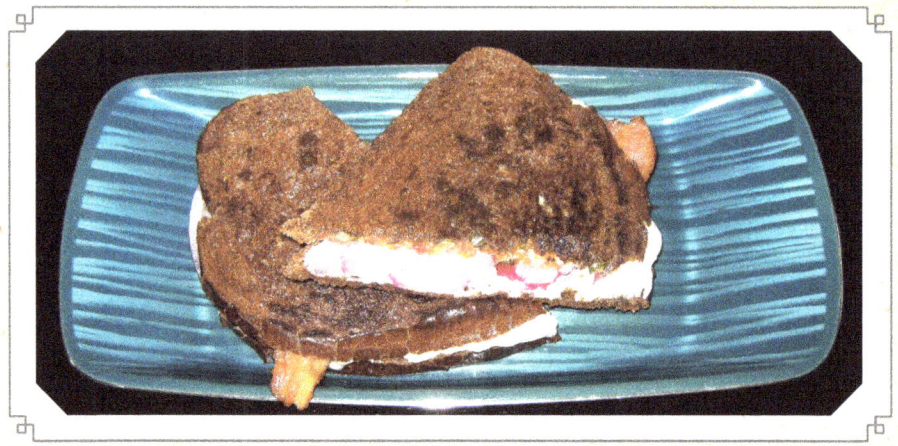

For this one, everything is the same with these exceptions:
- ☼ Use any kind of rye of pumpernickel for the bread

For the cheese, use:
- ☼ 2 ounces any sort of Bleu cheese—such as Gorgonzola (rather mild), Stilton, Bleu, or Roquefort (rather strong)—it just depends on your taste; crumbled.
- ☼ 3 ounces light cream cheese (Neufchâtel), softened

In a small bowl, mash the 2 cheeses together and spread equally on 2 slices of bread. Proceed with the directions in Pig & Curd on Bread. If you use pumpernickel, you will have to pay close attention to it, since it's already dark brown; you'll want it toasted but not burned. Cover and refrigerate leftovers. Serves 2-4.

 *My older daughter Chloë and I actually prefer this one; Bob hates rye breads and most sorts of Bleu cheeses. Gorgonzola seems to be the mildest of the Bleus, so sometimes I can get away with using this in various recipes.*

Glürbin's Gutless Wonders
(a.k.a. Curried Sausage Sandwiches)

I got this idea from food history reading. Apparently back in the day, sausages were quite popular—just as they are now. Unfortunately, one did not always have access to sterile intestines in which to encase your ground or chopped meat. So the idea of a "skinless sausage" became a trend. Obviously, this would save much time for a chef, who then wouldn't have to worry about sanitizing and then stuffing the casings (Wilson 313). I shudder to think of unclean intestines, don't you? Anyway, I immediately came up with the name "Gutless Wonders" and decided I had to create a spicy sandwich.

2 tablespoons plus 2 tablespoons salted butter
½ teaspoon plus 2 teaspoons hot Madras curry powder
1 teaspoon sugar
½ teaspoon dry thyme
¼ teaspoon plus ½ teaspoon salt
¼ teaspoon plus ½ teaspoon pepper
4 cups onion, cut into ½" slices
¼ cup all-purpose flour
1 pound hot bulk pork sausage
½ cup seasoned dry bread crumbs
1 extra large egg
½ cup low-sodium chicken broth
6 purchased good quality deli rolls
Maoglûrb's Mustard, recipe below

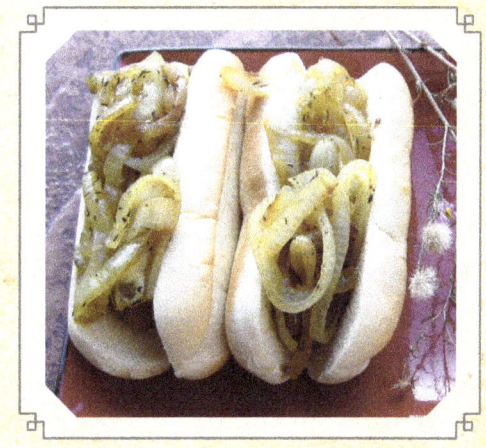

In a 3-quart deep skillet, melt 2 tablespoons butter over high heat. Add the ½ teaspoon curry, sugar, thyme, ¼ teaspoon salt, and ¼ teaspoon pepper. Separate the onion slices into rings and add to the skillet. Sauté over rather high heat 5 minutes, stirring frequently. Cover and cook over lowest heat 10 minutes; stir a couple of times. Let stand, covered.

Place the flour on a plate. Coat a 5-quart deep skillet with cooking spray. Place the sausage, bread crumbs, egg, 2 teaspoons curry, and the remaining salt and pepper in a medium bowl. With your hands, combine well. Divide the meat mixture into 6 portions and form each into a rough sausage; place on a plate. Melt 2 tablespoons butter over fairly high heat in the prepared skillet. Dredge sausages lightly in flour while still pressing the meat into cylinders about 6-7" long. Place in skillet and brown well on all sides. Add the chicken broth and bring to a boil. Cover and simmer over low heat 15 minutes, shaking the pan occasionally. Make mustard sauce now.

Meanwhile, lightly toast the rolls (or microwave briefly just to warm them). Place a sausage in a roll, spread with ½ tablespoon mustard, then top with onions. Serve immediately, while warm, or even at room temperature. Cover and refrigerate leftovers. Serves 6.

Maoglûrb's Mustard

2 tablespoons Dijon mustard
1 tablespoon mayonnaise
½ tablespoon prepared horseradish
½ teaspoon hot Madras curry powder

In a small bowl, whisk together all ingredients. Cover and refrigerate leftovers. Makes about 3 tablespoons, just enough for 6 Gutless Wonders. Double the recipe, if you want to make sure you have enough, then you can also use it on other sandwiches.

We've eaten these while watching the Super Bowl or other games (Bob is a longtime Vikings fan who lives in perpetual disappointment. I originally wrote this in 2010 and now I'm editing this again for a second edition in 2017. He is still disappointed…). They really do not look very pretty, which you'll notice when you make them; however, they do taste delicious. They are also fine without the onions. If you have leftovers, slice the meat, cook some wide noodles or pappardelle and combine with the mustard and onions (add some chicken broth to make a light sauce).

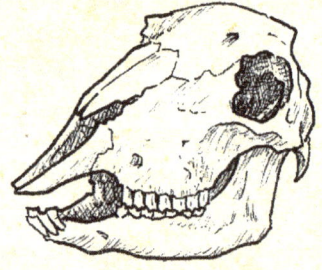

Meat on Metal Stick
(a.k.a. Lamb Kabobs with Mint Marinade)

Trolls love this dish, and the bit of mint in the marinade is often the only vegetable the average troll consumes. Often in the wilderness, the best a troll can get is a slow-moving bit of mutton. When they dine out, they prefer some tender lamb.

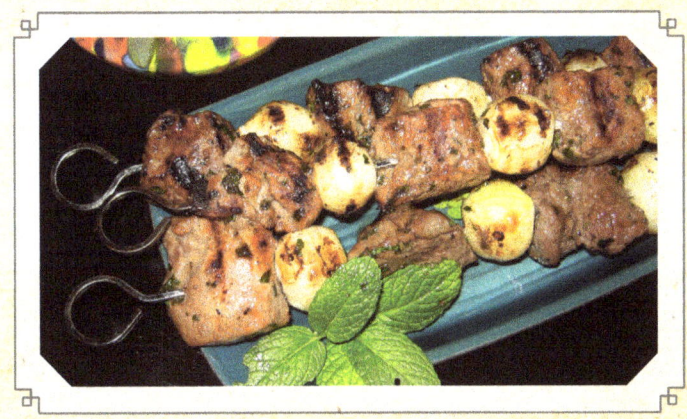

1 tablespoon each:
- honey
- walnut oil
- soy sauce
- red wine vinegar
- cream sherry
- Worcestershire sauce
- crushed ginger, fresh or from a jar

3-4 tablespoons fresh mint, minced
½ teaspoon salt
½ teaspoon pepper
1-1¼ pounds lamb (stew meat or from a roast), cut into 20 chunks, each about 2" or so[1]
3 cups water
16 pearl onions, any color (small boiler onions would also work)

[1] Other good protein choices are beef, pork (cuts such as tenderloin and sirloin are best), and chicken (preferably breast meat), and even large peeled shrimp (like tiger-size—tail on or not).

Combine the first 10 ingredients in a covered jar and shake well. Place lamb in a medium-sized bowl and pour the marinade over all. Refrigerate 2-3 hours (or even overnight); stir occasionally.

Meanwhile, in a 2-quart saucepan, combine 3 cups water and the onions. Bring to a boil and cook 1 minute. Drain and set aside until cool enough to handle. Cut off the ends and pull off the peel. On 4 metal skewers coated with cooking spray, alternately thread 5 chunks of lamb and 4 onions on each, beginning and ending with lamb; reserve marinade for basting. Place on a medium baking sheet. Coat grill with cooking spray and preheat to medium. Place kabobs on grill and liberally brush with half of the marinade. Cook 3-5 minutes. Turn the kabobs over and brush again with remaining marinade. Cook another 3-5 minutes or until meat is cooked to the desired temperature.[2] Let the kabobs rest for a couple of minutes on a clean baking sheet, then remove from skewers and serve. Cover and refrigerate leftovers. Serves 4.

[2] Cooking times will vary depending on your grill, your choice of meats, and your own taste.

Vegetarian Option—Simply replace the meat with various vegetables cut into 1" chunks or left whole. Good choices would be: bell peppers (any color), cherry tomatoes, mushrooms, and summer squashes (unpeeled). You could try falafel for a high protein option.

Actually, around our house, we're not too keen on lamb, let alone mutton (especially Bob). Happily, this recipe completely lends itself to the choices mentioned above. You can serve this over a rice pilaf or with crusty bread. Any sort of salad or vegetable goes well with this dish, though I doubt that trolls care much for green stuff.

Raskofim's Roadkill
(a.k.a. Braised Chicken & Pork with Artichokes)

Orcs probably eat on the run quite often and take advantage of whatever they find on their violent way to whatever battle they are attending…

750 ml. bottle dry white wine,
    such as Chardonnay
½ cup of a prepared lemony, garlicky,
    herby marinade
½ teaspoon each:
    salt
    pepper
    turmeric
¼ teaspoon cayenne pepper
1 cup onion, diced
1¾-2 pounds boneless country-style
    pork ribs
1¾-2 pounds boneless, skinless chicken thighs (trim off any large bits of fat)
½ cup heavy cream
⅓ cup all-purpose flour or Wondra
14-ounce can diced tomatoes, drained well
2 [14-ounce] cans tiny artichoke hearts, drained well (or medium hearts, cut in halves)
2 tablespoons small capers, drained well

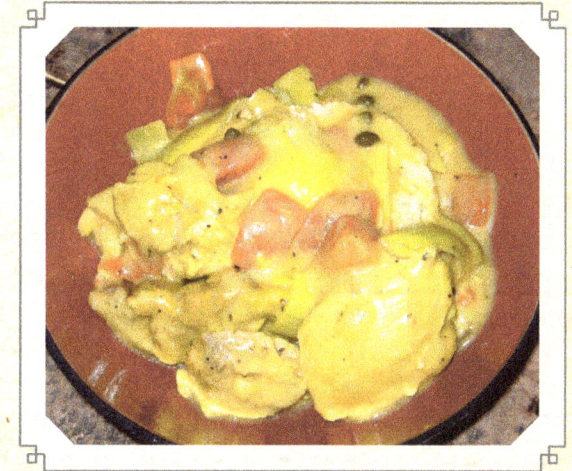

In a 6-quart saucepan, combine the wine, marinade, and the 4 seasonings. Add the onion and pork ribs. Bring to a boil, cover, then simmer at the lowest heat 1 hour. Add the chicken, bring to a boil again, cover, and simmer another 1½ hours at the lowest heat—the meat should be very tender. Stir a couple of times. With tongs, remove the meat to a plate and cover with the saucepan lid.

Pour the cream into a 2-cup glass measuring cup. Add ½ cup of the cooking sauce and the flour and whisk until smooth. Add to the saucepan and bring to a boil, whisking until thick and smooth. Lower heat to medium and add the remaining ingredients. Cook 5 minutes. Add back the meat and adjust seasonings, if desired. Cover and refrigerate leftovers. Serves 6-8.

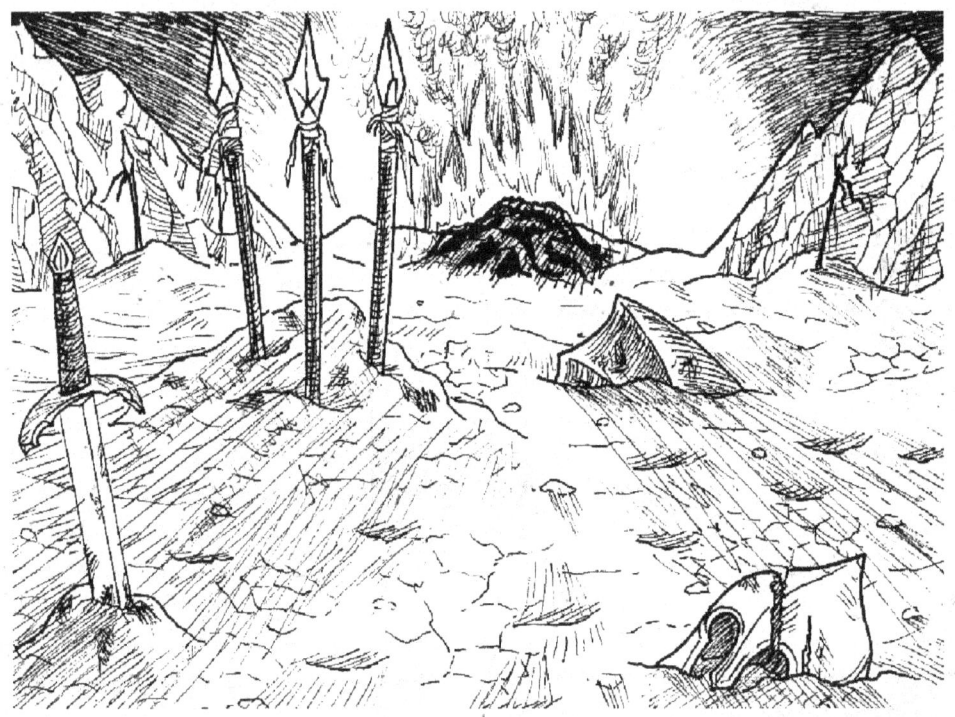

 *Serve this stew with a carbohydrate of your choice; the best ones are rice or couscous, though pasta and crusty bread are also nice. Beer is an excellent accompaniment... as usual...*

Gündürnüb's Grüb
(a.k.a. Seafood with Saffron Rice)

Here's an elegant dish which allows you a great amount of freedom in your protein choices, though being land-locked, my own choices are usually limited and expensive. Monsters certainly ate like gourmands around my house when I was testing these recipes. But I'm sure lots of people have completely different access to affordable seafood than I do. Serve with a salad, and some crusty bread is welcome on the side.

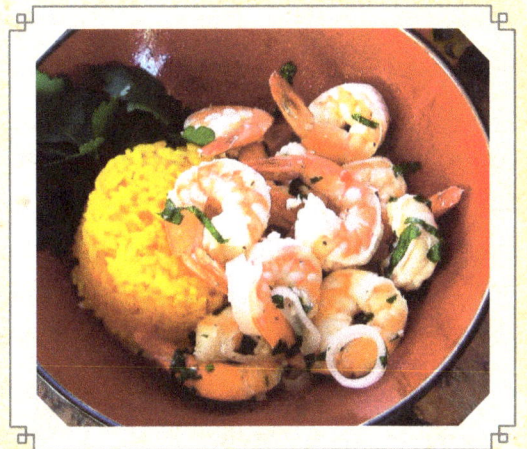

1 cup short grain rice
1⅓ cups water
1 teaspoon saffron, crushed
½ teaspoon plus ½ teaspoon salt
3 tablespoons plus 5 tablespoons salted butter
¾ cup shallots, cut into ¼" slices
2-3 tablespoons fresh garlic, minced or cut into paper-thin slices
2-2¼ pounds various raw shellfish[1]
½ cup dry white wine, such as Chardonnay
2 tablespoons lemon juice
½ teaspoon pepper
¼ cup fresh parsley, minced

In a 1½-quart saucepan, combine the rice, water, saffron, and ½ teaspoon salt. Bring to a boil and stir once. Cover and reduce heat to the lowest setting. Cook 15 minutes. Turn off heat and add 3 tablespoons butter. Cover again; let stand undisturbed 15-20 minutes.

[1] This reflects the weight without any shells, and you will need all your fish choices to be in bite-size pieces. This dish is free to interpret according to what is available to you—good choices are: bay scallops, lobster, or peeled shrimp (tail on or not); combinations are nice, or you can simply use one. If using frozen seafood, thaw according to package directions. I'll inevitably use the 2-pound bag of large, peeled, raw, tail-on frozen shrimp which I usually get from a place like—you guessed it—Costco.

Chapter Seven: Monstrous Morsels

Meanwhile, when your rice has cooked and while it is standing, melt the 5 tablespoons butter in a 5-quart deep skillet over very high heat. Add shallots and garlic and sauté 1 minute, just until the butter starts to brown. Add your seafood and cook over very high heat 2-3 minutes, stirring often, until fish is almost done (be careful not to overcook!). Add the wine, lemon juice, ½ teaspoon salt, and pepper. Sauté another minute or two. Season, as desired. Right before serving, stir rice and divide into bowls; pour fish and sauce over each. Sprinkle each with parsley. Cover and refrigerate leftovers. Serves 4-6.

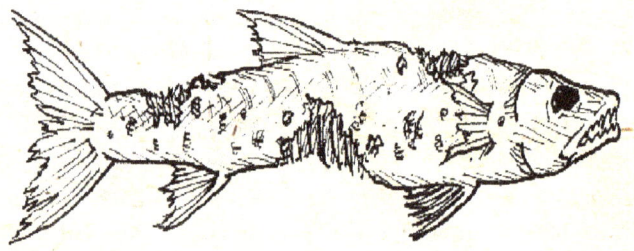

 **Vegetarian Option—**The rice is a completely separate item and requires no adjustment. To replace the fish, I would suggest any combination of bell peppers, onions, summer squashes, broccoli, cauliflower, or asparagus. You should have a total of 2-3 pounds worth of vegetables. All should be cut into relatively uniform 1" pieces; sauté just until they are crisp-tender, around 5-6 minutes.

 Bob actually enjoys this dish—so that's saying something! I would love to make this just with lobster, but I would probably need to refinance my house to do that.

Chunks & Gobbets
(a.k.a. Sauerkraut Sausage)

You know, reading a bit of food history will really change your perspective and make you glad you are living in the modern world, mostly. In older recipe books, however, you will actually read directions that sound positively monstrous, and put you in mind of modern horror movies, with zombie attacks or serial slashings. Colorful verbs such as hacking, ripping, smiting, and hewing are common in recipes (Tannahill 247). I was thinking instructions like these would have been fun to use if I had adopted that goblin persona, Zeldóshâkh.

When I originally made this up, I assumed one pound of sausage would be enough and, nutritionally, it should be (along with the one pound of pork). Yet I noticed that the sausage would always seem to disappear because *certain* people (you know who you are!) would come along and sneak pieces out while the stew was cooking. So, I decided to go ahead and call for two pounds of sausage. You can omit the sauerkraut if you like and just serve some crusty bread alongside the stew, like a sourdough.

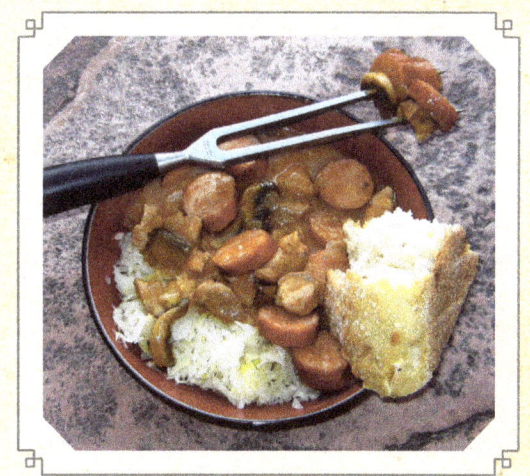

- ¼ cup salted butter
- 3-4 cups onion, coarsely ripped into ½" morsels
- 2 tablespoons minced garlic
- 1 pound pork tenderloin or sirloin, hewn into 1" gobbets
- ½ pound fresh mushrooms, slashed into ¼" slices
- ⅓ cup all-purpose flour or Wondra
- ½ teaspoon salt
- ½ teaspoon pepper
- 2 teaspoons paprika
- ⅓ cup spicy brown mustard
- 2 teaspoons Worcestershire sauce
- 2 [14½-ounce] cans low-sodium chicken broth
- 1-2 pounds Polish or smoked sausage (any variety), hacked into ¼" or ½" slices
- 2 pounds good quality sauerkraut

Coat a 6-quart saucepan with cooking spray. Melt the butter over high heat. Add the onion, garlic, pork, and mushrooms. Sauté until the pork loses its pink color. Add the flour, salt, pepper, and paprika and mix well. Then add the mustard, Worcestershire sauce, and broth and bring to a boil. Add the sausage, reduce heat to medium/low and cook, uncovered, 45 minutes, stirring frequently and scraping up the brown bits on the bottom of the pot. Adjust seasonings, if desired.

Meanwhile, put the sauerkraut in a 2-quart saucepan. Cover and cook over medium heat until fully heated. Drain or use tongs to place the sauerkraut in bowls. Ladle stew over all or serve on the side. Serve with some crusty bread. Cover and refrigerate leftovers. Serves 6-8.

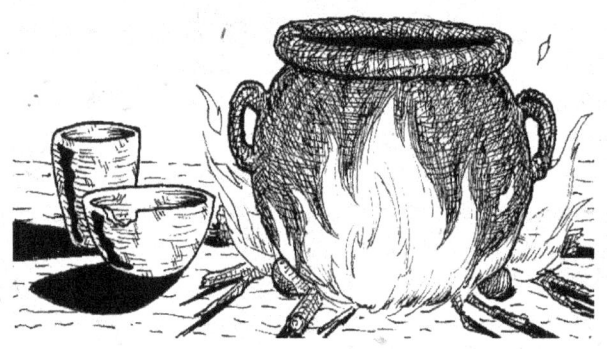

Now I must tell you, I was trying to remember an old recipe when I developed this. Bob loves sauerkraut (…though he hates cooked cabbage…) and pork and sausage. I had an old Better Homes and Gardens *cookbook with a stew recipe using those ingredients which I made a few times. This old cookbook is long gone from my house, having been replaced by a newer edition. This was not a recipe I liked much, since at the time I really disliked sauerkraut—now I can tolerate it, but only in small amounts.*

Anyway, I had an induction appointment to have Chloë in 1989, so I made up a batch of this stew for Bob to have while I was in the hospital. Then life interfered, plus a second daughter, Callista, and the original cookbook disappeared, probably in some garage sale. So this recipe hearkens back to the original, but I really can't remember all of the original ingredients. I do remember it used canned mushrooms. Bob likes this version just as well, if not better, especially since I increased the amount of sausage. And keep in mind, you can always omit the sauerkraut if you also dislike it; the stew alone with some bread makes a hearty meal.

Clôxiga's Crunchable Salmon
(a.k.a. Salmon with Sriracha)

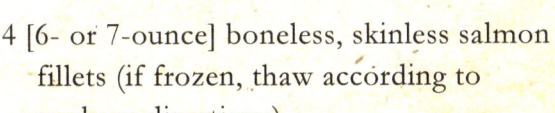

If you don't care for spice, substitute ketchup for the Sriracha or simply omit it entirely. These fillets are also good with tartar sauce (see Farsi's Tartar Sauce on page 117, if you would like a recipe).

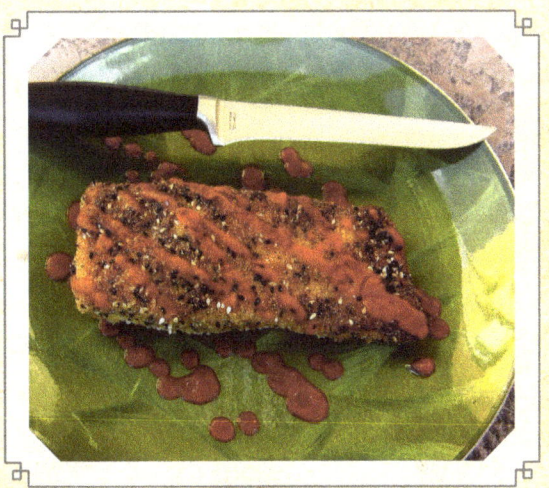

- 4 [6- or 7-ounce] boneless, skinless salmon fillets (if frozen, thaw according to package directions)
- ½ cup buttermilk
- 1 tablespoon Sriracha chili sauce
- ½ teaspoon plus ¼ teaspoon salt
- ½ teaspoon plus ¼ teaspoon pepper
- ⅓ cup seasoned dry bread crumbs
- 3 tablespoons cornmeal
- 2 tablespoons sesame seeds (any color)
- 1 teaspoon poppy seeds
- ¼ cup vegetable oil
- 4 teaspoons sesame oil
- Additional Sriracha chili sauce, if desired

Preheat oven to 450°. Coat a large baking sheet with cooking spray or grease lightly. In a shallow bowl, whisk together the buttermilk, Sriracha, ½ teaspoon salt, and ½ teaspoon pepper. In another shallow bowl, combine the bread crumbs, cornmeal, the remaining salt and pepper, and all the seeds. Pour the oil into a 5-quart deep skillet. Turn on a very high heat while you prepare the fish. Coat a fillet with the buttermilk mixture, then coat all over in the bread crumb mixture. Place in hot oil. Repeat with the remaining fillets (discard the extra buttermilk). Sprinkle leftover crumb mixture over fish if there are bare spots. Fry about 3-4 minutes until golden brown. Carefully turn over and fry an additional 3-4 minutes until golden brown. Place on prepared sheet and bake 10 minutes. Drizzle each with 1 teaspoon sesame oil and drizzle with extra Sriracha, if desired. Cover and refrigerate leftovers. Serves 4.

Tshigwí's Bit o' the Flank
(a.k.a. Savory Stuffed Flank Steak)

Inspired by a lovely scene in Peter Jackson's film version of *The Two Towers*, this goes well with any sort of carbohydrate you like—mashed potatoes are probably the best choice, but try rice, pasta, or even couscous.

½ teaspoon plus ¼ teaspoon salt
½ teaspoon plus ¼ teaspoon pepper
½ teaspoon plus ½ teaspoon paprika
¼ cup dry bread crumbs[1]
¼ cup minced onion
1 ounce Parmesan or Romano cheese, finely shredded
1 tablespoon minced garlic
A large beef flank steak (around 2¼ pounds)
2 tablespoons salted butter
1 cup dry red wine, such as Cabernet Sauvignon or Merlot
14½-ounce can low-sodium beef broth
¼ cup all-purpose flour or Wondra
1 tablespoon Worcestershire sauce
Kitchen twine

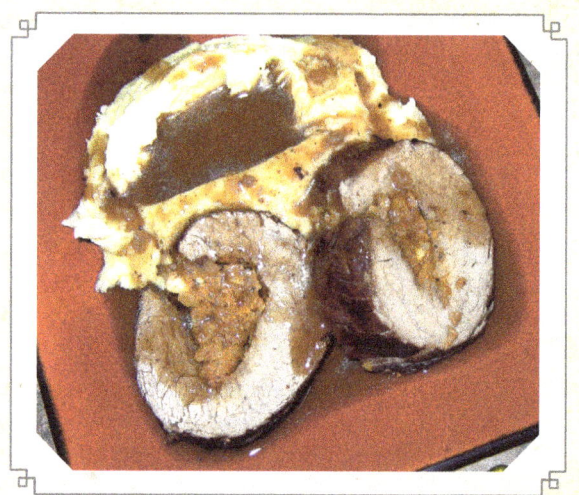

[1] Plain, seasoned, or try Panko bread crumbs.

Cut kitchen twine into 5 lengths, 15" each. For the rub, combine the ½ teaspoon each of salt, pepper, and paprika in a tiny bowl. In a small bowl, combine the bread crumbs, onion, cheese, garlic, and remaining seasonings; set aside. Place the steak on a large cutting board. Sprinkle half of the rub onto the steak and press in. Turn meat over and repeat with the remaining rub. Place crumb mixture down the center of the steak. Fold the sides up and secure snugly with the twine (any stuffing that falls out can just be added to the saucepan with the meat).

Coat a 6-quart saucepan with cooking spray, then melt the butter over rather high heat. Carefully place the steak in the saucepan and brown all over (again, it's okay if some stuffing falls out). Add the wine and broth and bring to a boil. Reduce heat to

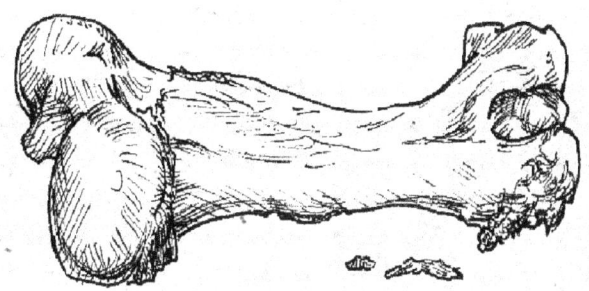

a very low gentle simmer, cover, and cook 2 hours. Turn meat over every 30 minutes. Remove meat to a clean cutting board and cover with the saucepan lid. Combine 1 cup cooking liquid, flour, and Worcestershire sauce in a 2-cup glass measuring cup with a whisk. Bring remaining cooking liquid to a boil, then whisk in the flour mixture. Cook over high heat, scraping up any brown bits until sauce thickens. Adjust seasonings, if desired. Cut the strings, then cut the steak into ½" or ¾" slices. Pour gravy over meat. Cover and refrigerate leftovers. Serves 4-6.

As usual, 4 ounces of drained, roasted, chopped green chile is a great addition to the gravy at the end.

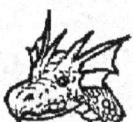

Cold Dead Livid Bread
(a.k.a. Blueberry Quick Bread)

Monsters sometimes like bizarre colors in their foods.

½ cup soft salted butter
¾ cup sugar
1 extra large egg, room temperature
2½ cups all-purpose flour
2 teaspoons baking powder
2 teaspoons cinnamon
¾ teaspoon salt
½ teaspoon baking soda
¼ cup 1% milk, room temperature
14½-ounce can blueberries in light syrup
1 teaspoon vanilla extract
1 cup dried blueberries
4 ounces walnuts, lightly toasted and coarsely chopped

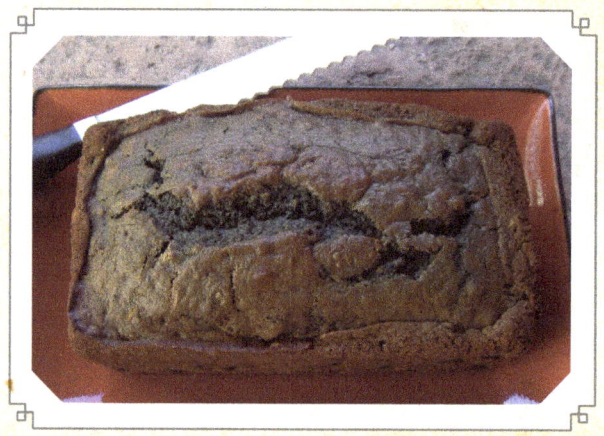

Preheat oven to 350°. Coat a 9" by 5" loaf pan with cooking spray or grease lightly. In a large bowl, combine the butter, sugar, and egg well on a medium speed. In a medium bowl, combine the flour, baking powder, cinnamon, salt, and baking soda. Place the milk, blueberries, and vanilla in a blender and blend until fully combined. Mix ⅓ of the dry ingredients into the butter, then half of the milk. Add alternately, beginning and ending with the dry ingredients and mixing well between each addition. Scrape sides, if needed. Add the dried blueberries and walnuts and combine well on medium speed. Spread into prepared pan and bake 60-70 minutes, until it tests done in the center. Place on a rack for 30 minutes. Turn out onto the rack and cool at least 4 hours before cutting. Store covered at room temperature. Serves 10-12.

This definitely has a scary and distinct color to it, more of a dark bluish-grey. If you really need a more authentic monster experience, let this loaf sit out uncovered on your counter for about a month—it's bound to change its texture and color and while that may be more appealing to monsters, you'd do better to eat it more quickly; it's delicious as a snack or serve as a dessert with ice cream.

Sweets for Sbileng
(a.k.a. Chocolate Raspberry Cake with Ganache)

You can think of blood and bones when you prepare this cake—at least, that's what true monsters would do...

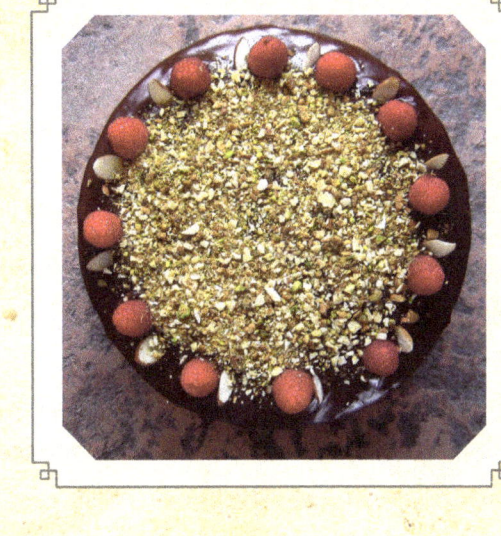

2 ounces pistachios; shelled, roasted, and salted
2 ounces sliced almonds
12 ounces fresh raspberries
1 cup water, room temperature
1 teaspoon vanilla extract
1 teaspoon almond extract
2¼ cups plus 3 tablespoons all-purpose flour
1 teaspoon baking soda
½ teaspoon salt
½ teaspoon cream of tartar
½ cup unsweetened cocoa powder
1 cup vegetable oil
1½ cups sugar
4 extra large eggs, room temperature
2 cups heavy cream
1 pound bittersweet chocolate (60-72%; broken into squares or use chips)
12 perfect sliced almonds

Lightly toast the pistachios and the 2 ounces sliced almonds. Cool 30 minutes, then grind them finely. Set aside ¼ cup and place the remainder in a medium bowl. Wash the raspberries and place on a couple of paper towels. Set aside 12 perfect ones for garnish. Combine the water and extracts and set aside. Add the 2¼ cups flour, baking soda, salt, cream of tartar, and cocoa powder to the ground nuts and mix well; set aside.

Preheat oven to 350°. Liberally coat three 9" heavy, round pans with cooking spray or grease lightly. Sprinkle 1 tablespoon flour in each and shake the pans to coat mostly the bottoms. Combine the oil, sugar, and eggs in a stand mixer and beat on medium speed until well combined. Add ⅓ of the flour mixture to the oil mixture, then add half of the water mixture; beat on medium speed about 30 seconds after each addition. Add another ⅓ of the flour, the remaining water, then end with the flour mixture, beating well on a medium speed; scrape down the sides. Add the raspberries and mix on low speed for a few seconds. Pour batter equally into the prepared pans. Bake 28-32 minutes, until the centers test done.

Meanwhile, prepare the ganache: Start when you put the cakes in the oven. Pour the cream into a 2-quart saucepan and cook over a medium/high heat until it starts to simmer. Take off the heat and add the chocolate. Whisk until the chocolate is completely melted and smooth. Cover and let stand.[1]

Place pans on racks and let stand 1 hour. If necessary, use a knife around the sides of the pans and remove cakes from pans; place on racks for another 15 minutes or until cool.

To assemble: place 1 cake layer on a platter. Spread with ⅓ cup ganache. Place another cake layer on top and spread with another ⅓ cup ganache. Place the last layer on top and spread about ¾ cup ganache all over the top and sides; working quickly, fill in bare spots with more ganache. Sprinkle the nuts evenly on the top. Place the reserved raspberries and the sliced almonds at equal intervals around the outer edge of the cake. Refrigerate about 30 minutes to set the ganache before serving. You may pour more ganache (reheat slowly) over the slices. For long-term storage, cover and store in the refrigerator; let stand at room temperature about an hour before serving it. Cover and refrigerate leftover ganache; reheat slowly. Serves 12.

---

[1] Keep this in mind as a simple ganache recipe, for those times when you need warm, chocolatey goodness for other desserts. You can let it cool and become more solid for use as a spreadable frosting. Cream and chocolate—paradise.

Queevhô's Bleedin' Treats
(a.k.a. Cherry Lava Cakes)

Your average goblin would savor these treats while relishing memories of past skirmishes in the wild.

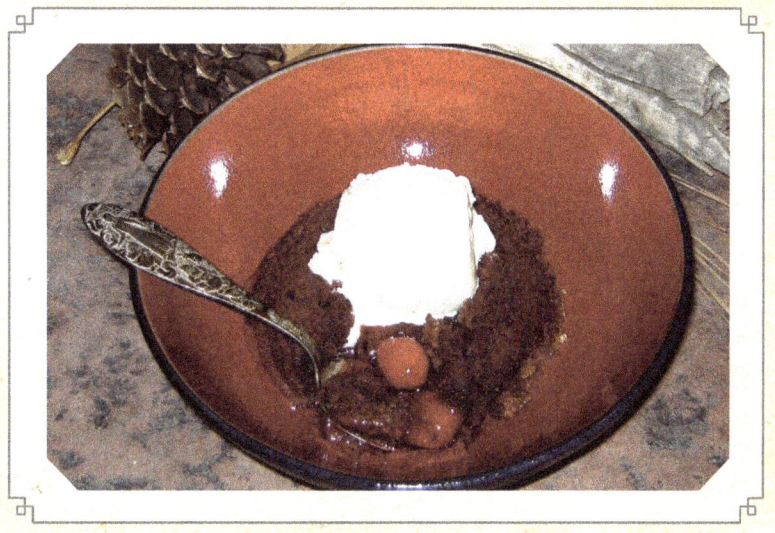

21-ounce can cherry pie filling (light or regular)
½ cup salted butter
8 ounces bittersweet chocolate (60-72%), broken into squares (chips are okay)
6 tablespoons turbinado (raw) sugar
¾ cup sugar
½ teaspoon salt
2 extra large eggs, room temperature
2 teaspoons vanilla extract
½ cup half-and-half, room temperature
1 cup all-purpose flour

Coat 6 regular-sized muffin cups with cooking spray. Divide the cherry pie filling evenly in each. Freeze about 3 hours, or until mostly firm.

Combine the butter and chocolate in a large glass bowl. Microwave on HIGH in 30-second intervals until fully melted. Let stand.

Preheat oven to 450°. Liberally coat six 1-cup ramekins with cooking spray, especially on the bottoms. Sprinkle 1 tablespoon turbinado sugar in each. Roll ramekin around to coat bottom and sides with the sugar. Place ramekins on a large baking sheet. Add the sugar, salt, eggs, and vanilla to the chocolate mixture and combine well with a whisk. Add the half-and-half and flour and whisk well. Divide equally into the ramekins. Use a sharp knife around the frozen cherries and place in each ramekin. Press down slightly. Bake 20-24 minutes. Let stand 10 minutes on the baking sheet. Use a sharp knife around the edge of each cake to invert into a dessert bowl. You can leave any leftover cakes in the ramekins; cover and keep at room temperature. Microwave about 45 seconds for fresh-out-of-the-oven cherry lava; don't bother inverting your cake, just eat it out of the ramekin. Makes 6.

This is **hardcore** *chocolate, to quote my son-in-law. If it's too intense, serve it with whipped cream, ice cream, or go crazy and intensify the chocolatey goodness by pouring some extra sauce all over the cakes—you could use the ganache in Sweets for Shileug, page 195, or just use a purchased fudge sauce. This is ideal to make around a Valentine's Day weekend of chocolate decadence.*

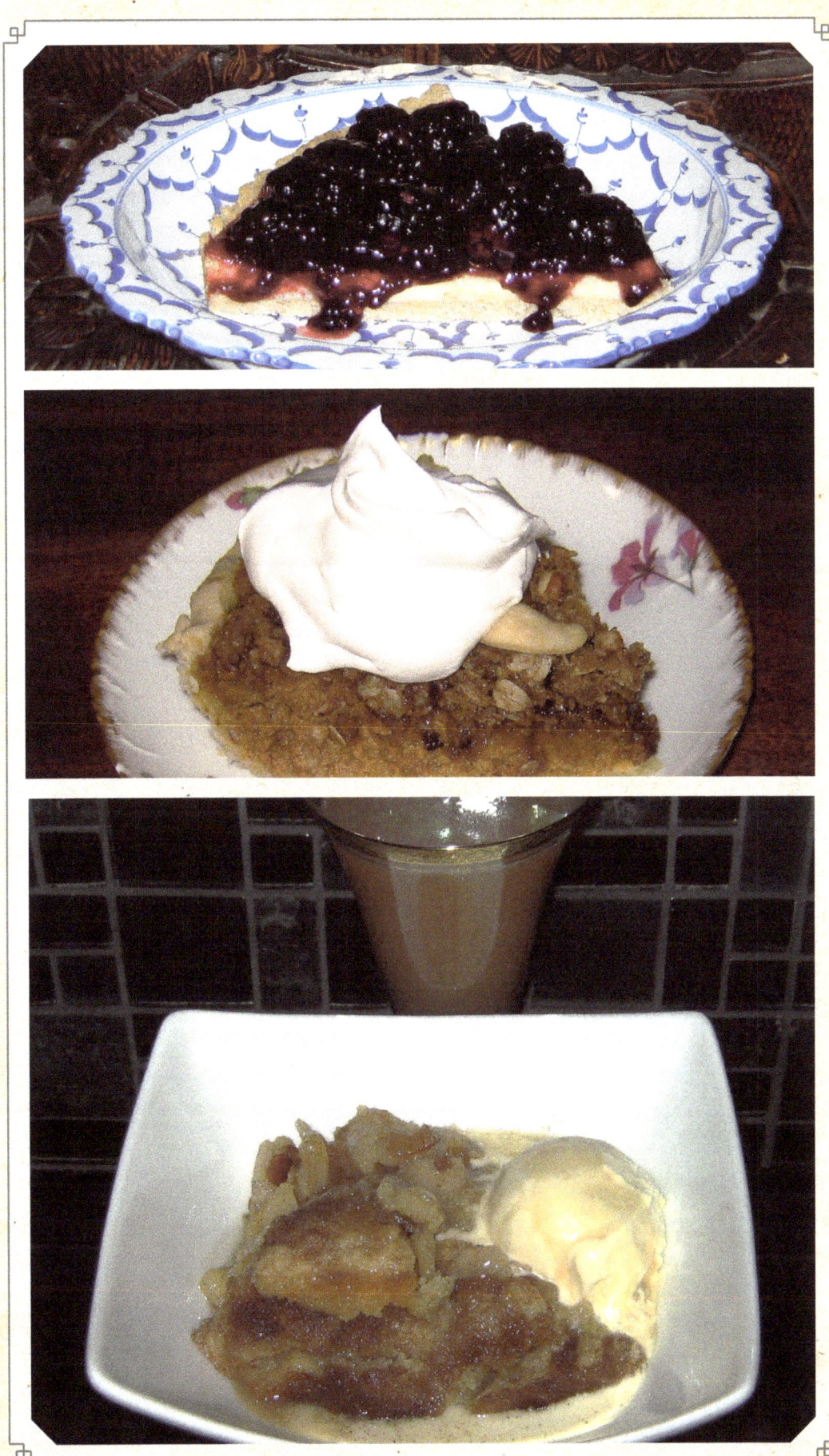

Chapter Eight

Nympha Nemorosa

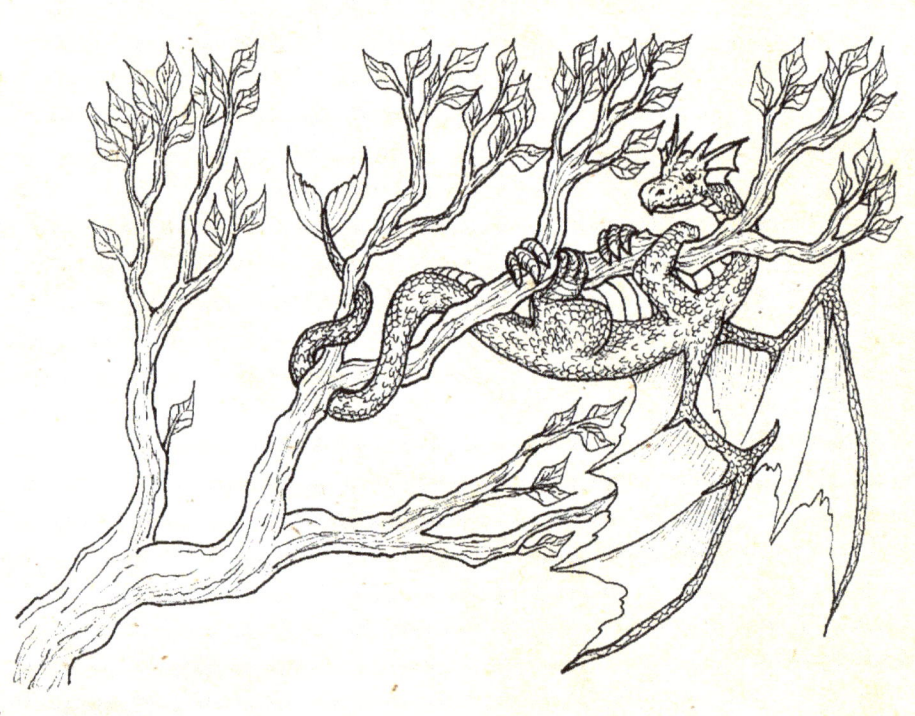

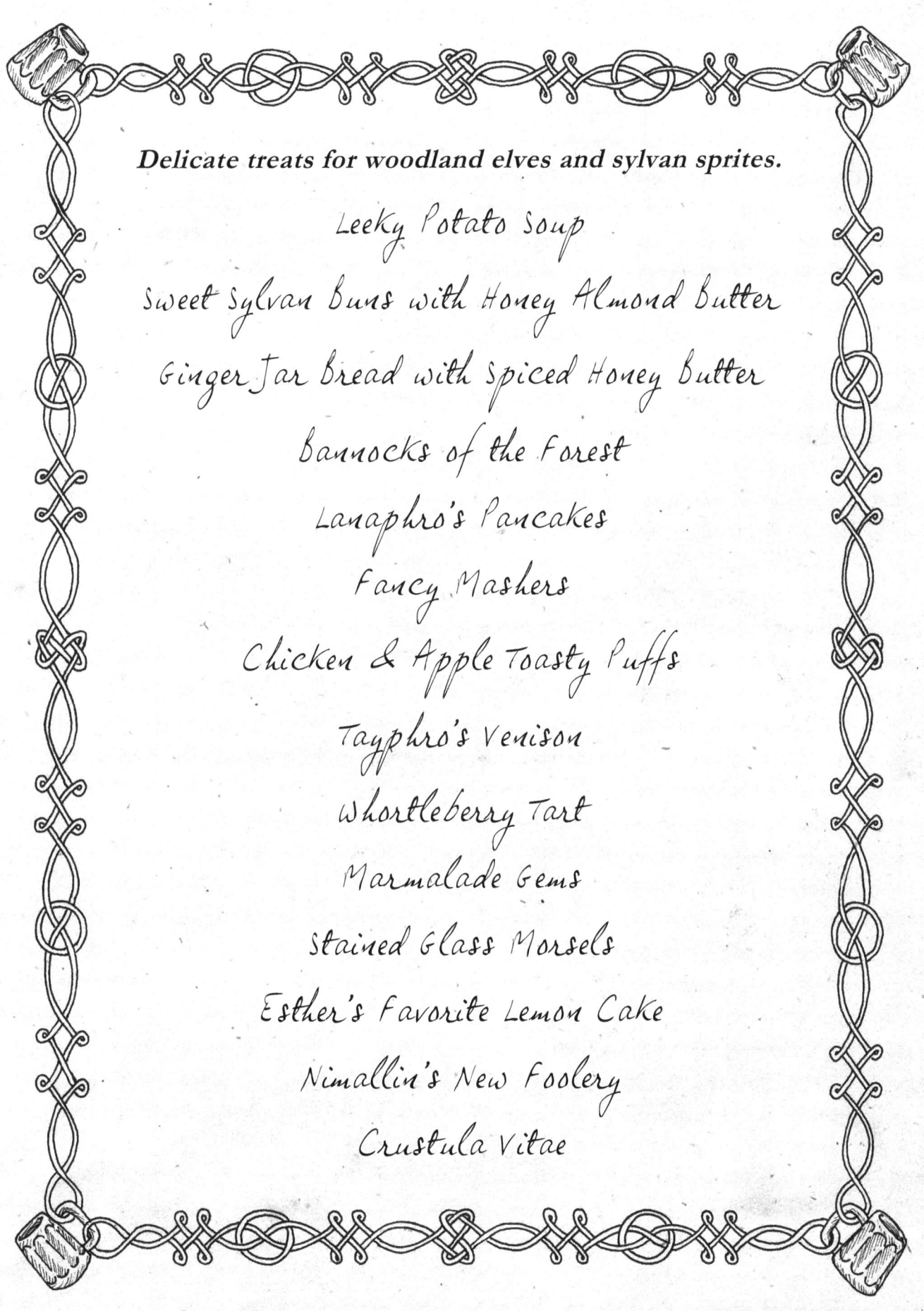

Delicate treats for woodland elves and sylvan sprites.

Leeky Potato Soup

Sweet Sylvan Buns with Honey Almond Butter

Ginger Jar Bread with Spiced Honey Butter

Bannocks of the Forest

Lanaphro's Pancakes

Fancy Mashers

Chicken & Apple Toasty Puffs

Tayphro's Venison

Whortleberry Tart

Marmalade Gems

Stained Glass Morsels

Esther's Favorite Lemon Cake

Nimallin's New Foolery

Crustula Vitae

Nympha Nemorosa

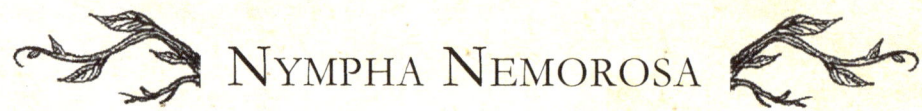

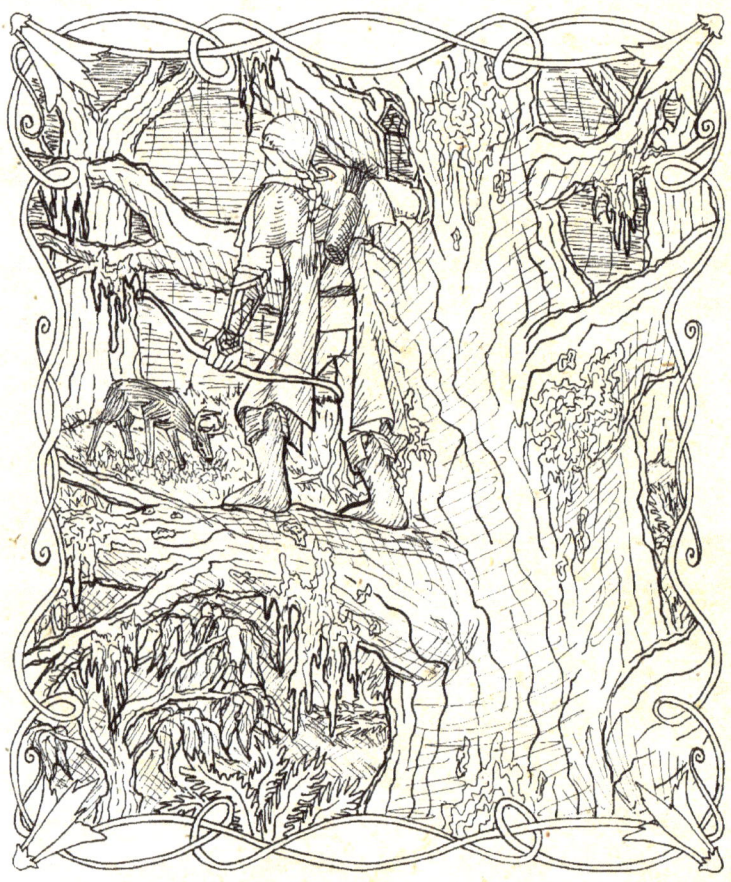

I'm just guessing what woodland elves and sylvan sprites (and fairies, pixies, kelpies, brownies, etc…) might like to eat. In Middle-earth, the only foods mentioned for elves are apples, wine, bannocks (oat-cakes), and venison; they are all here. You can imagine whatever type of elf you like when preparing these dishes; some of you might prefer them tall and arrogant, others might prefer them mischievous and diminutive. You could picture your favorite magical realm as a setting for this restaurant chapter; I would picture the Rivendell of the Jackson films.

Leeky Potato Soup

My mother frequently threw potatoes and leeks into a pot and made a creamy soup similar to this, but she never really told me her recipe. I have a feeling her basic formula probably evolved occasionally, but this one's just as good, if not better.

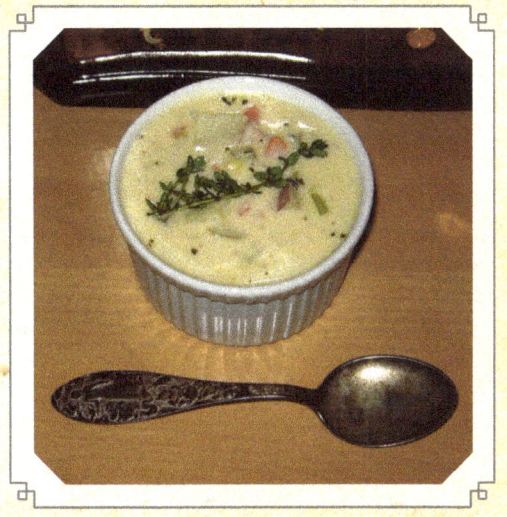

¼ cup salted butter
1 cup celery, cut into ¼" bits
1 cup carrot, peeled and cut into ¼" bits
4 cups very clean leeks, cut into ¼" slices
   (use only white and light green parts)
1 pound red potatoes, unpeeled and cut into
   ½" pieces
1 quart vegetable broth
2 large bay leaves
¾ teaspoon salt
¾ teaspoon pepper
½ teaspoon each:
   Savory Seasoning
   dry thyme
   dry marjoram
2 cups half-and-half
¼ cup all-purpose flour
8 ounces light sour cream, room temperature

Use a 4-cup glass measuring cup to prepare everything in this recipe (don't bother to rinse it out as you make the soup). Coat a 6-quart saucepan with cooking spray. Melt the butter over high heat. Add the celery, carrot, leeks, and potatoes and sauté 10 minutes, stirring frequently over rather high heat. Add the broth and seasonings; bring to a boil. Reduce to a simmer, cover, and cook 10 minutes. Stir a few times. Raise heat to medium and cook, uncovered, 10 minutes. Pour the half-and-half into the 4-cup glass measuring cup; add the flour and whisk together until well combined. Add to the soup and cook over medium heat for about 5 minutes.

Meanwhile, place the sour cream in the 4-cup glass measuring cup. Add about a cup of hot soup to this and whisk to combine. Pour sour cream mixture into the saucepan and cook over low heat for a minute or so; do not boil. Discard the bay leaves. Adjust seasonings, if desired. Cover and refrigerate leftovers; don't freeze. Serves 4-6.

 *You know, I like to have vegetarian days once or twice a week, though Bob always asks, "where's the meat?" Mostly he asks that just to bug me. If you need to convert this soup to satisfy a* **Meat Lover***, just change the broth to chicken or beef and add a cup or two of leftover cooked meat (chopped ham or chicken are nice) or about a cup of cooked bacon or sausage near the end of the cooking* 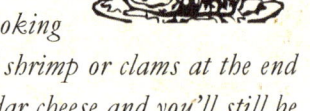 *time. Consider substituting clam juice for the broth and adding cooked shrimp or clams at the end of cooking. Consider just adding a half pound of shredded sharp Cheddar cheese and you'll still be vegetarian.*

Add anywhere from 4-8 ounces roasted and chopped green chile, drained, during the simmering.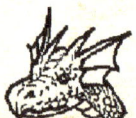

Sweet Sylvan Buns with Honey Almond Butter

Though currants are preferred in these dainty buns, you can certainly substitute any sort of small dried fruits: raisins, cherries, cranberries, or blueberries; chopped sugar dates or chopped apricots. Read my anecdotal material below for some fun facts about currants.

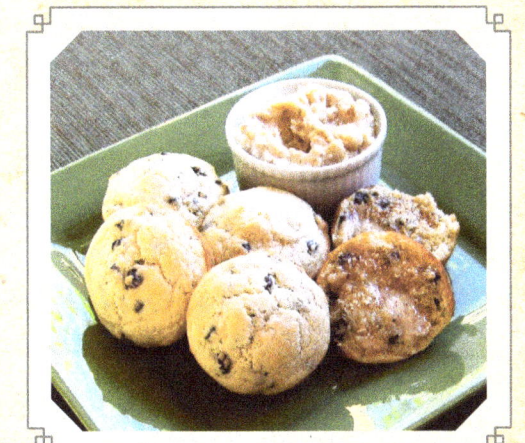

1½ cups all-purpose flour
¼ cup sugar
2 tablespoons cornmeal
2 teaspoons baking powder
¼ teaspoon salt
1 cup currants
½ cup very soft salted butter
1 cup half-and-half
Honey Almond Butter, recipe below

Preheat oven to 400°. Lightly coat 12 regular-sized muffin cups with cooking spray. In a large bowl, combine the flour, sugar, cornmeal, baking powder, and salt. Add the currants and combine. Add the butter and combine. Finally, add the half-and-half and mix until fully incorporated. Divide between the prepared cups. Bake 15-17 minutes. Let cool in pan for about 10 minutes before serving. Serve with Honey Almond Butter. Store covered at room temperature. Makes 12.

Honey Almond Butter

1 ounce sliced almonds; toast lightly and cool 30 minutes, then grind in a small food processor
½ cup soft salted butter
2 tablespoons honey

Combine in a medium bowl. Cover and refrigerate leftovers; bring to room temperature again for spreading. Makes about ⅔ cup.

These are delicate little buns and almost qualify as a dessert. The butter is great on other bread products. As I said above, I prefer currants in these buns. Way back when I was first developing these recipes for my college project, I was able to get currants easily. While I was working on the actual cookbook, however, I couldn't find currants

anywhere, even around the winter holiday season. This was really annoying to me, yet apparently a shortage of currants is not without precedent. In 1610, the British were faced with a reduction of currant exportation, and this threw the people into a tizzy. Apparently, currants were considered a beloved luxury, and if deprived, it is reputed that some people committed suicide from this lack of fruity goodness (Wilson 358-59).

So, although I was annoyed, I certainly never contemplated suicide. I talked to rather unhelpful store managers and then resorted to substituting other dried fruits. Who knew that currants could be such a treasured commodity? In November, 2010, I was looking for some odd vegetables in the supermarket and figured I would check the baking aisle just for kicks. Lo and behold! There were currants! I actually did a double-take in the store and bought three boxes. Of course, at the time, I was mostly done testing recipes. I bought them anyway, however, and I hoarded them away like dragon's gold…

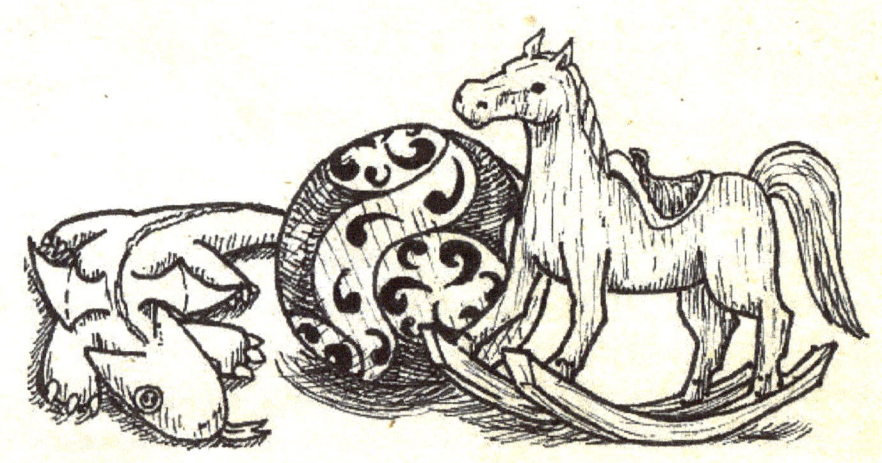

Ginger Jar bread with Spiced Honey Butter

This is a light, fragile gingerbread with a spicy, sweet butter. It's good any time of year, though it smells like the winter holiday season when you bake it. It's one of Chloë's favorites.

½ cup soft salted butter
½ cup sugar
1 extra large egg, room temperature
2 cups all-purpose flour
1 tablespoon baking powder
1 teaspoon ground ginger
½ teaspoon each:
  salt
  ground cloves
  nutmeg
1 cup 1% milk, room temperature
¼ cup molasses
1 teaspoon vanilla extract
2 ounces crystallized ginger, cut into ¼" bits
2 ounces pecans, chopped coarsely
Spiced Honey Butter, recipe below

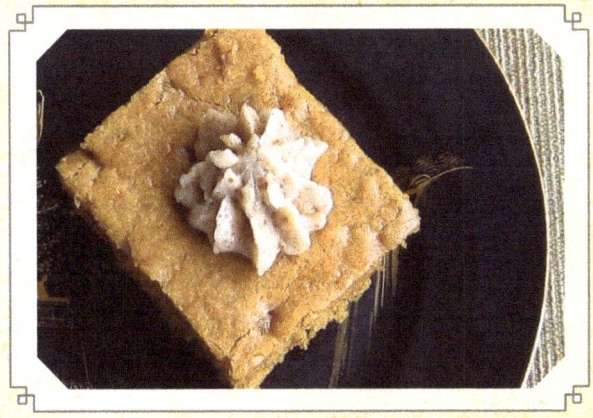

Preheat oven to 350°. Coat a 9" heavy aluminum square pan with cooking spray or grease lightly. In a large bowl, beat the butter, sugar, and egg on medium speed until creamy. In a medium bowl, combine the flour and the next 5 ingredients; set aside. In a 2-cup glass measuring cup, whisk together the milk, molasses, and vanilla. Add to the butter mixture starting with a third of the flour mixture and alternating with half of the liquid. Beat well after each addition, especially after the final one (don't be dismayed if this appears curdled at first). Scrape down sides. Mix in the crystallized ginger and pecans. Pour into the prepared pan and bake 31-35 minutes or until the center tests done. Let stand at least 2 hours on a rack before cutting. Serve with Spiced Honey Butter. Cover and store at room temperature. Serves 9-12.

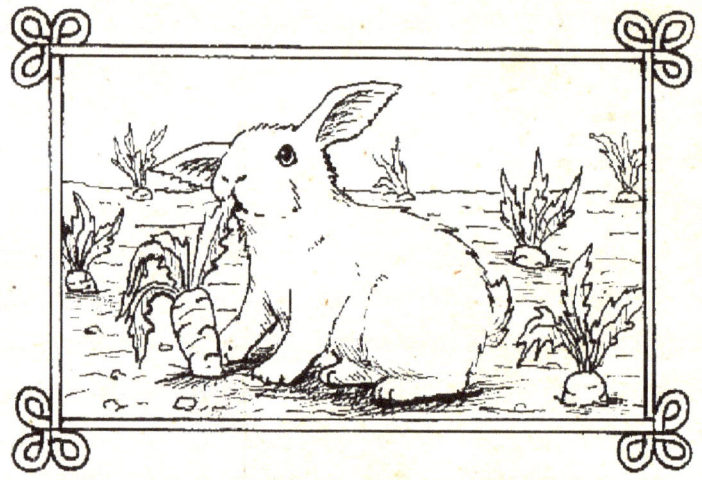

Spiced Honey Butter

1 ounce pecans; lightly toasted, cooled, then chopped finely or ground
½ cup soft salted butter
2 tablespoons honey
¼ teaspoon each:
    ground ginger
    ground cloves
    nutmeg

Combine all ingredients in a small bowl. Cover and refrigerate leftovers; soften at room temperature again for spreading. Makes about ¾ cup.

Bannocks of the Forest

These seem dense because of the oats, yet they are also light and delicate; best with butter and honey.

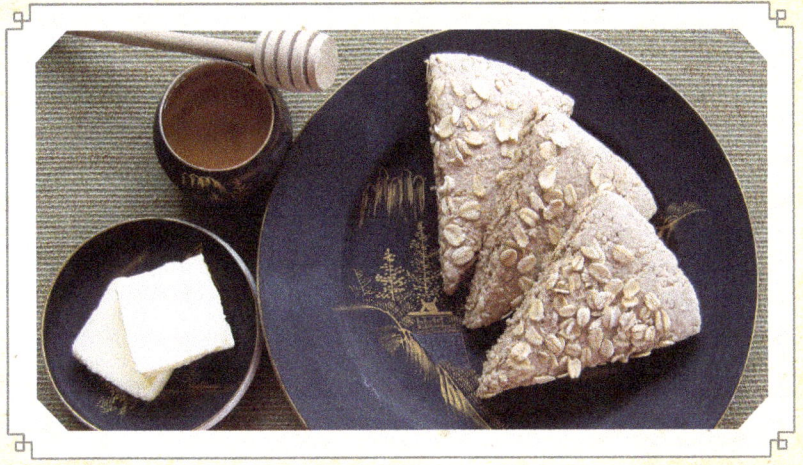

2 cups plus 1 tablespoon old-fashioned oats
⅓ cup all-purpose flour
2 tablespoons sugar
1 teaspoon each:
    salt
    baking powder
    cinnamon
¼ cup water
¼ cup salted butter

Preheat oven to 350°. Coat a large baking sheet with cooking spray or grease lightly. In a large food processor, pulse the 2 cups oats and the other dry ingredients until the oats are ground to a powder. In a 1-cup glass measuring cup, combine the water and butter. Microwave on HIGH in 20-second intervals to melt the butter. Add this to processor and pulse until well mixed. Turn onto a lightly floured surface and knead a couple times. Pat to a circle about 8" in diameter. Lightly spray the top of the dough with water and evenly sprinkle the 1 tablespoon oats all over. Press oats lightly into the dough. Cut into 8 wedges. Place on the baking sheet 1" apart. Bake 12-14 minutes, until they are barely brown on the bottom. Let stand on pan 5 minutes. Serve with plenty of butter, honey, and jam. Cover; keep at room temperature. Makes 8.

Chapter Eight: Nympha Nemorosa

Lanaphro's Pancakes

Elves who hunt might fry up some venison sausages to go with these pancakes for breakfast or brunch. You'll probably have to settle for bacon or pork sausages, but that's okay; it's tough for most of us living in the real world to practice our archery skills. Do elves like to eat second breakfasts? I really doubt it.

1¼ cups buttermilk
1 extra large egg
2 tablespoons walnut oil
2 tablespoons sugar
2 tablespoons cornmeal
1 tablespoon baking powder
1 teaspoon cinnamon
½ teaspoon salt
1 cup all-purpose flour
1¼ cups maple syrup[1]
3 ounces pecans, lightly toasted and finely chopped
Butter (optional)

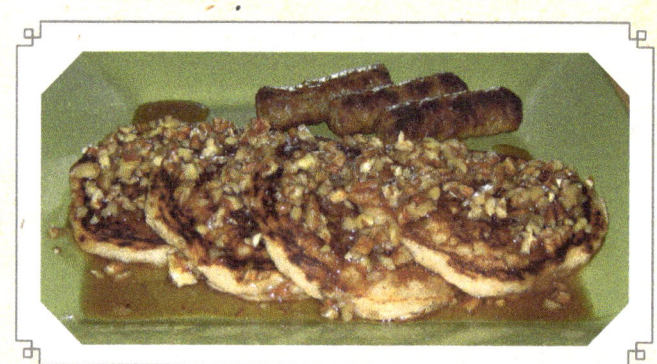

Whisk together the buttermilk, egg, and oil in a 4-cup glass measuring cup. In a 2-cup glass measuring cup, combine the sugar, cornmeal, baking powder, cinnamon, and salt. Add this to the buttermilk mixture and whisk together (rinse the 2-cup glass measuring cup well and use later on). Add the flour and combine well. Over a moderately high heat, heat a griddle that has been coated with cooking spray or melted butter. Drop batter in about 2 tablespoon portions onto heated griddle and cook until golden brown on the underside and some bubbles form on the topside. Turn and cook other side until golden brown. Place in a warming oven (250°), if desired. Continue with the remaining batter. Makes 12-16. Serves 3-4.

Meanwhile, measure the syrup in the 2-cup glass measuring cup and microwave on HIGH 45-60 seconds to warm. Mix in the pecans. Serve pancakes with butter, if desired, and pour syrup over all. Keep leftovers covered and refrigerated separately.

[1] You can use real maple syrup, if you like. I happen to use the light variety because I'm always trying to cut calories somewhere or other, and now I'm completely used to the lighter kind.

Fancy Mashers

An excellent side dish, but hearty enough to be the main course, with a salad on the side.

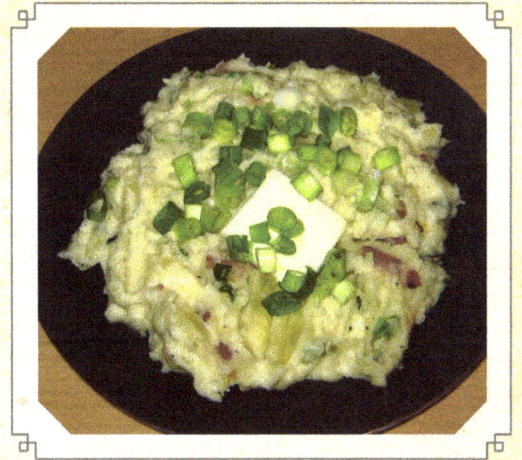

- 5 cups water
- 2 pounds potatoes, cut into 1" chunks (peeled or not; it depends on what kind you use)
- ½ cup plus about 2 tablespoons scallions, thinly sliced
- 2 ounces good quality precooked bacon, cut into ¼" slices
- ½ cup heavy cream
- ¼ cup light sour cream
- 1 teaspoon Savory Seasoning
- ½ teaspoon salt
- ½ teaspoon pepper
- ¼ cup plus 1 tablespoon salted butter

Combine the water and potatoes in a 3-quart saucepan. Bring to a boil and cook over medium/high heat, uncovered, about 15-20 minutes, or until fork tender. Drain and let stand in the strainer; don't wash the saucepan. Coat the saucepan with cooking spray and sauté the ½ cup scallions and the bacon 5-6 minutes over a medium/high heat, until the bacon becomes almost crispy; turn off heat and let stand. In a 2-cup glass measuring cup, combine the heavy cream, sour cream, and the seasonings with a whisk. Add to the bacon mixture, along with the ¼ cup butter. When the butter has mostly melted, add the potatoes and mash coarsely with a potato masher. Adjust seasonings, if desired. Place in a serving bowl; garnish with the remaining butter and scallions. Cover and refrigerate leftovers. Serves 4-6 as a side; 2-3 as a main dish.

Mix 4 ounces of drained, roasted, and chopped green chile to the bacon mixture.

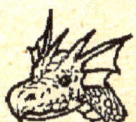

Chapter Eight: Nympha Nemorosa

Chicken & Apple Toasty Puffs

If you want to skip baking for a change, an easy alternative to making these puffs is to use 12 miniature croissants or some fun slider buns.

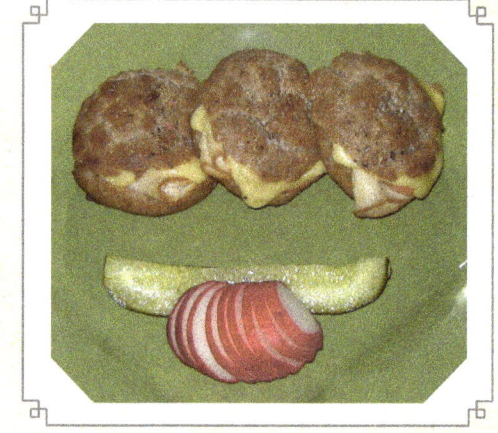

1 ounce walnuts, lightly toasted and cooled
¼ cup all-purpose flour
½ cup water
¼ cup salted butter
½ teaspoon salt
¼ teaspoon Savory Seasoning
¼ teaspoon pepper
2 extra large eggs, room temperature
2 tablespoons spicy brown mustard
1 tablespoon honey mustard
½ tablespoon apple butter
12 slices of cooked chicken breast, paper-thin slices
   (use lunch meat from ½-pound package)
1 giant apple, cored and cut in half lengthwise;
   cut each half into 12 slices, ¼" thick
12 slices Gouda cheese, cut into 2" squares, ¼" thick (about ⅓ pound total)
2 tablespoons salted butter, melted
Freshly ground pepper

In a small food processor, grind the walnuts and flour; set aside. In a 2-quart saucepan, combine the water, ¼ cup butter, salt, Savory Seasoning, and pepper. Bring to a boil, then whisk in the flour mixture once the butter has melted. Beat over medium heat until it is thick (kind of like mashed potatoes). Take off heat and cool 10 minutes. Preheat oven to 400° now.

Coat a large baking sheet with cooking spray or grease lightly. After the dough has cooled 10 minutes, beat the eggs into the flour mixture well with a whisk. Drop batter in 12 portions onto prepared sheet. Bake 25 minutes. Let stand on pan at least 30 minutes.

Preheat oven to 450°. Meanwhile, whisk mustards and apple butter in a small bowl and set aside. Prepare the apple and cheese slices and set aside. With a small, sharp knife, slice each puff in half horizontally. Spread bottom half with a generous ½ teaspoon of mustard mixture. Layer chicken next, folding each slice in quarters to fit. Place 2 slices of apple on each, then the cheese. Press lid on top and place back on baking sheet. Brush tops generously with melted butter, then top each with some freshly ground pepper. Bake 8 minutes. Let stand about 5 minutes before serving. Serve hot, warm, or even at room temperature. Cover and refrigerate leftovers. Makes 12.

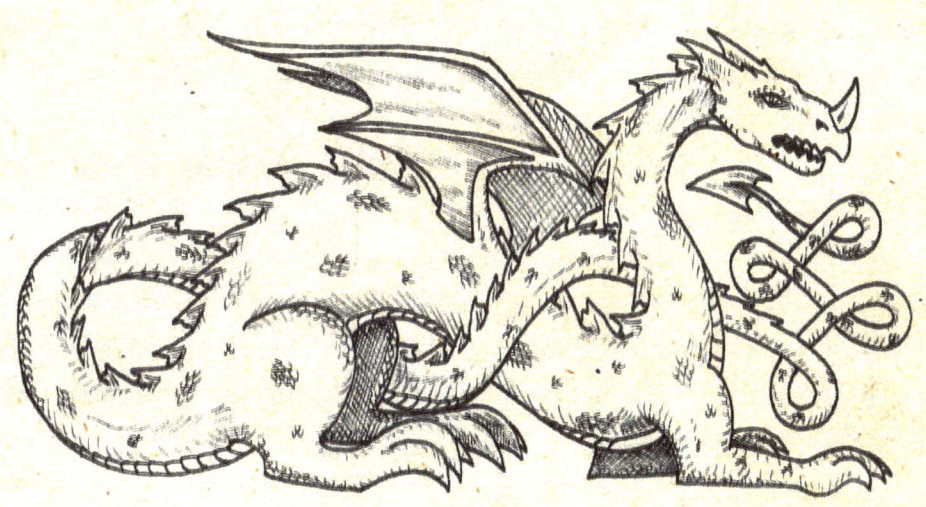

Tayphro's Venison

Serve these with any carbohydrate of your choice—rice, pasta, potatoes, bread. Elves would also probably like salads or vegetables alongside; unlike trolls, elves undoubtedly do appreciate lots of greenery in their diet.

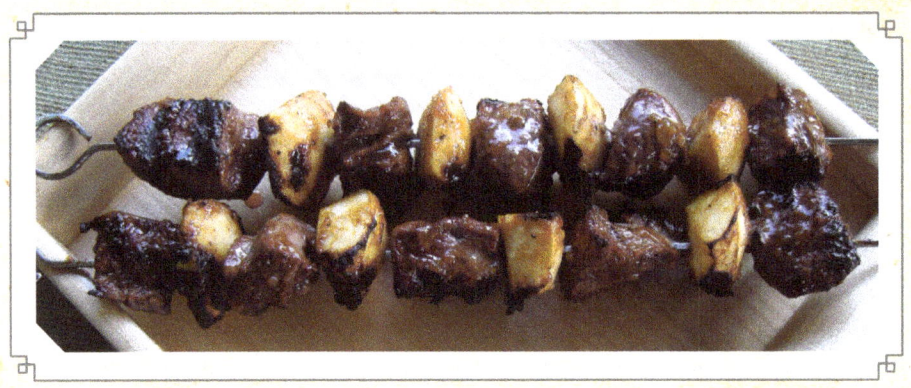

1-1¼ pounds venison (stew meat or from a roast), cut into 2" pieces
   (you'll need 20)[1]
½ cup dry red wine, such as Cabernet Sauvignon or Merlot
½ cup mango chutney
1 tablespoon each:
   soy sauce
   malt vinegar
   wine from marinade (discard the rest)
1 teaspoon Dijon mustard
1 teaspoon crushed ginger
½ teaspoon salt
½ teaspoon pepper
2 large apples; peeled and cored, each cut into
   8 chunks (for a total of 16 pieces)

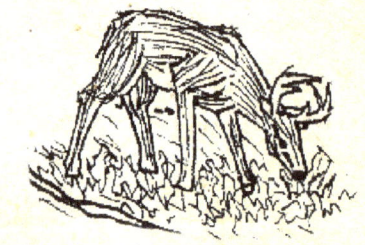

Combine the meat and wine in a medium-sized glass bowl. Refrigerate 2-4 hours and stir a couple of times. In a blender or small food processor, combine the next 8 ingredients and process until fully blended. Transfer to a small bowl and set aside. Coat a grill with cooking spray and preheat to medium. Coat 4 metal skewers with cooking spray and alternately thread each with 5 pieces of meat and 4 chunks of apple, beginning and ending with meat. Place on a medium baking sheet. Place kabobs on grill and liberally brush with half of the glaze. Grill 3-5 minutes. Turn kabobs over and brush the top sides; grill another 3-5 minutes, or until meat is cooked to the desired temperature.[2] Let the kabobs rest a couple of minutes on a clean baking sheet, then remove from skewers and serve. Cover and refrigerate leftovers. Serves 4.

> [1] You can easily use other proteins, such as beef or chicken, but the best alternative is pork tenderloin for that lovely pork/apple combination.
>
> [2] Cooking times will vary depending on your grill, your choice of meats, and your own taste.

 **Vegetarian Option**—You could replace the meat with various vegetables cut into 1" chunks or left whole. Good choices would be: onions, bell peppers (any color), cherry tomatoes, mushrooms, and summer squashes (unpeeled).

Whortleberry Tart

What is a whortleberry? It's also known as a bilberry. For this recipe, you can simply think of it as a blueberry. You could substitute raspberries, if you like, or use a combination (use a raspberry fruit spread, as well). Only use fresh berries!

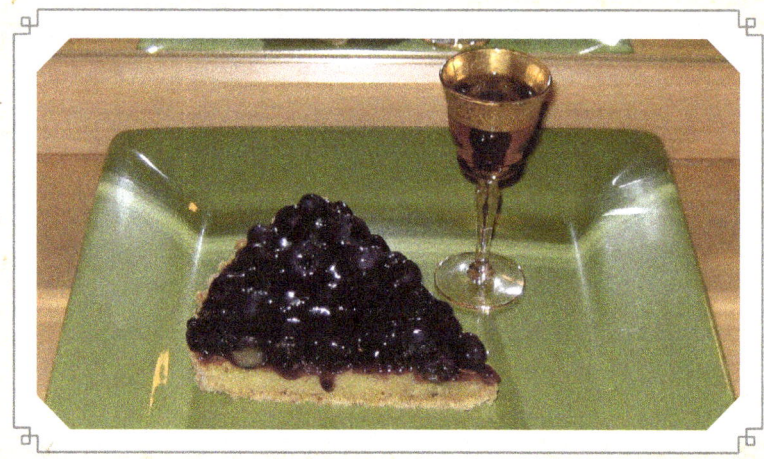

4 ounces whole almonds, toasted lightly and cooled for about 30 minutes
½ cup all-purpose flour
2 tablespoons plus ¼ cup sugar
¼ teaspoon salt
¼ cup soft salted butter
3 extra large eggs
1 teaspoon vanilla extract
7-8 ounces almond paste, broken into ½" pieces
12 ounces fresh blueberries
11-ounce jar blueberry fruit spread (a 9- or 10-ounce jar will also work)
2 tablespoons water
1 teaspoon almond extract

Preheat oven to 350°. Coat a 9½" tart pan with 1" removable sides with cooking spray or grease lightly. In a large food processor, process the almonds until ground. Add the flour, 2 tablespoons sugar, and salt and process. Add the butter and process well. Press evenly into the prepared pan, starting with the sides (don't bother washing the bowl or blade). Bake 10 minutes. Remove and place on a rack.

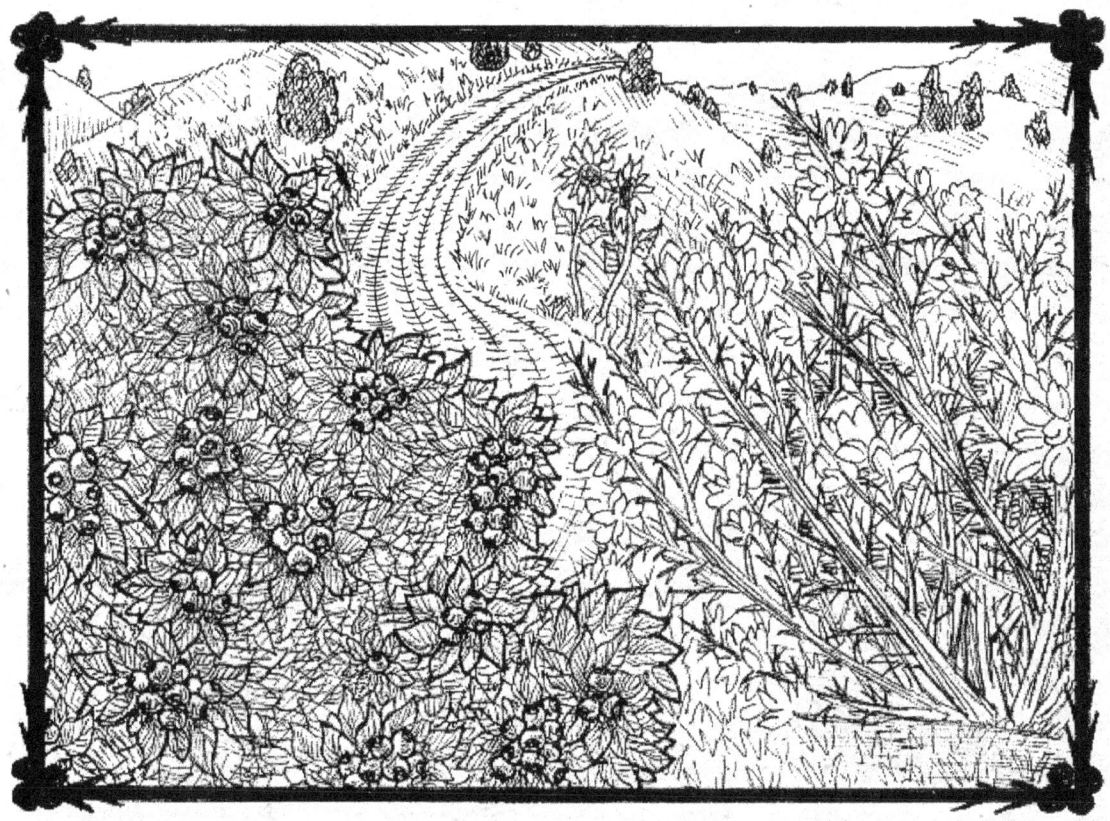

Meanwhile, place the eggs, ¼ cup sugar, vanilla, and almond paste in the bowl and process well. Pour onto baked crust and bake 26-30 minutes, until set. It will be puffy, but will deflate when you let it cool a bit. Cool on a rack 1 hour.

While tart cools, wash the blueberries and set on a clean towel or a couple paper towels to dry. In a 1-quart saucepan, combine the remaining ingredients. Over a medium heat, cook and stir with a whisk just until the fruit spread has melted and the mixture is smooth; cover and set aside. Remove the sides from the tart and set on a serving plate. Pile the blueberries on the top (they can overlap). Spoon the fruit spread all over, then use a pastry brush to fill in empty areas to the edge. Chill at least 2 hours or overnight before cutting. Cover and refrigerate leftovers. Serves 8-10.

Marmalade Gems

Other marmalade flavors will also be fine in these crisp little cookie/cake treats.

½ cup plus 1 tablespoon soft salted butter
2 tablespoons half-and-half
1 cup all-purpose flour
2 tablespoons plus ¼ cup sugar
½ teaspoon plus ¼ teaspoon mace
½ teaspoon plus ¼ teaspoon ground ginger
¼ teaspoon salt
3 ounces light cream cheese (Neufchâtel), softened
⅓ cup orange marmalade
1 extra large egg
¾ cup powdered sugar
2 tablespoons orange juice
1 teaspoon cinnamon sugar

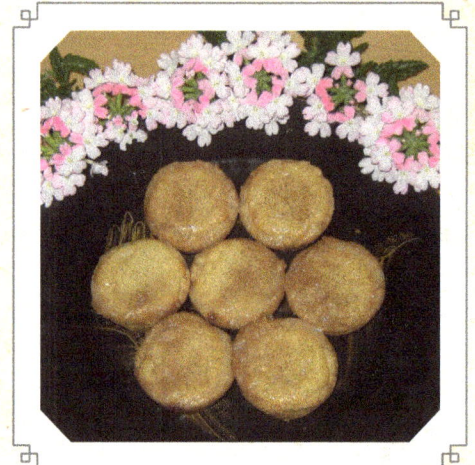

Preheat oven to 350°. Liberally coat 24 miniature muffin cups with cooking spray. Place the ½ cup butter, half-and-half, flour, 2 tablespoons sugar, ½ teaspoon mace, ½ teaspoon ginger, and salt in a very large bowl and combine well with a hand mixer. Divide dough into 24 portions and place in each cup (don't bother washing bowl or beaters). Press dough all the way up the sides, then bake 10 minutes. Remove and maintain oven temperature. Use a rounded spoon or a shot glass to press the dough down, if it ends up too puffy.

Meanwhile, place the cream cheese in the bowl. Beat until smooth. Add the ¼ cup sugar, marmalade, egg, ¼ teaspoon mace, and ¼ teaspoon ginger and combine well. Divide evenly into each baked cup, then bake 20 minutes. Cool 30 minutes. Set a rack over a large baking sheet. Use a sharp knife around the edges to remove the cookies from the pan, then place them on the rack. Combine the powdered sugar, 1 tablespoon butter, and orange juice in a medium bowl and whisk until fully mixed. Drizzle all over the pastries. Sprinkle evenly with the cinnamon sugar. Keep covered at room temperature or refrigerate. Makes 24.

Stained Glass Morsels

These fruity treats are crispy the first day and more like tiny pies on the second day.

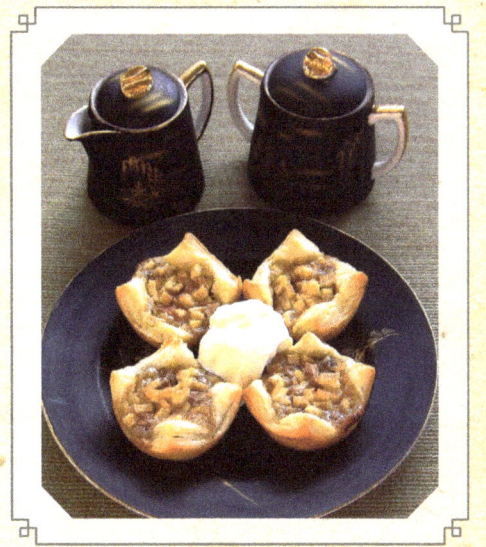

17.3-ounce package puff pastry, thawed according to package directions (such as Pepperidge Farm)
About 6 ounces dried cherries
2 ounces pecans, chopped finely
1¼ cups apple; peeled, cored, and chopped into ¼" bits
½ cup heavy cream
½ cup packed golden brown sugar
1 extra large egg
1 teaspoon vanilla extract
½ teaspoon each:
    mace   ground ginger
    ground coriander seed
⅛ teaspoon salt
2 teaspoons cinnamon sugar

Coat 2 regular-sized muffin pans with cooking spray or grease lightly. Place 1 sheet of puff pastry on a cutting board. Cut vertically along the 2 creases. Cut horizontally into 4 equal sections. Place each piece in a muffin cup, pressing lightly to fit while leaving the corners intact.

Preheat oven to 400°. Put 4 cherries in each cup. Sprinkle nuts evenly in each, then sprinkle apple bits evenly over all.

Place the cream, brown sugar, egg, vanilla, coriander, ginger, mace, and salt in a medium bowl. Use a whisk to combine well. Pour 1 tablespoon into each cup. Sprinkle evenly with the cinnamon sugar. Bake 17-19 minutes, until golden brown. Let stand 10 minutes. Use a sharp knife around the edges to facilitate removal from pans. Serve with whipped cream or ice cream. Cover and store at room temperature. Makes 24.

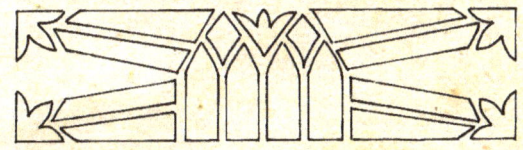 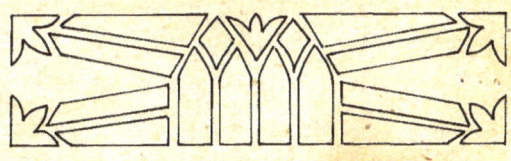

Esther's Favorite Lemon Cake

You could certainly substitute orange or lime flavors with good results in this lovely, light cake.

1 giant lemon (or 2 medium lemons)
About ¾ cup plus 1 tablespoon 1% milk, room temperature
¼ cup soft salted butter
¾ cup sugar
1 extra large egg, room temperature
1½ cups all-purpose flour
1 teaspoon baking powder
½ teaspoon baking soda
¼ teaspoon salt
1 tablespoon plus ½ teaspoon poppy seeds
1 teaspoon vanilla extract
½ cup plus 1 tablespoon soft lemon curd, room temperature
⅓ cup powdered sugar

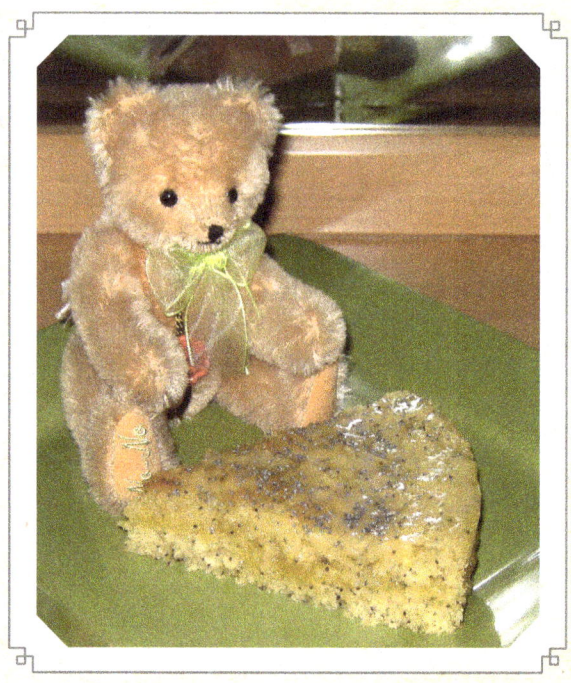

Preheat oven to 350°. Coat a 9" heavy aluminum round pan with cooking spray or grease lightly. Lightly flour bottom of pan. With a fine grater or microplaner, scrape as much zest as you can from the lemon; you should end up with 1-2 tablespoons—set aside. Then squeeze the lemon and measure out about ¼ cup of juice into a 2-cup glass measuring cup (remove any pits, of course). Add ¾ cup milk to this, or enough to measure 1 cup total. Add the zest and vanilla; whisk and set aside (it will most likely appear curdled—don't worry).

In a large mixing bowl, cream the butter, sugar, and egg on medium speed until thoroughly combined. In a medium bowl, combine the flour, baking powder, baking soda, salt, and 1 tablespoon poppy seeds. Add to butter mixture alternately with the lemon/milk mixture, beginning and ending with the dry ingredients. Mix well on medium speed; scrape down sides. Spread in prepared pan and bake 33-37 minutes, until cake tests done in the center. Cool in pan on a rack 15 minutes. Run a knife around edge and turn out onto the rack, bottom down—cool 1 hour.

Transfer to a serving plate and split in half horizontally; carefully set aside the top layer. Mix up the ½ cup lemon curd and gently spread on the cake. Replace top carefully. In the same bowl you mixed the flour in (don't bother washing it out), whisk together the 1 tablespoon lemon curd and 1 tablespoon milk, then add the powdered sugar and whisk until fully combined. Spread this evenly over the top—it's okay for some to drizzle over the sides. Sprinkle with the ½ teaspoon poppy seeds. Cover and store at room temperature or refrigerate. Serves 6-8.

 *Though I have named this for my mother, I could also call it Callista's Favorite Lemon Cake, after my youngest daughter, since she has informed me it is her favorite. But when I asked what her favorite recipe was in the cookbook, her first response was the Salmon Tartlets, so too bad; my mom got first dibs.*

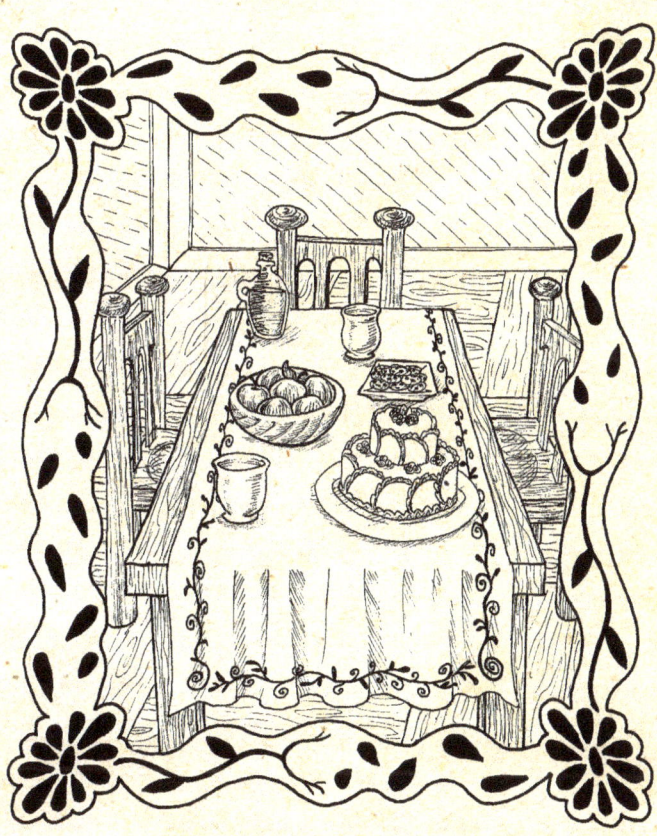

Nimallin's New Foolery

The simple, delicious taste of a beautiful, fresh strawberry and pure heavy cream—two ingredients combine in a bowl to produce an almost spiritual, even Platonic, representation of what food should be. While strawberries and cream in Jackson's *Lord of the Rings* film trilogy seem to represent a melancholic yearning for home, peace, and contentment, Tolkien instead closes his text of *The Lord of the Rings* by utilizing strawberry and cream imagery to express utter happiness and hope.

Besides apples and dried fruit, berries are extremely popular in Middle-earth; strawberries being the most popular variety. You can always serve an elf, a hero, or a halfling the simplest of desserts by putting a few fresh strawberries (sliced, quartered, halved, or whole, depending on their relative size) in a bowl, sprinkling them with a little sugar if you feel the need, and pouring a tablespoon or two of heavy cream over them. That's not much of a recipe… so I figured a new version of a "fool" would be an appropriate way to present this classic combination.

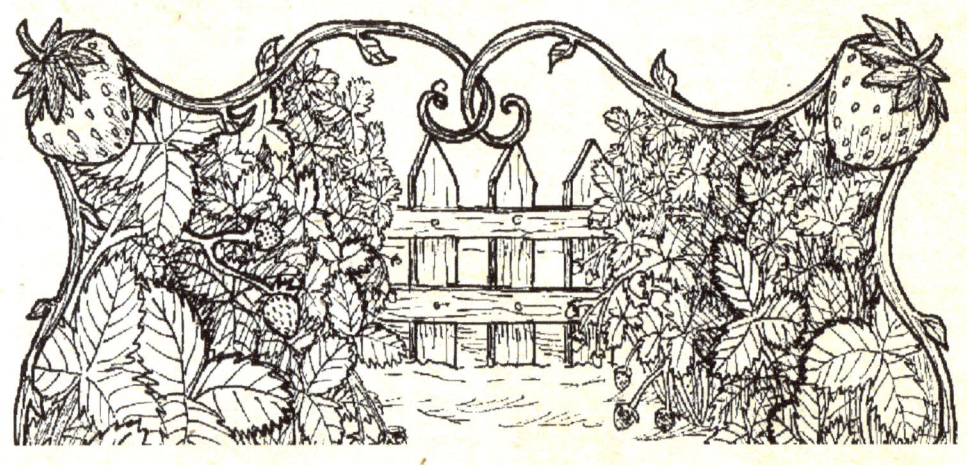

1 quart fresh strawberries
½ cup plus 2 tablespoons sugar
1½ cups heavy cream

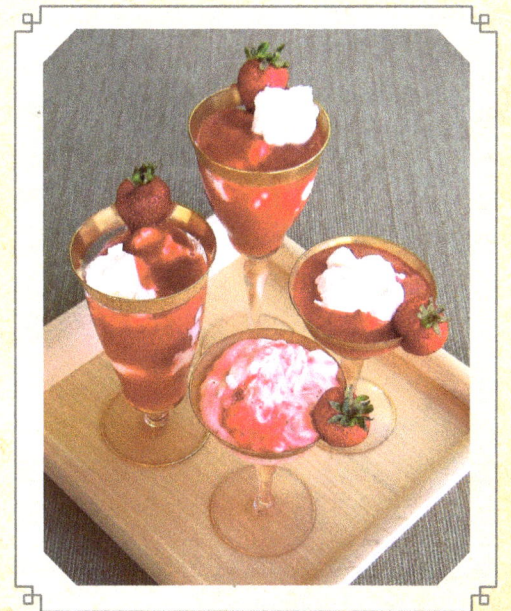

Reserve 6 or 8 small berries for garnish, if desired. Wash the remaining berries; stem them. Cut in halves or quarters and place all in a 3-quart saucepan. Turn the heat on rather high just until they start cooking, then lower the heat to medium and cook, uncovered, 20 minutes. Stir frequently so the strawberries don't burn. Remove from heat. Mix in the ½ cup sugar and let stand 1 hour. Puree in a blender or processor, then place in a 4-cup covered container. Refrigerate at least 4 hours or overnight.

In a very large bowl, combine the cream and 2 tablespoons sugar. With a hand mixer, whip the cream until fluffy, but not too dry. Layer with the strawberries in pretty glasses or dessert dishes as a parfait. Or, combine the strawberries in the large bowl with the cream and mix gently with a spatula, making sure to leave some differentiation between the two components. Wash the reserved berries and leave the stems on. Cut a vertical slit in each and place on the rim of each glass or dish, if desired. Refrigerate until serving time. Cover and refrigerate leftovers; this surprisingly lasts for quite a few days in the fridge. Serves 6-8.

Crustula Vitae

This final recipe is my version of the mysterious elvish food item Tolkien calls *lembas*. At first I was not going to bother making this, because *lembas* seemed to have sort of an elven magic (*not* as in Keebler) involved in their production that would be impossible to recreate in the real-world kitchen.

My decision not to attempt a *lembas* recipe was confirmed in April 2009, when I attended a lecture at UNM by the eminent Tolkien scholar, Dr. Verlyn Flieger. A member of the audience asked whether or not *lembas* could be a metaphor for the Eucharist, since through its consumption, the consumer finds strength and is sustained through hardship. Of course, no absolute conclusion was reached, nor could there have been. I believe this would be a fascinating topic for a conference paper or even a thesis. This would require research and scholastic writing which I am thankful I do not have to do anymore.

Yet old academic habits die hard, and thinking about this did lead me to consult Tolkien's letters, which are always fascinating to read. Sure enough, Tolkien does discuss the matter of *lembas*, and he assigns spiritual significance to its consumption; it goes beyond mere physical nourishment. I don't believe one can truly reproduce *lembas* exactly in the way Tolkien seems to be intending. Is it a bread, a biscuit, a cake, a cracker, a cookie? In some ways, he almost describes a treat that perhaps should be deep-fried, but I can't imagine that Tolkien's elves break out a deep-fryer to get that light brown exterior with a creamy interior; and anyway, he does say they are baked. I have a feeling Tolkien probably did not cook or bake very frequently, if ever. So I merrily composed all of my original recipes and made a conscious decision not to bother with the mysterious *lembas*.

However, a few months after I (thought I had) completed this cookbook, and after talking about the project with different people (mostly members of the UNM Hobbit Society), I realized it would be better simply to go ahead and interpret *lembas* in my own way. Everybody expected and hoped for a recipe. Then, of course, I had to come up with an appropriate name for them. I broke out the Latin dictionaries for a bit of research and settled on *Crustula Vitae*, or "Cookies of Life." *Crustula* can also mean biscuit. It seemed a good compromise.

I doubt these will stay fresh for weeks, mainly because we real-world humans do not have the benefit of special leaves (part of that elven magic Tolkien mentions), so we can't wrap up our *crustula* for longer storage. It's more likely that this will never be an issue, because these particular *crustula* will probably suffer a more hobbitish fate and be devoured pretty quickly. They might not sustain you spiritually or on long journeys, but on those days when you are being "good on your diet," you can wistfully remember eating these *crustula*; you can wish that you can eat them every day, and never have to think about calories in the real world. Now there's a fantasy. If I were more poetic, I would compose a sort of *ubi sunt* ("where are they…?") ode to *crustula* here. You'll just have to settle for a recipe composition.

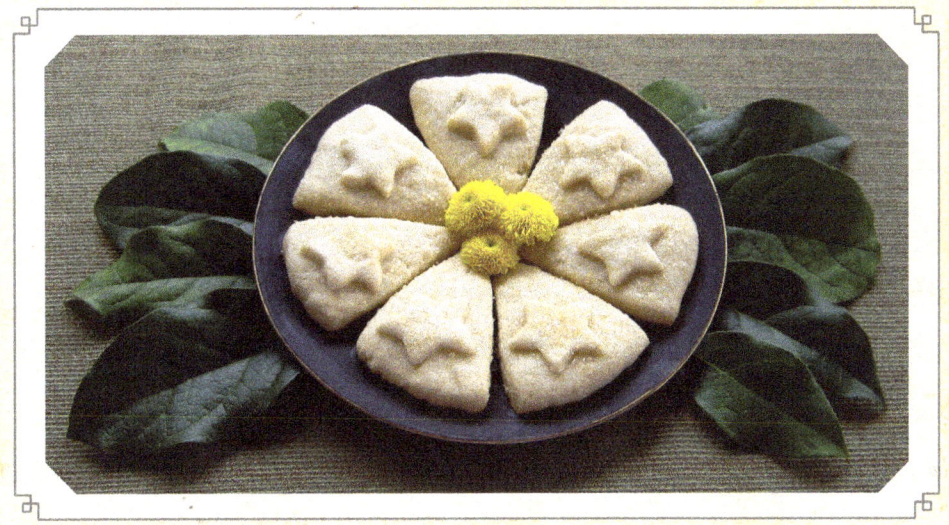

½ cup soft salted butter
⅓ cup sugar
1½ cups all-purpose flour
¼ teaspoon each:
    salt
    baking soda
    cream of tartar
¼ cup heavy cream
1 tablespoon turbinado (raw) sugar

Set oven rack to the level right above the middle level. Preheat oven to 375°. Coat a large baking sheet with cooking spray or grease lightly. In a medium bowl, combine the butter and sugar with a wooden spoon. Add the dry ingredients and mix well. Add the cream and mix with your hands until fully combined and smooth.

Break off about a fourth of the dough and place on a lightly floured surface. Roll this out to about ⅛". Cut 16 small decorations and carefully set these aside (I like to use a small star shape). Take the scraps and add to the other dough; knead a few times to incorporate. Divide this dough in half. Roll and pat 1 half to a circle measuring 6-7" and ¼" thick on a lightly floured surface. Cut into 8 wedges. Repeat with the other half of the dough. Lay the decorations near the wider edge of each wedge. Spray all lightly with water. Sprinkle evenly with the turbinado sugar.

Lay each carefully on the prepared sheet. Bake 12-14 minutes, until they are very lightly browned on the bottom. Let stand on sheet 2 minutes. Carefully place on a rack. Store covered at room temperature. Makes 16.

 *As I thought of the* ubi sunt *trope in various literary works (including Tolkien's...), suddenly I felt the urge to write a poem in Latin! Believe me, this has never happened before. Most likely, it will never happen again. And Bob keeps telling me Latin is a dead language. Here is a poem for you, and fortunately I have included a translation.*

Ubi sunt dies
quando edere poteramus crustula libere?
Heu! Sempiternum evanescunt.
Solum capilli cani et dolor articulorum,
exercitatio et inedia,
comitant nos nunc. Heu.

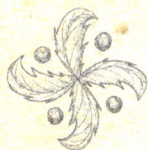

Where are the days
when we could eat cookies freely?
Alas! They are gone forever.
Only the grey hairs and the stiff joints,
the exercise and the starvation,
accompany us now. Alas.

A Typical Fantasy Meal

On a final note: sometimes you're too busy or tired to do any actual cooking, but you just want to evoke your favorite fantasy setting, or a Middle-earth (or Narnia, Westeros, Krynn, Fionavar, Earthsea, Hogwarts, Discworld; perhaps even Gallifrey, why not?) meal. You can set out a generous buffet (see photo on page 77) by purchasing various ingredients with absolutely no cooking involved. Or you can arrange to host an assigned potluck—it's just as easy to ask one of your guests to bring a bag of dried fruits instead of a bag of potato chips. Careful reading of Tolkien's texts led me to develop this shopping list for you, and you are free to exercise your own tastes here, regarding your particular choices (with this list, you can feed maybe six people; increase or decrease according to the appetites of your diners—maybe a pound of meat in your family only feeds two people…):

- A pound or two of "salted meats." I would use thinly sliced good quality delicatessen meats: roast beef, ham, turkey, chicken (then, of course, you could also use more "exotic" meats, if you are so inclined, such as salami or pastrami)
- A pound or two of good quality cheeses. Serve sliced, or set the cheeses out in block form and supply some slicers. Gouda and sharp Cheddar are great choices (keep them as non-processed as possible—they need to be *real* cheeses, if you know what I mean…)
- A loaf or two of rustic, whole-grain bread
- A dish with softened salted butter for spreading
- An assortment of dried fruits
- A few apples
- A bottle or two of wine (whatever you like, perhaps a red and a white)
- A few cans or bottles of beer (again, whatever you like)
- Plenty of water (filtered tap is best; those plastic bottles will bury us one day)
- You can't go wrong with coffee, tea, and options for these beverages

So, even if you can't find the time to cook, you can always set out a fantasy-themed smörgåsbord by following the basics in this list. While this shopping list is complete in itself, you could expand this menu somewhat by adding items such as shelled nuts and fresh berries, and also serving other condiments, such as mustards, mayonnaise, and prepared horseradish. As for greenery, various varieties of lettuces, sliced tomatoes, cucumber, onion, and pickles (dill and sweet) would be welcome and definitely in keeping with the fantasy spirit.

A Typical Fantasy Meal

MENU SUGGESTIONS

For a Rather Casual Family Supper that is still Good Enough for Guests, Try:

Hild's Mushroom Bacon Dish of Might
Herby Cabbage Sauté
Marcella's Cherries

Or, for Something Just a Bit More Elegant, Try:

Gündürnüb's Grüb
Ted's Spinach Mushroom Salad
Esther's Favorite Lemon Cake

For a Viewing of Your Favorite Fantasy Film, Try:

Beery Beef Stew
Ellen's Favorite Salad
Elfryda's Apple Crisp

Or Try:
Glürbin's Gutless Wonders
Keep-You-Awake Cauliflower
Queevhô's Bleedin' Treats

Or Try:
Chloë's *Macrows ond Chese*
Beets for Hypomur
Jan's Baked Apples

**For a Marathon Movie Day, whereby you Attempt
to Watch THREE Films, Try:**

Thrúd's Hearty Split Pea Soup
Bill's Spicy Nut Mix (a savory snack)
Quest Depot Deluxe Granola (a sweet snack)
(all can be made the day before you attempt such a foolhardy quest...)

For a Breakfast or Brunch, Try:

Journey Brunch Pie
Good-for-You Muffins
Fresh fruit on the side
And don't forget some butter, jams, and honey

For a Second Breakfast, Try:

Snorri's Special Ham & Eggs
Head-in-the-Clouds Biscuits
More butter, jams, and honey

**For a Reading of The Hobbit or
any of The Chronicles of Narnia, Try:**

Bon Voyage Biscotti
Comforting Chai

For a Summer Party, Try:

Meat on Metal Stick
Lise's Lentil Salad
Nimallin's New Foolery
Purchase some crusty bread, like sourdough—and don't forget the butter!

For a Nice Sunday Dinner, or even a Holiday, Try:

Sine Qua Non Chicken
Cress Composition
Pumpkin Streusel Pie for Randgrið
(make the pie in the morning or the night before—
be sure not to assemble the salad until right before serving)

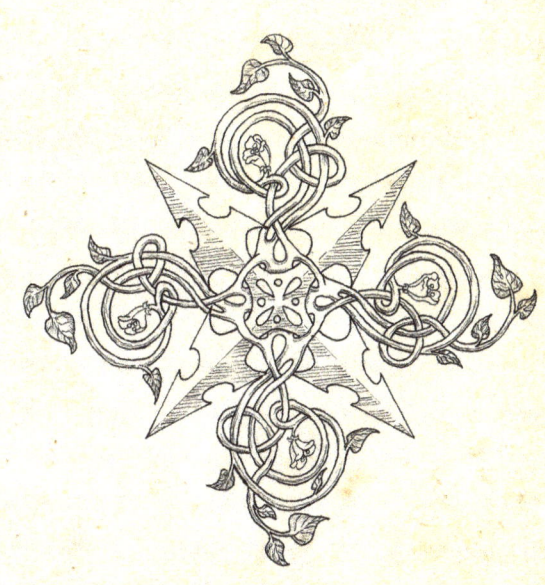

PRACTICAL MATTERS

Altitude

Living at a mile-high altitude, as I do, means I am baking and cooking at a mile-high altitude. If you live at sea level you might have to make some adjustments to a recipe. You might have to cook or bake for a little less time or put in less flour or a smidge more baking powder. You might not. You might have to experiment a bit, though I have given a range of cooking or baking times (my own personal baking time is right in the middle). It would have been impractical for me to test all of these items at sea level, since I am quite attached to my land-locked home near the mountains and usually reluctant to travel, sort of like a hobbit.

Substitutions

Some ingredients should not be substituted for others. Now obviously, you can be creative and change various items according to your own tastes or dietary requirements. I guess I really mean please do not use margarine instead of butter (see below for a discussion on butter). Or use milk when I list cream. I've listed light sour cream and cream cheese and I've used 1% milk throughout. If you prefer to use whole dairy products, you certainly may do so. I've never used the absolute skim or non-fat dairy varieties for any of the recipes within, however.

Mayonnaise is up to you—perhaps you make your own; perhaps you like an olive oil variety. Sometimes I've switched to a light variety and it also works well, then I've switched back to the original variety. I do think the high-fat variety usually produces a better result in general, but again, if you are truly trying to cut calories, you may use the low-fat and that should be fine (as with the dairy products listed above, I've never used the non-fat or so-called "vegan" varieties).

I can't guarantee the results of using egg substitutes, but you never know; sometimes using half real egg and half egg substitute can result in a good product. See below for more information on baking substitutions.

I use your basic type of soy sauce (Kikkoman), but you can definitely substitute different varieties—light, low-sodium, or even try Ponzu or Tamari. I use a variety of oils in the cookbook, such as almond and hazelnut, but you are free to use vegetable or olive oil instead.

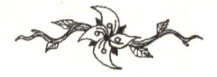

Measuring & Baking

All measurements should be level, unless specifically stated otherwise. This mainly refers to dry ingredients. So, scoop up a full cup of flour, then level it off with the back of a flat knife (I sometimes use the back of my cleaver if I'm using it). Liquids are generally exact. If I say something like "about ½ cup of chopped onion," you can go a little over or under. I'll often say that about vegetables or meats. I know sometimes you just want to chop up one carrot, but it doesn't happen to measure EXACTLY ½ cup. Should you cut up another carrot? Don't bother; the recipes can be rather flexible. Usually, you don't want to fiddle with baked goods, however. Do you need to sift various dry ingredients? Only if the recipe specifically says to do so. Actually, I can't remember the last time I used my sifter. Sometimes, items like powdered sugar can be a bit lumpy, but if I want to sprinkle some of that on a sweet, I'll just use a fine-mesh strainer.

Speaking of baking in general: I have a conventional gas oven. My own personal baking time is always right in the middle, in recipes where I have given a range of baking times. If you have a convection oven, you'll have to experiment with your own personal adjustments regarding decreases in total baking time and/or temperature. Your rack should be placed in the middle of the oven, unless otherwise specified. For items such as cookies that might occupy two racks, I use the middle and the lower level, then I switch the pans halfway during my baking to assure more even browning. Perhaps my next oven will be a convection model, but for now, I have been getting along pretty well with my conventional model.

When it comes to baked goods, be careful with your substitutions. As I mentioned above, you might be able to get away with using half real eggs and half egg substitute. You might be tempted to try using powdered buttermilk. I haven't been satisfied with the results; your batter or dough ends up too thin or too sticky, then you end up having to add more flour just to work with it. I am not conversant with sugar or flour substitutions, but if you are, you are welcome to experiment and make adjustments as necessary.

Salt & Butter

Salt is a big issue in the modern culinary world, and it seems like many restaurants are becoming heavier-handed with salt. I am generally moderate about seasoning, but if you have a concern about salt in particular, you might want to put in less. You can always add more, but you can't take it away. I know I'll make something and think it is perhaps too salty or just right, then Bob will add salt at the table. I'll see chefs adding a whole handful of salt to pasta water, yet I don't usually do this. When I do, I use it minimally, especially compared to what you'll see on your average cooking show. Aren't doctors always telling people to cut back on salt consumption? You will probably find the recipes within will taste good—only you can judge whether you can go without salt or use a salt substitute. In baked goods, you should stick with whatever salt is required, however.

Salt is so subjective. I did invent a dry seasoning mix called "Savory Seasoning" (see the Essential Seasoning Mixes on page xxi) that is a combination of flavors—this is the first official recipe in the cookbook and would be handy to make immediately (if you haven't already done so) since it is incorporated into quite a few recipes. It has less sodium content than plain salt and can be used on plenty of other items outside of the cookbook.

All recipes using butter call for a salted variety, but you can probably substitute unsalted if you are terribly concerned about sodium. I use salted sweet cream butter (yes, it's the Costco kind), which has 90mg of sodium per one tablespoon serving. Salted butter is a more traditional ingredient historically (see Tannahill, 28; Wilson, 153). I'm afraid the junk food industry has used *so* much fat, sugar, and sodium *so* excessively, that people in general have forgotten about the term *moderation*.

Herbs & Spices

Tolkien often mentioned herbs when he wrote about Middle-earth. Fresh is usually best. If you can grow them successfully, you are lucky. In the recipes, I will often give you two measurements for herbs: one for fresh and one for dry. Sometimes I will ask you only to use fresh herbs; at other times, only dry. I find that when I buy certain fresh herbs, especially parsley, some of it goes to waste, so sometimes it is convenient to use dried ones. I had never grown my own herbs because I have been busy and I don't have great soil nor a particularly green thumb, but four summers ago, I actually grew a few herbs in my backyard containers as well as some tomatoes. My flat-leaf parsley was almost more like a shrub and my dill, mint, and rosemary were doing well. The next summer, pretty much all of it was a flop and my tomatoes were attacked by plump worms. Callista and I let them devour the plants and observed them as a sort of casual science experiment. The summer after that, I didn't bother with anything. I try not to be an herb snob, so I give you options in the recipes.

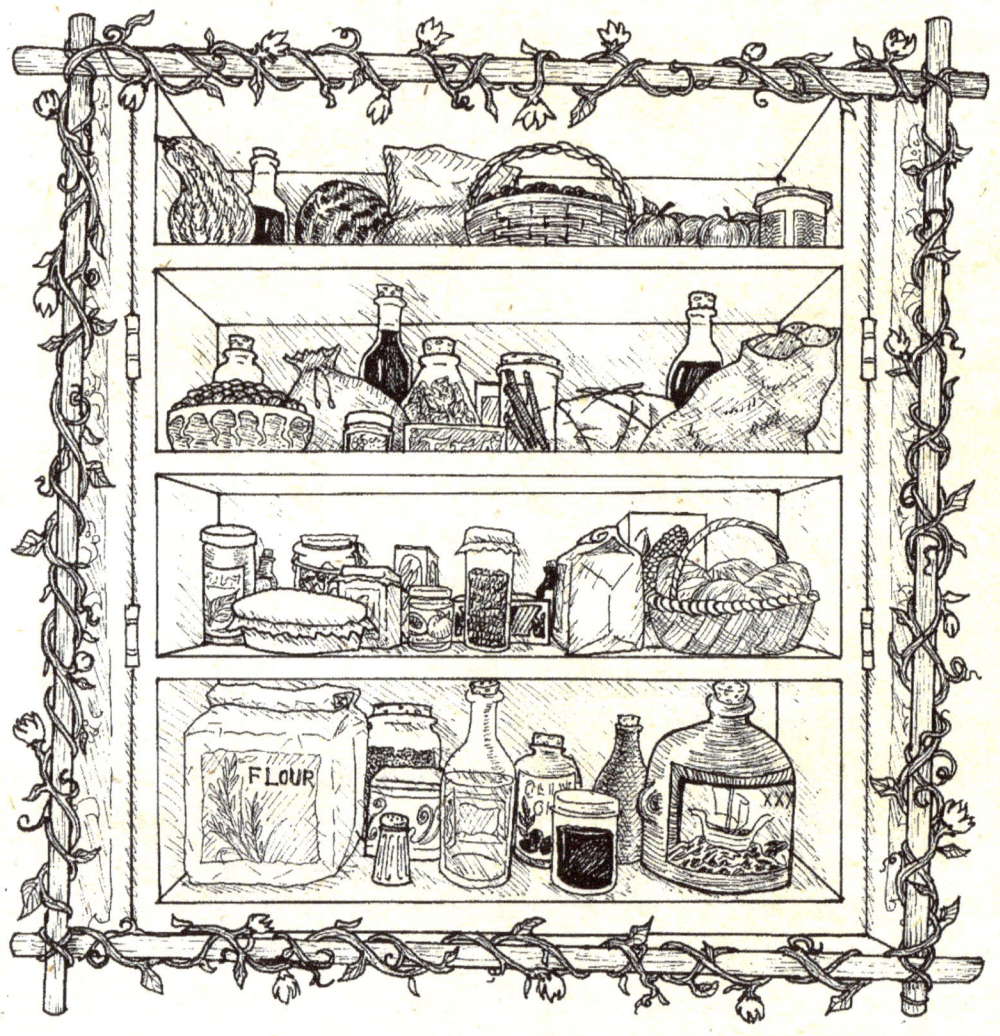

If you are interested in stocking your dried herb and spice cabinet, however, here is a listing of all the items you would want to have on hand to make all the recipes within. Again, I'll specify in each recipe whether you need to use fresh or dry:

- ☼ Allspice, ground
- ☼ Bay leaves, whole
- ☼ Cardamom, pods and ground
- ☼ Cinnamon, sticks and ground
- ☼ Cinnamon sugar (see page xxiii for a recipe)
- ☼ Citric acid
- ☼ Cloves, whole and ground
- ☼ Coriander, seeds and ground
- ☼ Cumin, ground (roasted is fine)
- ☼ Dill, weed and seed
- ☼ Garlic
- ☼ Ginger, fresh (either the root or from a jar) and ground
- ☼ Herbes de Provence (see page xxii for a recipe)
- ☼ Hot Madras Curry Powder
- ☼ Mace, ground
- ☼ Marjoram
- ☼ Mint, fresh only
- ☼ Nutmeg, ground
- ☼ Paprika (smoked is fine)
- ☼ Parsley
- ☼ Peppers—regular coarse ground black pepper, whole peppercorns, and cayenne
- ☼ Poultry Seasoning
- ☼ Rosemary, fresh and preferably crushed in dried form
- ☼ Saffron
- ☼ Sage, rubbed Dalmatian
- ☼ Salts—regular salt, sea salt; garlic, onion, and celery
- ☼ Seeds—mustard, celery, poppy, sesame, and anise; pumpkin and sunflower (both preferably salted and dry-roasted)
- ☼ Star Anise
- ☼ Thyme
- ☼ Turmeric, ground

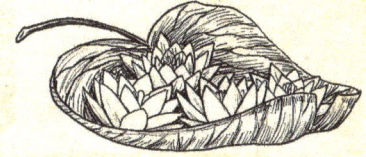

Mushrooms

The character of Frodo Baggins admits a weakness for mushrooms. I, too, love mushrooms and my original cookbook had an entire chapter showcasing our favorite fungi. These recipes have now been redistributed throughout the current cookbook (many ended up in Chapter Six, which caters to dwarves). Mushrooms come in myriad forms, but for all of these recipes, you will only need common types easily found at grocery stores. Hobbits might pluck mushrooms right out of the ground, but I would not suggest going out to your yard and harvesting unknown fungi (unless you happen to be a fungi expert, or mycologist—I once had a particularly phallic fungus growing out of my lawn that even my dog would not touch, though this looked quite similar to something Andrew Zimmern was eating on *Bizarre Foods*—so do not eat mystery mushrooms, NEVER, EVER). In general, you will be using plain whites (*Agaricus bisporus* or *Champignons*), brown mushrooms known as Portobellos (sometimes spelled Portabellas), or Creminis (sometimes spelled Criminis). You could certainly experiment with Morels and Chanterelles in some of the recipes. None of the recipes are appropriate for dried, canned, or jarred mushrooms. All mushrooms should be firm, clean, and very fresh.

Pie Crusts

I have purposely been generous with my pie crust proportions so you will have enough scraps to decorate your pie, whether it be single- or double-crust. It just seems right that the pies included here should have some sort of decoration on top and often some sort of glaze. In a pinch, of course, you can skip this. You can even use purchased crusts if pressed for time (the rolled-up, refrigerated kind is best and not broken as frozen crusts often are). I have found that lard, indeed, is usually your best bet for shortening in a crust, or a combination of lard and butter. Vegetable shortening can be used as a substitute for the lard, if you prefer.

Another tip: try not to take too many shortcuts with your pie crusts. It really does help to have chilled shortening and ice water. It really does help to refrigerate your crust for 30-60 minutes. You can mix up your pie crusts in a food processor or a stand mixer if you prefer, but I have been experimenting. Usually I resort to the stand mixer since I find that a food processor seems too harsh on the dough. But lately I have had flakier results with simply mixing up the dry ingredients, cutting in the shortening with a pastry blender, adding in the liquid and mixing with a spatula or a wooden spoon, then smooshing it all together—all by hand. Yes, this all takes a little extra time and preparation, but your end result will be worth it.

If you use ready-made crusts, you will usually not have any extra for decorations since these crusts seem to fit just barely into a 9½" glass pie dish, but this is fine when you're really not in the mood or too busy. I decorated a recent pie for this cookbook with three strips of dough to represent stems and cut other scraps into leaf shapes and tulips. Callista told me it looked like a pie Snow White made in the old Disney film, just as if I had help from efficient woodland creatures (I did not, though if they did the dishes that would be worth it). It's fun to watch childhood movies again with college-age children (excuse me, I mean young adults)—they have a completely different perspective on themes that never bothered them before…

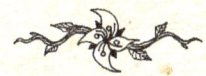

A Listing of Kitchen Utensils

I'm assuming you have equipped your kitchen the way you want it, but I thought it would be handy for me to list all of the pots, pans, gadgets, and small appliances I have used to make all of the recipes in this cookbook, including dimensions or capacities. I'm also listing miscellaneous, various items that are utilized in the cookbook. Sometimes, I've listed a brand name—this is not any sort of endorsement, it is just for your information. This looks like a lot of stuff, but you probably have all or many of these items already in your own kitchen (or your study, your linen closet, your junk drawer, your sewing basket, etc…). If you don't, then here's your chance to buy that electric ice cream maker or sushi kit you've always wanted!

Cooking Utensils & Miscellaneous Items

- ☼ Measuring spoons (⅛, ¼, ½, ¾, 1 teaspoon, ½ tablespoon, and 1 tablespoon)
- ☼ Measuring cups for dry ingredients (⅛, ¼, ⅓, ½, ⅔, ¾, and 1 cup)
- ☼ Glass measuring cups for liquid ingredients (1-, 2-, and 4-cup—Pyrex)
- ☼ Kitchen scale (a minimum of 1-pound—I have a digital 11-pound, which I love)
- ☼ Knife set (a few good, sharp knives, including a serrated one; I also use a cleaver)

- ☼ Towels / cloth napkins / potholders
- ☼ Wax paper / parchment paper / plastic wrap / aluminum foil (heavy and light)
- ☼ Cutting boards—medium and large
- ☼ Tape measure / scissors / kitchen twine / waxed dental floss
- ☼ Timer / candy thermometer / meat thermometer
- ☼ Plastic ice cube trays (3)
- ☼ Strainers and colanders, assorted sizes
- ☼ Toothpicks / cake tester
- ☼ Whisks—small, medium, and large
- ☼ Pastry bag with various basic tips / snack-size Ziploc bags
- ☼ Rolling pin / pastry blender / bent (or recessed) spatula
- ☼ Small cookie cutters / pastry brush
- ☼ Bamboo mat and paddle (for making sushi)
- ☼ Box grater / microplaner / zester / lemon juicer / egg slicer
- ☼ Spray bottle for water / shaker jar with tight-fitting lid for salad dressings
- ☼ Vegetable peeler / pizza slicer / potato masher
- ☼ Long metal skewers (4)
- ☼ Cocktail shaker for alcoholic beverages
- ☼ Spatulas / tongs
- ☼ Storage containers with lids (various sizes; plastic and glass)
- ☼ Nested mixing bowls, both glass and stainless (various sizes)
- ☼ Punchbowl / cake dome and pedestal
- ☼ Serving platters / dishes / utensils

Small & Large Appliances

- ☼ Toaster oven / 4-slice toaster
- ☼ 5-quart stand mixer (KitchenAid—with the regular attachments)
- ☼ Small food processor (Cuisinart "Mini-Prep"—3-cup variety)
- ☼ Large food processor (Cuisinart—12-cup variety)
- ☼ Hand mixer / Blender (Oster—5-cup variety)
- ☼ 6-cup electric ice cream maker (Cuisinart)
- ☼ Gas stove and outdoor grill (just to let you know I'm cooking with gas)
- ☼ Microwave (never used for cooking, just for melting various items)

Pots & Pans

- Saucepans (pots) with lids (1-, 1½-, 2-, 3-, 4-, and 6-quart)
- Skillets (small 8", medium 10", large 12"—I use lids from my saucepans here)
- Griddle (I just use a portable one for the stove burners)
- 3-quart (medium), 2" deep skillet with lid
- 5-quart (large), 2" deep skillet with lid

Baking Pans & More Miscellaneous Items

- 2 Half sheet (large) pans (Nordicware—18" by 13"—heavy aluminum, with 1" rims)
- 2 Quarter sheet (medium) pans (13" by 9"—heavy aluminum, with 1" rims)
- Cooling racks (a few, plus I have a very handy one that fits over my half sheet pan)
- 9" round cake pans (2" deep, heavy aluminum; you'll need 3)
- 9" square pan (2" deep, heavy aluminum or glass)
- 8" square pan (2" deep, heavy aluminum or glass)
- 13" by 9" glass baking dish
- 11" by 7" glass baking dish
- 15" by 11" glass baking dish
- 9½" glass pie dish
- 9" by 5" glass loaf pan (metal is okay)
- 8½" by 4½" glass loaf pan (metal is okay)
- 9" springform pan (2" sides)
- 1-cup ramekins (you'll need 6)
- Tart pans with removable sides (1" deep—you'll need a 9½" one and an 11" one)
- Muffin pan—regular size (you'll need 2 pans to make 24 muffins)
- Miniature muffin pan (you'll need to be able to make 24 mini-muffins)
- Broiler-proof casserole-type dishes (1-, 2-, and 3-quart; also a 11" by 7" type)

Conversion Charts

I'm including some basic measurement conversions in the following charts. I haven't developed any of the recipes using metric measure since, for good or ill, I'm a product of the American public school system. If you need to convert these recipes, you might note slight variations. I consulted many sources for this information—some charts convert one ounce dry weight to 28 grams; others convert to 30 grams. The math is obviously easier using the 30 gram increments, but the 28 gram option for dry ingredients seems more accurate (although how 4 ounces ends up being 113 grams and not 112 is a mystery to me, but rounding when converting seems common). All equivalents are approximate.

Dry Ingredients by Weight

Multiply number of ounces by 28 to convert to grams.

⅛ teaspoon	a pinch			
3 teaspoons	1 tablespoon			
⅛ cup	2 tablespoons	1 ounce		28 grams
¼ cup	4 tablespoons	2 ounces	⅛ pound	56 grams
⅓ cup	5 tablespoons plus 1 teaspoon	3 ounces		84 grams
½ cup	8 tablespoons	4 ounces	¼ pound	113 grams
⅔ cup	10 tablespoons plus 2 teaspoons	5⅓ ounces	⅓ pound	150 grams
¾ cup	12 tablespoons	6 ounces		168 grams
1 cup	16 tablespoons	8 ounces	½ pound	230 grams
1¼ cups		10⅔ ounces	⅔ pound	300 grams
1½ cups		12 ounces	¾ pound	340 grams
2 cups		16 ounces	1 pound	450 grams
4 cups		32 ounces	2 pounds	900 grams
			2.2 pounds	1 kilogram

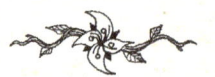

Liquid Ingredients by Volume

The column with parenthetical measurements on the right is for rounding up, if you don't need very precise conversions. Multiply number of ounces by 30 to convert to milliliters.

¼ teaspoon				
½ teaspoon				
1 teaspoon			5 ml	
1 tablespoon	3 teaspoons	½ ounce	15 ml	
1 fluid ounce	2 tablespoons	⅛ cup	30 ml	
2 ounces	¼ cup		60 ml	
3 ounces	⅓ cup		80 ml	
4 ounces	½ cup		120 ml	
5⅓ ounces	⅔ cup		160 ml	
6 ounces	¾ cup		180 ml	
8 ounces	1 cup	half a pint	240 ml	(250 ml)
12 ounces	1½ cups		350 ml	
16 ounces	2 cups	1 pint	475 ml	(500 ml)
24 ounces	3 cups		700 ml	(750 ml)
32 ounces	4 cups	1 quart	1 liter	
128 ounces	16 cups	1 gallon	3.8 liters	(4 liters)

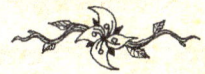

Lengths & Widths

Multiply number of inches by 2.5 to convert to centimeters.

1 inch			2.5 cm	
6 inches	½ foot		15 cm	
12 inches	1 foot		30 cm	
36 inches	3 feet	1 yard	90 cm	
40 inches			100 cm	1 meter

Practical Matters

TEMPERATURES

Fahrenheit	Celsius	Gas Mark
32°	0°	(freezes water)
212°	100°	(boils water)
225°	110°	¼
250°	130°	½
275°	140°	1
300°	150°	2
325°	160°	3
350°	180°	4
375°	190°	5
400°	200°	6
425°	220°	7
450°	230°	8
475°	240°	9

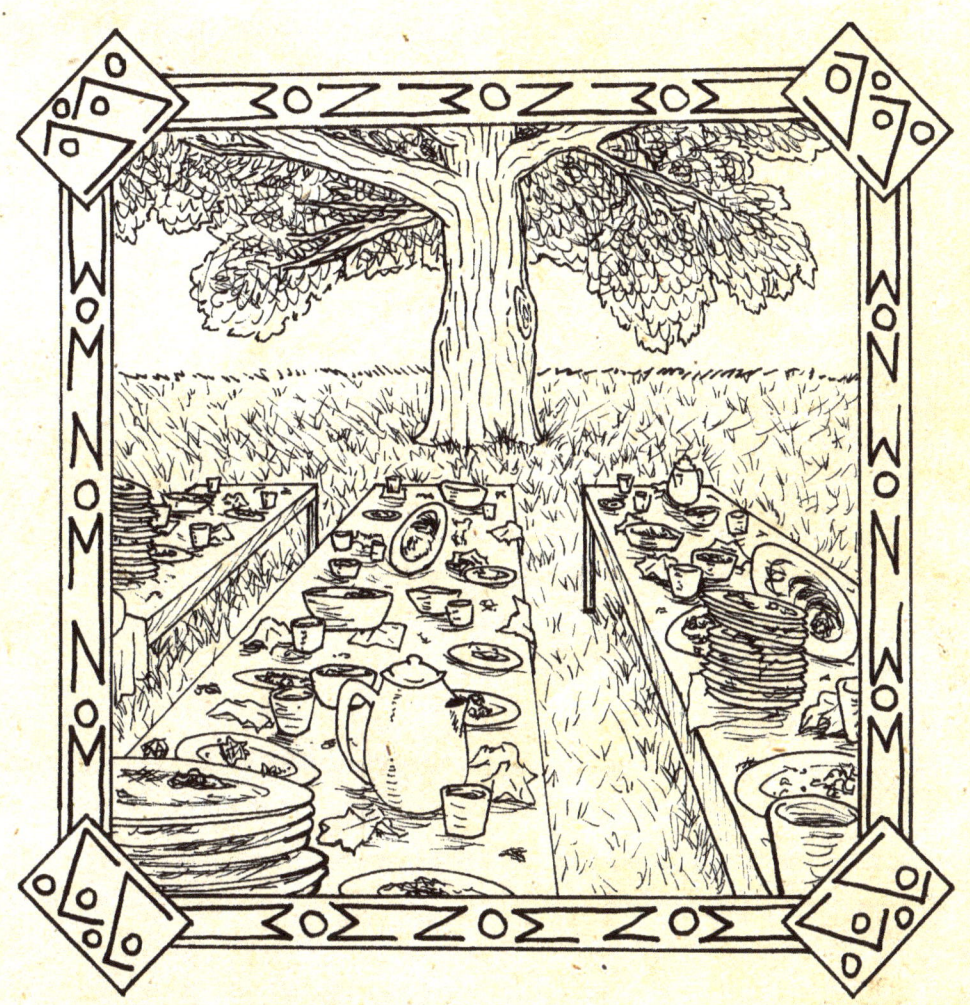

conclusion

This has been quite a quest. I have never eaten so much bacon, potatoes, and apples in my entire life as I did between the years 2009 and 2011. I have also consumed a lot more beer than I usually would. These were sacrifices I was willing to make in order to get authentic photographs for my Facebook page. Oddly enough, the first year, my weight stayed mostly the same; the second year, I actually lost 20 pounds (then the holidays came around and I gained back seven—but there was a net loss of 13 pounds for the year, which is better than nothing, I suppose…). I felt like wearing a button: Hobbit Diet—Ask me how!

Explaining that in detail would be tedious and can mostly be summed up by saying "eat significantly less food and move rather a bit more." You also need to catch a wretched stomach flu… twice… and now you know why I'm not going to go into further detail here.

Well, during the year 2011, I learned that instead of a stomach flu, I was really having gallbladder attacks. And this is another exciting story for another time and perhaps another book… we shall see.

We were pasta- and spice-deprived and, especially near the end of recipe development, Callista said we had eaten so much hobbit food she was afraid her feet would become hairy. When I get new cookbooks or magazines (which hasn't happened in about five years now), I use a check mark to indicate recipes that sound good enough to try. Afterwards, I rank recipes with "yuck" which means "what were they thinking? This will never be made in my house ever again." Or I'll write "OK" which means "(obviously) okay—but we don't care enough to make it again, unless I completely doctor the recipe to change it; but then, what's the point of doing that?" It's always surprising to me how many recipes, even by professional chefs and gourmet magazines, fall into these two categories, but I suppose that food is perhaps the most subjective subject in the world (even more subjective than music, comedy, movies, or cars…).

My best ranking is a "star" which means "this is a new favorite and we hope to see it again—it doesn't even require tinkering (or so little as to be negligible)." I am hopeful that you will find many star recipes in this cookbook and reconnect with more genuine food products. Real, true foods and drinks not only nourish the body, but also the soul—this sounds like a cliché you may have heard many times. However, next time you shop, examine the foods you are buying. Can you pronounce everything listed as an ingredient? If not, try putting it back on the shelf. Perhaps all our foods should have capital letters: Strawberry. Cream. Tomato. Apple. Butter. Then we might appreciate food's innate virtues. One time, I brought a bizarre vegetable to the checkout at my local super-grocery store. It was a light green sphere, about 7" in diameter, with tight leaves. The clerk, who seemed to be about 23 or so, wondered what it was. I said, "cabbage." Would you or your children know what a cabbage is? I can't speak for Tolkien, of course, but I think he would like everyone to appreciate Good Food and Drink. I hope this cookbook has helped you to do just that.

Fantastic Cooking!

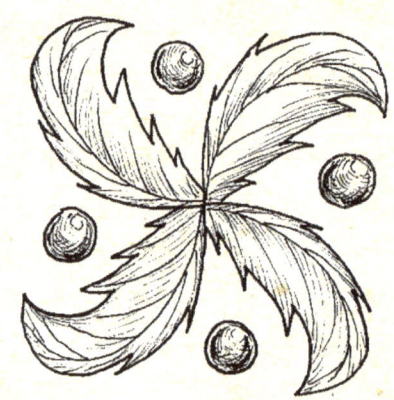

Acknowledgments

Thanks to Dr. Leslie Donovan, for remembering
undergraduate projects from long ago.
You embody all the best qualities inherent in the word "Mentor."

Thanks to the UNM Hobbit Society.

Thanks to Geneva Harstine, for her lovely artistic interpretations
of the Middle-earth universe.

A special shout-out to Steve "Rifflo" Fitch, for somehow finding me
madly tweeting away in the Twitterverse.
Oh Bearded One, the Force is strong with you.

Thanks to Lara Sookoo and all of her fellow nerds/geeks at the now defunct
Oloris Publishing, for thoughtful design and layout: "It's a gift!"
The Great Tales have ended, but the Road goes ever on.

A final word of thanks to my eagle-eyed editor, Stephanie Chan, who respected
and nurtured the cookbook. She is a kindler of stars, indeed.

The Fellowship of the Recipe Testers

Thanks very much to the following people who tested these recipes:

Bethany Abrahamson
Megan Abrahamson
Elizabeth Barteau
Stephanie Cottrell
Troy & Chloë Garrett
John Harstine
Masato Kaida

Maurice Prada
Dana Reinhardt
Adela Smith
Mark & Ellen Sturmer
Kaci Watkins
Walter & Callista Winegar-Valdez

Works Cited & Sourced

Better Homes and Gardens New Cook Book. Ed. Jennifer Dorland Darling. Des Moines: Meredith Corporation, 1996.

Bizarre Foods. Television series, created by Andrew Zimmern. Travel Channel: 2006-2011.

Everybody Loves Raymond. Television series, created by Philip Rosenthal. Perf. Ray Romano et al. Warner Bros.: 1996-2005.

Gies, Frances and Joseph. *Life in a Medieval Castle*. New York: Harper & Row, 1974.

Lewis, C. S. *The Chronicles of Narnia*. Seven volumes. New York: The Macmillan Company, 1950-1956.
—. *The Horse and His Boy*. New York: The Macmillan Company, 1954.
—. *The Lion, the Witch and the Wardrobe*. New York: The Macmillan Company, 1950.
—. *The Magician's Nephew*. New York: The Macmillan Company, 1955.

The Lord of the Rings: The Fellowship of the Ring. Special Extended DVD Edition. Dir. Peter Jackson. Screenplay by Peter Jackson, Fran Walsh, and Philippa Boyens. Perf. Elijah Wood et al. United States: New Line Home Entertainment, 2002.

The Lord of the Rings: The Return of the King. Special Extended DVD Edition. Dir. Peter Jackson. Screenplay by Peter Jackson, Fran Walsh, and Philippa Boyens. Perf. Elijah Wood et al. United States: New Line Home Entertainment, 2004.

The Lord of the Rings: The Two Towers. Special Extended DVD Edition. Dir. Peter Jackson. Screenplay by Peter Jackson, Fran Walsh, and Philippa Boyens. Perf. Elijah Wood et al. United States: New Line Home Entertainment, 2003.

Monty Python's Flying Circus. Television series, created by Graham Chapman, John Cleese, Terry Gilliam, Eric Idle, Terry Jones, and Michael Palin. BBC: 1969-1974.

Snow White. Walt Disney Home Video, 1994.

Sturluson, Snorri. *The Prose Edda*. Trans. Jean I. Young. Los Angeles: University of California Press, 1954.

Tannahill, Reay. *Food in History*. New York: Three Rivers Press, 1988.

Tolkien, J. R. R. *The Fellowship of the Ring, Being the first part of The Lord of the Rings*. 2d ed. Boston: Houghton Mifflin, 1965.
—. *The Return of the King, Being the third part of The Lord of the Rings*. 2d ed. Boston: Houghton Mifflin, 1965.
—. *The Two Towers, Being the second part of The Lord of the Rings*. 2d ed. Boston: Houghton Mifflin, 1965.
—. *The Hobbit*. Boston: Houghton Mifflin, 1966.
—. *The Letters of J. R. R. Tolkien*. Ed. Humphrey Carpenter. New York: Houghton Mifflin, 2000.
—. *Roverandom*. Boston: Houghton Mifflin, 1998.

Top Chef. Television series. Magical Elves Productions, 2006-unknown.

Wilson, C. Anne. *Food and Drink in Britain*. Chicago: Academy Chicago Publishers, 1973.

Woolf, Virginia. *A Room of One's Own*. New York: Harcourt, Inc., 1929.

Wikipedia. Multiple articles. www.wikipedia.org

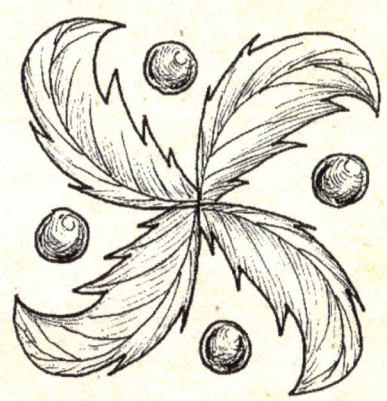

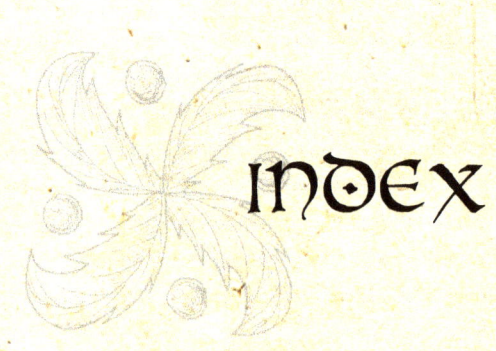INDEX

A

Apple & Raspberry Jam Tart, 22
Aradosa's Cheese, xxiv
Aradosa's Rustic Bread & Cheese, 109
Asbjorn's Fish, Chips, and Sauce, 116

B

Bannocks of the Forest, 209

BEEF
    Beery Beef Stew, 40
    Epic-Urean Stew, 119
    Golden Barley Beef Soup, 29
    Hearty Lunch Pie, 11
    Mellow Mushroom Meatloaf, 67
    Mushroom Steaks, 18
    Roast Beef Toasties, 31
    Savory Stuffed Flank Steak (a.k.a. Tshigwú's Bit O' the Flank), 192
    Tshigwú's Bit O' the Flank (a.k.a. Savory Stuffed Flank Steak), 192

Beery Beef Stew, 40
Beets for Hypomur, 113

BEVERAGES
    Comforting Chai, 24
    Healing Chocolate Chai, 52
    Spring-in-Your-Step Punch, 76
    Turquoise Tipple, 144

Bill's Spicy Nut Mix, 83
Blancmange Puffs, 88
Bleu & Bacon Panini (a.k.a. Want Stinkier Sandwich), 180
Blueberry Quick Bread (a.k.a. Cold Dead Livid Bread), 194
Bob's Obsession, 114
Bon Voyage Biscotti, 101
Braised Chicken & Pork with Artichokes (a.k.a. Raskofím's Roadkill), 185
Brave Blackberry Tart, 47

BREADS/CEREALS
    Aradosa's Rustic Bread & Cheese, 109
    Bannocks of the Forest, 209
    Blueberry Quick Bread (a.k.a. Cold Dead Livid Bread), 194
    Cheddar Sage Scones, 7
    Cold Dead Livid Bread (a.k.a. Blueberry Quick Bread), 194
    Crunchable Croutons, 108
    Crustula Vitae, 224
    Dilly Bread & Butter, 33
    Ginger Jar Bread with Spiced Honey Butter, 207
    Göll's Gorgeous Seed Cake, 152
    Good-For-You Muffins, 87
    Head-in-the-Clouds Biscuits, 59
    Herfjötur's Fancy Bread Pudding, 167
    Lanaphro's Pancakes, 210
    Marmalade Gems, 218
    Quest Depot Deluxe Granola, 86
    Spicy Breadsticks (a.k.a. Zeldóshâkh's Gnarly Bones), 175
    Sweet Sylvan Buns with Honey Almond Butter, 205
    Walter's Special Cinnamon Rolls, 111
    Zeldóshâkh's Gnarly Bones (a.k.a. Spicy Breadsticks), 175

BREAKFAST/BRUNCH
SUGGESTIONS
    Aradosa's Rustic Bread & Cheese, 109
    Bannocks of the Forest, 209
    Blueberry Quick Bread (a.k.a. Cold Dead Livid Bread), 194
    Cheddar Sage Scones, 7
    Cold Dead Livid Bread (a.k.a. Blueberry Quick Bread), 194
    Comforting Chai, 24
    Crustula Vitae, 224
    Dilly Bread & Butter, 33
    Doughty Hero Casserole, 38
    Ginger Jar Bread with Spiced Honey Butter, 207
    Göll's Gorgeous Seed Cake, 152
    Good-For-You Muffins, 87
    Head-in-the-Clouds Biscuits, 59
    Healing Chocolate Chai, 52
    Herfjötur's Fancy Bread Pudding, 167
    Hild's Mushroom Bacon Dish of Might, 156
    Journey Brunch Pie, 95
    Lanaphro's Pancakes, 210
    Marmalade Gems, 218
    Quest Depot Deluxe Granola, 86
    Snorri's Special Ham & Eggs, 158
    Spicy Breadsticks (a.k.a. Zeldóshâkh's Gnarly Bones), 175
    Sweet Sylvan Buns with Honey Almond Butter, 205
    Walter's Special Cinnamon Rolls, 111
    Zeldóshâkh's Gnarly Bones (a.k.a. Spicy Breadsticks), 175

Brie & Bacon Panini (a.k.a. Pig & Curd on Bread), 178
Busy Day Rice Pudding, 49
Button Pickles, 61

C

CAKES
    Cherry Lava Cakes (a.k.a. Queevhô's Bleedin' Treats), 197
    Chocolate Raspberry Cake with Ganache (a.k.a. Sweets for Sbileug), 195
    Council Catering Celebration Cake, 73
    Crustula Vitae, 224
    Esther's Favorite Lemon Cake, 220
    Etta-Evelyn's Angelic Treats, 132
    Göll's Gorgeous Seed Cake, 152
    Queevhô's Bleedin' Treats (a.k.a. Cherry Lava Cakes), 197
    Spidery Spice Cake, 134
    Sweets for Sbileug (a.k.a. Chocolate Raspberry Cake with Ganache), 195
Callista's Salmon Tartlets, 84
Candied Almonds, 89
CANDY
    One Wizard's Precious Delight, 140
Cardamom Berries with Honey Vanilla Ice Cream, 136
Cauliflower Cheese (a.k.a. Must Eat Brain Food...), 177
Cheddar Sage Scones, 7
Cherry Lava Cakes (a.k.a. Queevhô's Bleedin' Treats), 197

CHICKEN
> Blancmange Puffs, 88
> Braised Chicken & Pork with Artichokes (a.k.a. Raskofím's Roadkill), 185
> Chicken & Apple Toasty Puffs, 212
> Courageous Low-Carb Chicken, 36
> Grape & Chicken Cups, 6
> Raskofím's Roadkill (a.k.a. Braised Chicken & Pork with Artichokes), 185
> Reginleif's Favorite Chicken, 162
> Sine Qua Non Chicken, 121
> Six of One Half a Dozen Soup, 3
> Stout & Sturdy Chicken & Dumplings, 16
> Troy's Springtime Pie, 91
> Wisdom Chicken Soup, 57

Chicken & Apple Toasty Puffs, 212
Chloë's Macaroni and Cheese (a.k.a. Chloë's *Macrows ond Chese*), 14
Chloë's *Macrows ond Chese* (a.k.a. Chloë's Macaroni and Cheese), 14
Chocolate Raspberry Cake with Ganache (a.k.a. Sweets for Sbileug), 195
Chunks & Gobbets (a.k.a. Sauerkraut Sausage), 189
Clôxiga's Crunchable Salmon (a.k.a. Salmon with Sriracha), 191
Cold Dead Livid Bread (a.k.a. Blueberry Quick Bread), 194
Comforting Chai, 24

COOKIES
> Bon Voyage Biscotti, 101
> *Crustula Vitae*, 224
> Donald's Cinnamon Sticks, 70
> Hrist's Nutmeggers, 165
> Marmalade Gems, 218
> Nutty Honey Bars, 20
> Richard's Orange Biscuits, 99
> Skögul's Spice Cookies, 166

Council Catering Celebration Cake, 73
Courageous Low-Carb Chicken, 36
Crackling Caramel Sauce, 139
Cress Composition, 32
Cress Dress, xxv
Crunchable Croutons, 108
Crustula Vitae, 224
Curried Sausage Sandwiches (a.k.a. Glürbin's Gutless Wonders), 181

D

DESSERTS
> Apple & Raspberry Jam Tart, 22
> Blueberry Quick Bread (a.k.a. Cold Dead Livid Bread), 194
> Bon Voyage Biscotti, 101
> Brave Blackberry Tart, 47
> Busy Day Rice Pudding, 49
> Cardamom Berries with Honey Vanilla Ice Cream, 136
> Cherry Lava Cakes (a.k.a. Queevhô's Bleedin' Treats), 197
> Chocolate Raspberry Cake with Ganache (a.k.a. Sweets for Sbileug), 195
> Cold Dead Livid Bread (a.k.a. Blueberry Quick Bread), 194
> Council Catering Celebration Cake, 73

Crustula Vitae, 224
Donald's Cinnamon Sticks, 70
Elfryda's Apple Crisp, 51
Essential Mocha Tart, 71
Esther's Favorite Lemon Cake, 220
Etta-Evelyn's Angelic Treats, 132
Ginger Jar Bread with Spiced Honey Butter, 207
Göll's Gorgeous Seed Cake, 152
Good-For-You Muffins, 87
Hasty-One-Pot-Cobbler-Pie, 138
Herfjötur's Fancy Bread Pudding, 167
Honey Vanilla Ice Cream, 137
Hrist's Nutmeggers, 165
Jan's Baked Apples, 45
Marcella's Cherries, 21
Marmalade Gems, 218
Nimallin's New Foolery, 222
Nutty Honey Bars, 20
One Wizard's Precious Delight, 140
Pumpkin Streusel Pie for Randgrid, 163
Queevhô's Bleedin' Treats (a.k.a. Cherry Lava Cakes), 197
Quest Depot Deluxe Granola, 86
Richard's Orange Biscuits, 99
Skögul's Spice Cookies, 166
Spidery Spice Cake, 134
Stained Glass Morsels, 219
Sweet Sylvan Buns with Honey Almond Butter, 205
Sweets for Sbileug (a.k.a. Chocolate Raspberry Cake with Ganache), 195
Walter's Special Cinnamon Rolls, 111

Whortleberry Tart, 216
Dill Mayonnaise, 85
Dilly Bread & Butter, 33
Dilly Butter, 34
Donald's Cinnamon Sticks, 70
Doughty Hero Casserole, 38

E

Easy Herbes de Provence, xxii
EGGS
    Hideaway Sandwich, 8
    Lise's Lentils, 35
    Journey Brunch Pie, 95
    Marvelous Mushroom Pie, 97
    Mosaic Tart, 93
    Snorri's Special Ham & Eggs, 158
    Troy's Springtime Pie, 91
Elfryda's Apple Crisp, 51
Ellen's Favorite Salad, 5
Ellen's Dressing, xxvi
ENTRÉES
    Asbjorn's Fish, Chips, and Sauce, 116
    Beery Beef Stew, 40
    Blancmange Puffs, 88
    Bleu & Bacon Panini (a.k.a. Want Stinkier Sandwich), 180
    Braised Chicken & Pork with Artichokes (a.k.a. Raskofím's Roadkill), 185
    Brie & Bacon Panini (a.k.a. Pig & Curd on Bread), 178
    Callista's Salmon Tartlets, 84
    Chicken & Apple Toasty Puffs, 212
    Chloë's Macaroni and Cheese (a.k.a.

Chloë's *Macrows ond Chese*), 14
Chloë's *Macrows ond Chese* (a.k.a. Chloë's Macaroni and Cheese), 14
Chunks & Gobbets (a.k.a. Sauerkraut Sausage), 189
Clôxiga's Crunchable Salmon (a.k.a. Salmon with Sriracha), 191
Courageous Low-Carb Chicken, 36
Curried Sausage Sandwiches (a.k.a. Glürbin's Gutless Wonders), 181
Doughty Hero Casserole, 38
Epic-Urean Stew, 119
The Exquisite Soup of Master Mage Stormgutz, 107
Fancy Mashers, 211
Fungus Liquid (a.k.a. Mushroom Bacon Bisque), 173
Garlic Seafood with Saffron Rice (a.k.a. Gündürnüb's Grüb), 187
Geirahod's Pork Pie of Battle, 160
Glürbin's Gutless Wonders (a.k.a. Curried Sausage Sandwiches), 181
Golden Barley Beef Soup, 29
Good Harvest Pumpkin Soup, 81
Grape & Chicken Cups, 6
Gündürnüb's Grüb (a.k.a. Garlic Seafood with Saffron Rice), 187
A Halfling Hero's Dream (a.k.a. Rabbit Braised with Herbs), 42
Halfling Home-Style Fish, 9
Hearty Lunch Pie, 11
Hideaway Sandwich, 8
Hild's Mushroom Bacon Dish of Might, 156
Hlökk's Trenchers, 155
Journey Brunch Pie, 95
Lamb Kabobs with Mint Marinade (a.k.a. Meat on Metal Stick), 183
Lanaphro's Pancakes, 210
Leeky Potato Soup, 203
Marvelous Mushroom Pie, 97
Meat on Metal Stick (a.k.a. Lamb Kabobs with Mint Marinade), 183
Mellow Mushroom Meatloaf, 67
Mosaic Tart, 93
Mushroom Bacon Bisque (a.k.a. Fungus Liquid), 173
Mushroom Steaks, 18
Pig & Curd on Bread (a.k.a. Brie & Bacon Panini), 178
Rabbit Braised with Herbs (a.k.a. A Halfling Hero's Dream), 42
Rádgrid's Stuffed Mushrooms, 151
Raskofím's Roadkill (a.k.a. Braised Chicken & Pork with Artichokes), 185
Reginleif's Favorite Chicken, 162
Roast Beef Toasties, 31
Salmon with Sriracha (a.k.a. Clôxiga's Crunchable Salmon), 191
Sauerkraut Sausage (a.k.a. Chunks & Gobbets), 189
Savory Stuffed Flank Steak (a.k.a. Tshigwú's Bit O' the Flank), 192
Sine Qua Non Chicken, 121
Six of One Half a Dozen Soup, 3
Skeggjöld's Boozy Beans, 153
Snorri's Special Ham & Eggs, 158
Stout & Sturdy Chicken & Dumplings, 16
Sushi, 128
Sweet & Savory Pork Roast, 68

Tayphro's Venison, 214
Thrúd's Hearty Split Pea Soup, 149
Treasured Tidbits, 125
Troy's Springtime Pie, 91
Tshigwú's Bit O' the Flank (a.k.a. Savory Stuffed Flank Steak), 192
Want Stinkier Sandwich (a.k.a. Bleu & Bacon Panini), 180
Wisdom Chicken Soup, 57

Epic-Urean Stew, 119
Essential Mocha Tart, 71
Esther's Favorite Lemon Cake, 220
Etta-Evelyn's Angelic Treats, 132
The Exquisite Soup of Master Mage Stormgutz, 107

F

Fancy Mashers, 211
Farsi's Tartar Sauce, 117
FISH
- Asbjorn's Fish, Chips, and Sauce, 116
- Callista's Salmon Tartlets, 84
- Clôxiga's Crunchable Salmon (a.k.a. Salmon with Sriracha), 191
- The Exquisite Soup of Master Mage Stormgutz, 107
- Garlic Seafood with Saffron Rice (a.k.a. Gündürnüb's Grüb), 187
- Gündürnüb's Grüb (a.k.a. Garlic Seafood with Saffron Rice), 187
- Halfling Home-Style Fish, 9
- Salmon with Sriracha (a.k.a. Clôxiga's Crunchable Salmon), 191
- Sushi, 128

Treasured Tidbits, 125
Fungus Liquid (a.k.a. Mushroom Bacon Bisque), 173

G

Gari (pickled ginger), 126
Garlic Seafood with Saffron Rice (a.k.a. Gündürnüb's Grüb), 187
Geirahod's Pork Pie of Battle, 160
Ginger Jar Bread with Spiced Honey Butter, 207
Glaze of Enchantment, 133
Glürbin's Gutless Wonders (a.k.a. Curried Sausage Sandwiches), 181
Golden Barley Beef Soup, 29
Göll's Gorgeous Seed Cake, 152
Good-for-You Muffins, 87
Good Harvest Pumpkin Soup, 81
Grape & Chicken Cups, 6
Gündürnüb's Grüb (a.k.a. Garlic Seafood with Saffron Rice), 187

H

A Halfling Hero's Dream (a.k.a. Rabbit Braised with Herbs), 42
Halfling Home-Style Fish, 9
Hasty-One-Pot-Cobbler-Pie, 138
Head-in-the-Clouds Biscuits, 59
Healing Chocolate Chai, 52
Hearty Lunch Pie, 11
HEARTY PIES
- Geirahod's Pork Pie of Battle, 160
- Hearty Lunch Pie, 11
- Journey Brunch Pie, 95

Marvelous Mushroom Pie, 97
Mosaic Tart, 93
Troy's Springtime Pie, 91
Herby Cabbage Sauté, 63
Herfjötur's Fancy Bread Pudding, 167
Hideaway Sandwich, 8
Hild's Mushroom Bacon Dish of Might, 156
Hlökk's Trenchers, 155
Honey Almond Butter, 205
Honey Vanilla Ice Cream, 137
Hrist's Nutmeggers, 165

J

Jan's Baked Apples, 45
Journey Brunch Pie, 95

K

Keep-You-Awake Cauliflower, 62

L

Lamb Kabobs with Mint Marinade (a.k.a. Meat on Metal Stick), 183
LAMB
    Lamb Kabobs with Mint Marinade (a.k.a. Meat on Metal Stick), 183
    Meat on Metal Stick (a.k.a. Lamb Kabobs with Mint Marinade), 183
Lanaphro's Pancakes, 210
Leeky Potato Soup, 203
Lise's Lentils, 35
Lise's Tangy Vinaigrette, xxvi

M

Maoglûrb's Mustard, 182
Marcella's Cherries, 21
Marmalade Gems, 218
Marvelous Mushroom Pie, 97
Meat on Metal Stick (a.k.a. Lamb Kabobs with Mint Marinade), 183
Mellow Mushroom Meatloaf, 67
Mini-Mashers, 11
MISCELLANEOUS
    Aradosa's Cheese, xxiv
    Bill's Spicy Nut Mix, 83
    Candied Almonds, 89
    Crackling Caramel Sauce, 139
    Cress Dress, xxv
    Crunchable Croutons, 108
    Dill Mayonnaise, 85
    Dilly Butter, 34
    Easy Herbes de Provence, xxii
    Ellen's Dressing, xxvi
    Farsi's Tartar Sauce, 117
    Glaze of Enchantment, 133
    Honey Almond Butter, 205
    Honey Vanilla Ice Cream, 137
    Lise's Tangy Vinaigrette, xxvi
    Maoglûrb's Mustard, 182
    Mini-Mashers, 11
    Pickled Ginger (*gari*), 126
    Savory Seasoning, xxi
    Simple Cinnamon Sugar, xxiii
    Spiced Honey Butter, 208
    Sushi Rice, 127
    Ted's Dressing, xxvii
    Vinegar Water, 127

Mosaic Tart, 93

MUSHROOMS
    Button Pickles, 61
    Chunks & Gobbets (a.k.a. Sauerkraut Sausage), 189
    Epic-Urean Stew, 119
    Fungus Liquid (a.k.a. Mushroom Bacon Bisque), 173
    Golden Barley Beef Soup, 29
    Hearty Lunch Pie, 11
    Hild's Mushroom Bacon Dish of Might, 156
    Hlökk's Trenchers, 155
    Marvelous Mushroom Pie, 97
    Mellow Mushroom Meatloaf, 67
    Mushroom Bacon Bisque (a.k.a. Fungus Liquid), 173
    Mushroom Steaks, 18
    Mushrooms of Mist, 154
    Rádgrið's Stuffed Mushrooms, 151
    Reginleif's Favorite Chicken, 162
    Sauerkraut Sausage (a.k.a. Chunks & Gobbets), 189
    Ted's Spinach Mushroom Salad, 58
Mushroom Bacon Bisque (a.k.a. Fungus Liquid), 173
Mushroom Steaks, 18
Mushrooms of Mist, 154
Must Eat Brain Food… (a.k.a. Cauliflower Cheese), 177

N

Nimallin's New Foolery, 222
Nutty Honey Bars, 20

O

One Wizard's Precious Delight, 140

P

PASTA
    Chloë's Macaroni and Cheese (a.k.a. Chloë's *Macrows ond Chese*), 14
    Chloë's *Macrows ond Chese* (a.k.a. Chloë's Macaroni and Cheese), 14
    Wisdom Chicken Soup, 57
Pickled Ginger (*gari*), 126
PIES/TARTS/CRISPS
    Apple & Raspberry Jam Tart, 22
    Brave Blackberry Tart, 47
    Elfryda's Apple Crisp, 51
    Essential Mocha Tart, 71
    Hasty-One-Pot-Cobbler-Pie, 138
    Marcella's Cherries, 21
    Pumpkin Streusel Pie for Randgrið, 163
    Stained Glass Morsels, 219
    Whortleberry Tart, 216
Pig & Curd on Bread (a.k.a. Brie & Bacon Panini), 178
PORK/SAUSAGE/HAM/BACON
    Bleu & Bacon Panini (a.k.a. Want Stinkier Sandwich), 180
    Braised Chicken & Pork with Artichokes (a.k.a. Raskofím's Roadkill), 185
    Brie & Bacon Panini (a.k.a. Pig & Curd on Bread), 178

Chunks & Gobbets (a.k.a. Sauerkraut Sausage), 189
Curried Sausage Sandwiches (a.k.a. Glürbin's Gutless Wonders), 181
Doughty Hero Casserole, 38
Fancy Mashers, 211
Fungus Liquid (a.k.a. Mushroom Bacon Bisque), 173
Geirahod's Pork Pie of Battle, 160
Glürbin's Gutless Wonders (a.k.a. Curried Sausage Sandwiches), 181
Hideaway Sandwich, 8
Hild's Mushroom Bacon Dish of Might, 156
Journey Brunch Pie, 95
Mushroom Bacon Bisque (a.k.a. Fungus Liquid), 173
Pig & Curd on Bread (a.k.a. Brie & Bacon Panini), 178
Rádgrid's Stuffed Mushrooms, 151
Raskofím's Roadkill (a.k.a. Braised Chicken & Pork with Artichokes), 185
Sauerkraut Sausage (a.k.a. Chunks & Gobbets), 189
Skeggjöld's Boozy Beans, 153
Snorri's Special Ham & Eggs, 158
Sweet & Savory Pork Roast, 68
Thrúd's Hearty Split Pea Soup, 149
Troy's Springtime Pie, 91
Want Stinkier Sandwich (a.k.a. Bleu & Bacon Panini), 180

Potentially Pungent Potatoes, 65
Pumpkin Streusel Pie for Randgrid, 163

Q

Queevhô's Bleedin' Treats (a.k.a. Cherry Lava Cakes), 197
Quest Depot Deluxe Granola, 86

R

RABBIT
    Rabbit Braised with Herbs (a.k.a. A Halfling Hero's Dream), 42
Rabbit Braised with Herbs (a.k.a. A Halfling Hero's Dream), 42
Rádgrid's Stuffed Mushrooms, 151
Raskofím's Roadkill (a.k.a. Braised Chicken & Pork with Artichokes), 185
Reginleif's Favorite Chicken, 162
Richard's Orange Biscuits, 99
Roast Beef Toasties, 31
Roasted Asparagus with Mustard Sauce, 64

S

SALADS/DRESSINGS
    Beets for Hypomur, 113
    Bob's Obsession, 114
    Button Pickles, 61
    Courageous Low-Carb Chicken, 36
    Cress Composition, 32
    Cress Dress, xxv
    Ellen's Favorite Salad, 5
    Ellen's Dressing, xxvi
    Grape & Chicken Cups, 6
    Keep-You-Awake Cauliflower, 62

Lise's Lentils, 35
Lise's Tangy Vinaigrette, xxvi
Ted's Spinach Mushroom Salad, 58
Ted's Dressing, xxvii
Salmon with Sriracha (a.k.a. Clôxiga's Crunchable Salmon), 191

SANDWICHES
Bleu & Bacon Panini (a.k.a. Want Stinkier Sandwich), 180
Brie & Bacon Panini (a.k.a. Pig & Curd on Bread), 178
Chicken & Apple Toasty Puffs, 212
Curried Sausage Sandwiches (a.k.a. Glürbin's Gutless Wonders), 181
Glürbin's Gutless Wonders (a.k.a. Curried Sausage Sandwiches), 181
Hideaway Sandwich, 8
Hlökk's Trenchers, 155
Pig & Curd on Bread (a.k.a. Brie & Bacon Panini), 178
Roast Beef Toasties, 31
Want Stinkier Sandwich (a.k.a. Bleu & Bacon Panini), 180

Sauerkraut Sausage (a.k.a. Chunks & Gobbets), 189
Savory Seasoning, xxi
Savory Stuffed Flank Steak (a.k.a. Tshigwú's Bit O' the Flank), 192
Simple Cinnamon Sugar, xxiii
Sine Qua Non Chicken, 121
Six of One Half a Dozen Soup, 3
Skeggjöld's Boozy Beans, 153
Skögul's Spice Cookies, 166
Snorri's Special Ham & Eggs, 158

SOUPS
The Exquisite Soup of Master Mage Stormgutz, 107
Fungus Liquid (a.k.a. Mushroom Bacon Bisque), 173
Golden Barley Beef Soup, 29
Good Harvest Pumpkin Soup, 81
Leeky Potato Soup, 203
Mushroom Bacon Bisque (a.k.a. Fungus Liquid), 173
Six of One Half a Dozen Soup, 3
Thrúd's Hearty Split Pea Soup, 149
Wisdom Chicken Soup, 57

Spiced Honey Butter, 208
Spicy Breadsticks (a.k.a. Zeldóshâkh's Gnarly Bones), 175
Spidery Spice Cake, 134
Spring-in-Your-Step Punch, 76
Stained Glass Morsels, 219

STEWS
Beery Beef Stew, 40
Braised Chicken & Pork with Artichokes (a.k.a. Raskofím's Roadkill), 185
Chunks & Gobbets (a.k.a. Sauerkraut Sausage), 189
Epic-Urean Stew, 119
A Halfling Hero's Dream (a.k.a. Rabbit Braised with Herbs), 42
Rabbit Braised with Herbs (a.k.a. A Halfling Hero's Dream), 42
Raskofím's Roadkill (a.k.a. Braised Chicken & Pork with Artichokes), 185

Sauerkraut Sausage (a.k.a. Chunks & Gobbets), 189
Stout & Sturdy Chicken & Dumplings, 16
Stout & Sturdy Chicken & Dumplings, 16
Sushi, 128
Sushi Rice, 127
Sweet & Savory Pork Roast, 68
Sweet Sylvan Buns with Honey Almond Butter, 205
Sweets for Sbileug (a.k.a. Chocolate Raspberry Cake with Ganache), 195

T

Tayphro's Venison, 214
Ted's Dressing, xxvii
Ted's Spinach Mushroom Salad, 58
Thrúd's Hearty Split Pea Soup, 149
Treasured Tidbits, 125
Troy's Springtime Pie, 91
Tshigwú's Bit O' the Flank (a.k.a. Savory Stuffed Flank Steak), 192
Turquoise Tipple, 144
A Typical Fantasy Meal, 228

V

VEGETABLES
Cauliflower Cheese (a.k.a. Must Eat Brain Food…), 177
Fancy Mashers, 211
Good Harvest Pumpkin Soup, 81
Herby Cabbage Sauté, 63
Hlökk's Trenchers, 155
Leeky Potato Soup, 203
Mini-Mashers, 11
Mushrooms of Mist, 154
Must Eat Brain Food… (a.k.a. Cauliflower Cheese), 177
Potentially Pungent Potatoes, 65
Roasted Asparagus with Mustard Sauce, 64
Skeggjöld's Boozy Beans, 153
VENISON
Tayphro's Venison, 214
Vinegar Water, 127

W

Walter's Special Cinnamon Rolls, 111
Want Stinkier Sandwich (a.k.a. Bleu & Bacon Panini), 180
Whortleberry Tart, 216
Wisdom Chicken Soup, 57

Z

Zeldóshâkh's Gnarly Bones (a.k.a. Spicy Breadsticks), 175

Author's Biography

Astrid Tuttle Winegar has been cooking, baking, and reading fantasy literature for over 40 years. She has a bachelor's degree in English and Latin and a master's degree in Comparative Literature and Cultural Studies from the University of New Mexico. Astrid lives with her husband in Albuquerque; she is also a mother and a grandmother. All photographs were taken by the author (in her non-professional capacity) with a Canon PowerShot A470. You may see additional photographs and artwork on Facebook (facebook.com/astridtuttlewinegar). For more information, visit her website: astridwinegar.com.

Illustrator's Biography

Geneva Harstine has been known by many names, making appearances in the *dies natalis* festivities of many a stranger. With a fondness for all manner of fantastic critters, she finds inspiration in nature and the landscapes surrounding her native state of New Mexico.

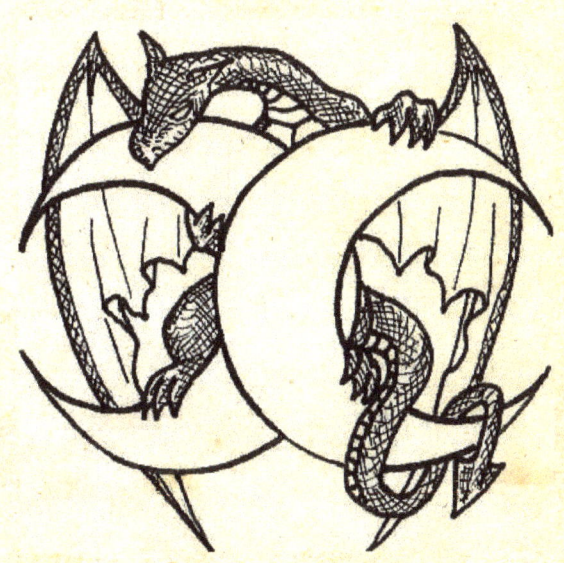

www.ingramcontent.com/pod-product-compliance
Lightning Source LLC
Chambersburg PA
CBHW061935290426
44113CB00025B/2914